Moral Responsibility in Prolonging Life Decisions

CONTRIBUTORS TO THIS VOLUME

Rev. Benedict M. Ashley, O.P., Ph.D.
Professor of Moral Theology
The Aquinas Institute of Theology
St. Louis, Missouri

Gary M. Atkinson, Ph.D.
Assistant Professor of Philosophy
The College of St. Thomas
St. Paul, Minnesota

Joseph M. Boyle, Jr., Ph.D.
Assistant Professor of Philosophy
Center for Thomistic Studies
University of St. Thomas
Houston, Texas

Paul A. Byrne, M.D.
Director/Neonatology
Archbishop Bergan Mercy Hospital
Omaha, Nebraska

Rev. John R. Connery, S.J., S.T.D.
Professor of Moral Theology
Loyola University of Chicago
Chicago, Illinois

Dennis J. Horan, J.D.
Attorney at Law
Hinshaw, Culbertson, Moelmann,
Hoban and Fuller
Chicago, Illinois

Oscar B. Hunter, M.D.
Director, Hunter Laboratory
Bethesda, Maryland

Rev. Donald G. McCarthy, Ph.D.
Director of Education
Pope John XXIII Medical-Moral
Research and Education Center
St. Louis, Missouri

William J. Monahan, Jr., Ph.D.
Associate Professor of Sociology
St. Louis University
St. Louis, Missouri

Rev. Albert S. Moraczewski, O.P., Ph.D.
Vice President for Research
Pope John XXIII Medical-Moral
Research and Education Center
St. Louis, Missouri

Rev. Lawrence T. Reilly, S.T.D.
Director, Office of Medical Morals
Providence Health Care Corporations
Seattle, Washington

Rev. Richard R. Roach, S.J., Ph.D.
Professor of Moral Theology
Marquette University
Milwaukee, Wisconsin

Rev. Patrick J. Sena, C.PP.S., S.S.L.
Professor of Biblical Studies
Mt. St. Mary Seminary
Cincinnati, Ohio

Kenneth R. Smith, Jr., M.D.
Professor of Surgery
St. Louis University Medical School
St. Louis, Missouri

Moral Responsibility in Prolonging Life Decisions

Edited by
Donald G. McCarthy, Ph.D.
and
Albert S. Moraczewski, O.P., Ph.D.

Pope John Center
St. Louis

Nihil Obstat:
   Rev. Robert F. Coerver, C.M., S.T.D.
   Censor Deputatus

Imprimatur:
   The Rev. Monsignor Edward J. O'Donnell, V.G.
   Archdiocese of St. Louis   November 21, 1981

The Nihil Obstat and Imprimatur are a declaration that a book or pamphlet is considered to be free from doctrinal or moral error. It is not implied that those who have granted the Nihil Obstat and Imprimatur agree with the contents, opinions, or statements expressed.

Copyright 1981
by
The Pope John XXIII Medical-Moral
Research and Education Center
St. Louis, Missouri 63134

Library of Congress Catalog Card Number: 81-83158
ISBN 0-935372-08-3

Distributors for the Trade:
   FRANCISCAN HERALD PRESS
   1434 West 51st St.
   Chicago, IL 60609

Contents

v

vi

Preface

The last decade has seen an amazing proliferation of books and articles on medical ethics, particularly on life and death issues. This volume, however, is intended to fulfill a previously unmet need. We have assembled here a comprehensive resource book analyzing all facets of prolonging life decisions from the perspective of Catholic teaching and the Judeo-Christian heritage. As these decisions multiply during the 1980s, the value of this volume can only increase.

The year 1982 marks the 25th anniversary of the famous allocution of Pope Pius XII to an international gathering of anesthesiologists when the Holy Father outlined officially the Catholic teaching about ordinary and extraordinary means of prolonging life. The Vatican *Declaration on Euthanasia*, found in Appendix I of this volume, reviewed and systematized that teaching in 1980. The twenty chapters of this volume reflect it within the theological, medical, and legal context of the United States today.

The many authors who contributed the first 12 chapters of this volume did not work in isolation from each other. They presented their material to an Institute for 240 health care professionals and pastoral care persons in St. Louis, MO, Sept. 19-21, 1980. Subsequently, their essays were each circulated to at least ten specially chosen readers for critical comments. Many of the authors participated in the two subsequent Institutes in Tampa and Phoenix in the spring of 1981. Their final manuscripts reflect the interdisciplinary dialogue of these Institutes.

Furthermore, the last eight chapters of this book, although written by ourselves, actually contain the essence of the clinical/pastoral seminars held at each Institute. In a sense, then, these chapters were written by the resource persons who led those seminars and by the 550 persons who took part in them.

Who can use this volume? The persons whose responsibilities are discussed in the final four chapters — administrators of health care facilities, physicians, nurses, and pastoral care persons — will profit from every single chapter. Furthermore, the pastoral care persons addressed in the last chapter include all those who render pastoral help to sick and dying persons, especially the parish clergy.

Readers of this book, who are not health care professionals or pastoral care persons, still will at some time make or participate in prolonging life decisions. So it is their book, too. They will find chapter 8 by Father Benedict M. Ashley a straightforward review of the essential ethical or moral principles they need to know. The following chapter, by Father John R. Connery, pursues these principles more specifically into the difficult questions of identifying when burdensome life-prolonging procedures become ethically optional. In the next chapter, Father Lawrence T. Reilly outlines an approach to personal conscience formation.

Readers who are active in the pro-life movement will find several chapters especially helpful and relevant to current controversies. In chapter 2, Father Roach argues strongly against consequentialism, the ethical theory which can justify mercy killing and the omission of ordinary means of prolonging life for reasons of alleged mercy to the suffering. Chapter 3 presents the medical approach to the determination of death by brain criteria and includes a response which seeks to indicate medical uncertainties within this approach. Chapter 12 documents the increasing acceptance of mercy killing by American public opinion. Chapter 15 carefully analyzes the ethical objections to using a prospective quality of life standard in selecting severely defective newborn infants for therapeutic care.

This book has been prepared as a resource contribution to the Church's ministry to suffering and dying persons and to the healing and caring ministry of countless health care professionals. As chapter 7 indicates, the theological tradition of a limited responsibility for prolonging life in the face of burdensome medical treatments has a long and honorable history in the Church. The Pope John XXIII Center for Medical-Moral Research and Education, which has dedicated itself to the task of applying Church teaching to contemporary medical-moral issues, offers this resource volume as a continuation of that history.

This volume, for the service of human life and those who care for life, is dated on a feast of Mary, who gave earthly life to the Lord of life. We happily dedicate it to her as Mother of Christ and Mother of the Church.

December 8, 1981   Donald G. McCarthy
             Albert S. Moraczewski, O.P.

Acknowledgements

Literally hundreds of people participated in preparing this volume. We are grateful to them all, recognizing that without their assistance the book would be less adequate, while we assume responsibility for whatever deficiencies it contains. We appreciate, first of all, the assistance of the staff of the Catholic Health Association which co-sponsored with Pope John Center the three Institutes at which this subject material was presented and discussed.

Obviously, this volume would not exist without the work of the contributors listed on a previous page. They submitted willingly to our editorial process, which included seeking written reactions from at least ten readers for the chapters they prepared. We are especially grateful to Fathers Benedict M. Ashley, O.P., and John R. Connery, S.J., both Senior Research Fellows of the Pope John Center, who served on our Editorial Committee and reviewed the entire manuscript.

This volume does not always and in every way represent the opinions and suggestions of the many persons who were involved in its preparation. Nevertheless, we wish to acknowledge by name those who were resource persons for our seminars and the seminar moderators, as well as those who read various chapters of the manuscript and those persons who gave suggestions at the very initiation of the project.

The resource persons for the seminars that led to chapters 13 through 20 of this book are unsung heroes. Their wisdom and insights found their way into our text, usually without explicit attribution. The resource persons for chapters 13 through 16 were: Gary Arthur, M.D.; Sr. Roberta Francis Bronner, O.S.F., R.N.; William J. R. Daily, M.D.; William J. Dunn, M.D.; Mrs. Mary Lou Hess, R.N.; Mrs. Yvonne Hoefer, R.N.; Ms. Mary Honich, B.S.W.; Alice D. Kitchen, M.D.; Mrs. Jeannette Kowalski, R.N., M.S.N.; Sr. Kathleen Krekeler, C.C.V.I., R.N., Ph.D.; John Lawton, M.D.; Daniel Luedke, M.D.; Thomas W. McDonald, M.D.; William Malette, M.D.; Sr. Jeanne Meurer, S.S.M., C.N.M., M.S.; Jeffrey O'Connor, M.D.; John Reis, M.D.; Sr. A. Teresa Stanley, R.N., D.N.Sc.; Mrs. Marty Templin, R.N., B.S.N.; Sr. Clara Ternes, A.S.C., C.R.N.A., M.A.; Paul Williams, M.D.; Ms. Barbara Joan Wisniewski, R.N.

The resource persons for chapters 17 through 20 were: Rev. Thomas Beischel, C.PP.S.; Sr. Loretta Geringer, C.D.P.; Sr. Kathleen Krekeler, C.C.V.I., R.N., Ph.D.; Sr. Rita McCormick, C.S.J.; Sr. M. Mercy McGrady, R.S.M.; Sr. M. Anthony Power, L.S.P.; Raymond Rustige, M.A., F.A.C.N.H.A.; Sr. A. Teresa Stanley, R.N., D.N.Sc.; Sr. Clara Ternes, A.S.C., C.R.N.A., M.A.; Rev. Timothy J. Toohey, M.Div.; Sr. Elizabeth Ann Webb, S.C.N., M.A.

We add also our appreciation to the moderators who directed our seminars at the three Institutes, including: Sr. Benedict Armstrong, L.S.P.; Sr. M. Laurice Beaudry, O.S.F., R.N., M.A.; Rev. Robert D. Boisaubin; Sr. Maria Fidelis, S.C.; Rev. William M. Gallagher; George P. Giacoia, M.D.; Sr. Margaret John Kelly, D.C., Ph.D.; Rev. Robert L. Kramer, C.PP.S.; Sr. Mark Neumann, S.C.; Rev. James Reinert, S.J.; Ms. Ronda Russick; Stuart Showalter, J.D.; Sr. Mary Lenora Weier, O.S.F.; Rev. Eugene J. Weitzel; Sr. M. Antoinette Yelek, C.S.J.

Among the many kind persons who reviewed some of the chapters in this book we are happy to acknowledge: Sr. Corrine Bayley, C.S.J.; Robert Bertram, Ph.D.; Donald Brinkman, M.D.; Gerald D. Coleman, S.S., Ph.D.; Sr. Theresa Daly, C.C.V.I.; John E. Dineen, M.D.; Rev. Thomas M. Gannon, S.J., Ph.D.; Stanley Hauerwas, Ph.D.; Dr. Read F. McGhee, Jr.; Rev. John Meier, S.S.D.; Rev. George Montague, S.M.; Rev. Timothy E. O'Connell, Ph.D.; Rev. Raymond H. Potvin, Ph.D.; William W. Quick, M.D.; Henry F. Rohs, M.D.; Richard T. F. Schmidt, M.D.; Sr. Sandra M. Schneiders, I.H.M.;

Rev. Carroll Stuhlmueller, C.P., S.S.D.; Garth F. Tagge, M.D.; Leonard Weber, Ph.D.; John Zipprich, J.D.

In the winter of 1979-1980, before inaugurating this project, we sent a survey to many national leaders in the field of bioethics. In addition to benefitting from the advice of many of the persons listed above, we also received helpful suggestions from the following: Rev. Clarence Deddens, S.T.D.; Rev. Gerald Fath, O.P.; Emil J. Freireich, M.D.; Germain Grisez, Ph.D.; Sr. M. Michelle Holland, S.P., M.A.; Sr. Mary Jenkins; Rev. Ronald D. Lawler, O.F.M.Cap., Ph.D.; Rev. Edwin L. Lisson, S.J., S.T.D.; Sr. Francesca Lumpp, C.S.J.; Rev. Richard A. McCormick, S.J., S.T.D.; Rev. John M. McDermott, S.J., S.T.D.; Sr. Carlos McDonnell, D.C., M.S.N.; Rev. Msgr. James T. McDonough, A.C.S.W.; Rev. Eugene Maly, S.S.D.; Rev. Paul Marx, O.S.B.; William E. May, Ph.D.; Rev. Douglas A. Morrison; Rev. Gerald R. Niklas; Rev. Paul M. Quay, S.J., Ph.D.; Rev. Kevin D. O'Rourke, O.P., J.C.D.; Bernard J. Pisani, M.D.; Rev. William B. Smith, S.T.D.; John Stehlin, M.D.; Robert M. Veatch, Ph.D.

We are grateful to *Linacre Quarterly* for permission to include in chapter 9 some parts of the article by Father John R. Connery, S.J., which appeared in the May, 1980, issue of *Linacre Quarterly*. Our work in preparing this book was lightened by the cheerful assistance of Dr. Rita Adams, Mrs. Lucy Diefenbach and Mrs. Jo Anne Probst, secretaries of the Pope John Center, and Mrs. Joanne Lanser, secretary of the Long Term Care Division of the Catholic Health Association.

Unfortunately, making any list like the above risks unintended omissions. We regret any such omissions and can only hope that all who are listed here, and all who should be listed, have been properly entered in the Lord's own records for their share in furthering our common sense of responsibility for the gift of life.

D.M.C.
A.S.M.

Part I

Life and Death

Introduction

The four chapters comprising the first part of this resource book lay the necessary groundwork for the remaining sixteen chapters. Those remaining chapters make a multi-faceted approach to decisions of prolonging or not prolonging human life. They all reflect, however, the well-founded conviction within Western civilization and the Judeo-Christian tradition that human persons must not destroy their own lives or the lives of sick and suffering persons. On the other hand, those chapters all reflect the conviction that the obligation to prolong life extends only to treatments and procedures which are useful and

1

accessible without excessive hardship. These four preliminary chapters in Part I focus on human life and death as the points of reference for all decisions about prolonging life.

In chapter 1, Father Patrick J. Sena, C.PP.S., writing with a profound knowledge of the Bible, paints a picture of life and death as portrayed there. He sees each human life understood to reflect the life of the Living God and to enjoy His providential care. He finds the truth of life after death gradually revealed in the Bible and definitively proclaimed in the resurrection of Jesus Christ. Father Sena's particular study of the meaning of human blood in the Scriptures relates to his membership in the Society of the Precious Blood. He finds clear teaching in the Scriptures opposing the shedding of innocent blood, which includes a prohibition of mercy killing. Death, however, cannot be avoided, although Christians believe Jesus opened a path to eternal life after death.

In chapter 2, Father Richard R. Roach, S.J., of Marquette University, presents a forceful argument against compromising the prohibition of killing the innocent through the ethical methodology of consequentialism. He supports the Catholic tradition which finds the act of killing an innocent person contrary to the moral order, regardless of the weight of desirable consequences or compensating values.

Dr. Kenneth R. Smith, a neurosurgeon teaching at St. Louis University School of Medicine, defends in chapter 3 a new approach to the determination of human death by brain criteria, when circulatory and respiratory functions are artificially supported. Paul A. Byrne M.D. responds by questioning whether cessation of brain function always indicates death, and whether the irreversibility of that cessation can be reliably determined.

Dennis J. Horan J.D., a well-known lawyer-author from Chicago, recounts in chapter 4 the legal developments which are building a consensus that medical testimony to total and irreversible cessation of all brain functions, including the brain stem functions, should be acceptable for a legal pronouncement of death.

Hence these four chapters offer a biblical vision of life and death, an ethical and theological reflection on the prohibition of killing the innocent, and an analysis of the medical-legal trend to accept brain criteria for human death in the rare circumstances where respiration and circulation are artificially supported.

2

Chapter 1

Biblical Teaching
On Life and Death

The Reverend Patrick J. Sena, C. PP. S. , S. S. L.

Introduction

It would be rash to attempt to give a complete, detailed account of the concepts of life and death as the Bible presents them in so few pages and with so few words. Books and articles in the *Select Bibliography* will be of assistance to the general reader in the pursuit of a personal detailed study. The Bible is not just one book, but it is many books written over a time span of many centuries by various sacred authors; in the Bible they are not listed necessarily in the chronological order in which they were written.[1] Each commentator must make sound decisions based upon solid scholarship as to the probable dating of the scripture passages being cited. Unfortunately, scholars do not always agree. Thus a development of any biblical theme is rather difficult and tenuous; there are always presuppositions which the commentator must take into consideration — e.g. the dating of the selection. Nevertheless, despite

3

these pitfalls, this writer will attempt to give an overall view of the Bible's presentation of life and death in both the Old and New Testaments.

Old Testament

A common way of picturing God in the Bible is to point out that he is living and full of life. In fact, the Eastern culture of the ancient Hebrews, as far as language is concerned, was based upon the use of the verb; and so the people in that culture expressed themselves not in terms of definitions which are of primary importance in Western cultures which more frequently use nouns, but in terms of activity and experience.[2] At least 80 times in the Old Testament, the God of Israel is invoked by the expressions "living God" or "God lives". God is experienced as lively and active. It is fitting to point out some scripture texts which manifest this concern. It should be noted that the following texts, with the exception of the New Testament text, were all written roughly within the same historical period — a period revolving around the Babylonian Exile (587-536 B.C.), several decades before and several succeeding decades.

Ezekiel depicts God speaking in these words: "As I live, says the Lord God, surely with a mighty hand and an outstretched arm, and with wrath poured out, I will be king over you" (20:33).[3] To be sure, there were many other ways of designating God, but many of them speak about his activity: God leads, God comes, etc.[4] The understanding of God as one who is alive was very important for Israel's appreciation for life itself. In presenting the account of the reception of the Ten Commandments by Moses, the Deuteronomist points out the uniqueness of the God of Israel:

> I am the Lord your God, who brought you out of the land of Egypt, out of the house of bondage. You shall have no other gods before me. You shall not make for yourself a graven image, or any likeness of anything that is in heaven above, or that is on the earth beneath, or that is in the water under the earth (Dt 5:6-8).

Israel was not to have many gods, nor was she to worship the gods of other nations. The unique character of the active God of Israel prompted the people to observe a practical monotheism. Monotheism *per se* necessarily denies the existence of all but one god; this does not appear to be taught clearly in the Bible until the time of Deutero-Isaiah.

4

The composition of a significant part of Deuteronomy probably comes from the same exilic and post-exilic period.[5] By the time of the second and third century B.C., monotheism appears to be accepted as a fact of life and taken for granted.[6]

As the Living God, God was not only considered as having more power than the pagan deities, but also was considered as the champion of his people; the one who saw to it that they remained in the right. He accomplished a great work for Joshua and his people when he led them dryshod across the River Jordan to enter the land of Promise (Jos 3:10-13).[7] The idols of the pagans are seen to be both stupid and foolish; they are made from wood (Jer 10:8), and cannot take care of their own as God does for Israel (Jer 10:12-16). Israel's God gives to his people a certain quality of life which is an impossibility for the gods of the pagans. "All who make idols are nothing, and the things they delight in do not profit; their witnesses neither see nor know, that they may be put to shame" (Is 44:9-10). Such idols are manufactured and thus lifeless, but Yahweh, the God of Israel, is living. He is the author of all life, and the priestly tradition of Genesis points out that God created life on the fifth day when he created life in the seas (Gn 1:20), followed by living animals and birds and finally by the crown of his creation — man and woman. These he created in his own image and likeness (Gn 1:26). God breathed into his human creation "the breath of life; and man became a living being" (Gn 2:7). Not only did the Living God create and give life, but he also sustains life. Job reminds us that God holds all life in the very palm of his hands (12:10): this text is one of the "clearest statements of the divine origin of life;"[8] the same imagery is used in the New Testament pointing out the sovereignty of Christ who is called the Son of Man, holding the seven churches in his strong right hand (Rev 1:16). Ps 104:29-30 addresses itself to the same theme: the divine origin of life. God sends forth his spirit to create and to renew the very face of the earth. Yahweh is alive and shares his life with creation. As a living God, he cannot be captured in pictures, icons, or any type of image. He is unlike the gods of the pagans and he is unlike his human creation which is of flesh. Yet, it is the Living God who instills into his human creation that spark of life causing humankind to be a living entity.

Biblical Anthropology
Life Principles

The people of the Bible were men and women of their day; they did not live in a vacuum, but did have contact with other civilizations, other ideas, with ways of doing things other than their own. Their theology did not develop in an isolated manner apart from these other cultures. Among the ancients, blood always had a special place in religious practice and thought; for blood was perceived as the bearer of life.

In the Hebrew Old Testament, Masoretic Text (MT), the word blood, *dam,* is found approximately 350 times. It is first mentioned in Genesis 4:10 where the murdered Abel speaks through his spilled out blood and cries out to God for vengeance; the last usage is to be found in the prophet Zechariah 9:11 where it is the blood of the covenant which accomplishes union with God and which brings freedom and liberation to the oppressed. Between these two citations, the word *blood*[9] is employed in various ways,[10] not least among which is the context of blood sacrifices.[11] However, as regards the function of blood, the Old Testament is quite clear — blood is life; blood which has been shed signifies that life has been poured out. The Deuteronomist states: "Only be sure that you do not eat the *blood*; for the blood is life (*nepes*), and you shall not eat the life (*nepes*) with its flesh (*basar*)" (Dt 12:23). The Priestly author concurs: "Only you shall not eat the *flesh* with its *life,* that is, its *blood*" (Gn 9:4). And still, "For the *life* of every creature is its *blood*; whoever eats it shall be cut off" (Lev 17:14). Blood is thus clearly understood to be a life principle of living beings.

There was no dichotomy between body and spirit for the ancient Hebrews.[12] In fact, they had no specific word for body. The individual was viewed as a whole. It is only the later writings, above all in the later Wisdom literature and especially among the deuterocanonical books (Apocrypha), that we first run into the familiar body/soul concept (Wis 1:4-5).[13] In an attempt to demonstrate that Hebrew wisdom was just as good as the wisdom of the Greeks, the sacred author borrows Hellenistic concepts: "For a perishable body weighs down the soul, and this earthly tent burdens the thoughtful mind" (Wis 9:15). Among the ancient Hebrews, the term *basar,* flesh, is in no way contrasted with *nepes* (life/spirit). Whenever a contrast with flesh is implied, then *basar* refers to that which is weak in contrast to God who has power: "Hast thou eyes of flesh? Dost thou see as man sees?" (Job 10:4). The expected answer is, of course, "certainly not". In Isaiah 40:6-7, there is a contrast between *flesh* and the breath (*ruah*) of the Lord — a contrast between a human being who is weak and God who has power. The word *ruah* will be explained shortly.

However, the term which most frequently is employed in the Old Testament to designate the very life principle of a person is *nepes* which at its root signifies throat, and then the breathing substance or being of an individual. It is used in conjunction with the word blood in Dt. 12:23 cited above. Inasmuch as *nepes* is connected with breathing, it carries the meaning of that which makes a person alive. The people of the Bible saw that as long as a person actually breathed, that individual was alive — thus they made the connection of breath with life just as they saw the relationship of blood with life. In Genesis, when Rachel breathes her last breath, her life departs; thus the Elohist says: "And as her soul (*nepes*) was departing (for she died), she called his name Benoni" (35:18). Jeremiah, in his oracle against Jerusalem, (15:9) speaks about Jerusalem's death as the surrendering of *nepes*. So, from the meaning of breath of life, *nepes* often means life itself (I Sam 19:11).

It has already been noted (Is 40:6-7) that there is a third term dealing with life principles; that term is *ruah* and it means breath, wind, or spirit. Confusion arises in the English translations of the bible as it does in many other modern language translations when *ruah* is used in a similar way as is *nepes* when speaking of a life principle (Gn 6:17); nevertheless, *ruah* has one basic difference — it indicates the vital influence of God upon human beings whether this be in a natural way through creation or some supernatural way by God's direct intervention. God is indeed a living God and he does exercise a dynamic living influence upon his human creation. A human being's life principle, *nepes,* lives and dies; not so the *ruah*. The *ruah* is God's living force communicated to human beings; but of itself does not belong to the human being as such. *Nepes* conveys life; *ruah* conveys power — God's sustaining power. Thus the *ruah* of a living, breathing being dwelling in the *basar* (flesh) is a gift of God (Zech 12:1), is preserved by God (Num 27:16), and departs at death to return to God (Is 38:16; Ps 78:39).

Thus the biblical authors give us three principles of life: *dam* (blood), *nepes* (life/breath/spirit), *ruah* (God's sustaining power). When breathing ceases and when blood is poured out, there is no life left in the individual — that individual has died. But when an individual suffers physical death, God's *ruah* does not die, but returns to him because it is the Living God's sustaining influence in and upon the individual. Mistakenly and inaccurately, God's *ruah* has been equated with what moderns call soul. However, the people of the Bible did not think in those categories; they had a wholistic understanding of what it meant to be human. Human beings were described on the basis of the relationship which they had with God the creator and not in terms of a western bi-partite division of body/soul.[14] God's *ruah* is not to be understood as an equivalent to what we call soul.

Blood is Life

Because of the relationship of blood to life, blood must be reserved to Yahweh alone, the sole Master of all life. In the sacrificial ritual, what is important is not the death of the animal victim, but "the offering of its life, released in the form of blood, to God."[15] The regulation against the eating of blood is seen as having a religious basis: ". . .do not sin against the Lord by eating with the blood" (1 Sam 14:34). Life is in the blood and thus must be reserved for God — to eat blood is to take upon oneself the position of God as the communicator and giver of life. If the life of an animal belongs to God — the role of blood in animal sacrifices indicates this belief — then the reasoning follows that no human being has a right over the life of any other. Human life is so precious a possession that even an animal bloodletter must be punished. Ex 21:18f prescribes death for an ox which fatally gores either a man or a woman; even its flesh cannot be eaten for the animal has shed human blood and is thus contaminated.

In this context, it should be noted that Jehovah Witnesses refuse to submit to and to allow blood transfusions. One of the key texts in their position is Leviticus 17:14 as cited above. Certainly the idea of a blood transfusion did not enter the mind of the sacred author; it was not a medical practice of the time. The prohibition of the eating of blood may have been due in the shrouded past to hygenic reasons,[16] but, as recounted in the word of God which has been handed down to us in the Bible, it is seen clearly in the light of religious belief. Nowhere in the Bible is there any notice that one living human being with no discernible injury to self must not give blood to another so that others might continue to live. The Bible does maintain that God is sovereign over life — and life is to be found in the blood.

The legal codes of the Pentateuch list várious penalties for murder, the unjust taking of life. In Exodus 20:7-17, we have the content of the Ten Commandments of which one stipulation (v 13) is "You shall not kill", or in the *New English Bible* "Do no murder". In the passages which follow in Exodus 21:12-31, along with Leviticus 24:17 and Numbers 35:9-34, there are various occasions listed when the death penalty is to be exacted; all are serious occasions and most are in retribution for an innocent life which has been taken. Thus the statement "You shall not kill" is not an absolute imperative. It does not mean that the killing of a human being is always wrong under every circumstance; rather in the light of the other aforementioned cited passages, it is evident that the sacred writer is saying that it is not permitted to take an innocent life. The other passages inform us that there are occasions when a guilty individual's life may be taken. Human life is inviolate and those who take it must be punished — a punishment which often consists in the taking of their lives.

Because of the sacred character of life, blood revenge is taken for granted (Ex 21; Dt 19). Members of a tribe or clan or family all share the same life blood in their veins. If a member's blood has been shed, then the next of kin must bring about punishment and mete out measure for measure. Some primitive societies permitted the killing of a murderer's family or tribe — not so under the Mosaic Law; the murderer alone was to be punished (Dt 24:16; 2 Kgs 14:6). Blood revenge rested in the concept of corporate personality[17] — as a family, tribe, or nation, the members were one and thus any harm done to one individual was really harm being wrought upon all the members of the group. In the New Testament, God himself is portrayed as the avenger of blood (Rev 6:10). He is also the vindicator/redeemer (*go'el*) of whom Job speaks (19:25).

Human sacrifices and the practice of offering human blood had been forbidden to the Hebrew people although there is the one example from Israelite history of Jephthah offering his daughter as a holocaust (Jdg 11:31-40); he was severely punished for his misdeed. The story of Abraham and Isaac (Gn 22) tells us that only God has dominion over human life and thus human sacrifice is strictly forbidden by God himself. The whole account is a polemic against human sacrifice because God does not want any human life to be taken for an offering to him, even in ritual. Among the pagans, the emphasis in sacrifice was often on what human beings could do for their gods. Among the Israelites, the emphasis was upon what God could do for his covenanted people (Ex 19:5-6).

Death

The understanding that death was the common lot of all human creation was universally maintained by the ancient Hebrews: "We must all die, we are like water spilt on the ground, which cannot be gathered up again . . ." (2 Sam 14:14). Based on the Old Testament presentation we find a debatable question as to whether human beings were created to be mortal or immortal.[18] "Then the Lord God formed man of dust from the ground, and breathed into his nostrils the breath of life; and man became a living (*nepes*) being" (Gn 2:9). Later in 3:19 the man and woman are expelled from the garden after they have eaten the fruit from the forbidden tree of the knowledge of good and evil; they are told that they will return to the ground from which they were made — dust will return to dust. The impression conveyed is that they were created to be mortal. Gn 2:17 recounts that man in the garden was given free range of it and could eat of any fruit tree with one exception — the tree of the knowledge of good and evil. To eat of this tree will result in death — thus this tradition gives the impression that humanity was created to be immortal and not to see death. As both traditions were merged in cc 2-3 of Genesis, death is presented as coming into the world because of sin and it is a true punishment for disobedience. Nevertheless, it would appear that this is not the mainstream of Old Testament thought, at least not until the Maccabean/Hasmonean[19] period when the deuterocanonical books (The apocrypha[20]) were written; the burden of the Old Testament teaching is that human beings were created to be mortal and to see death.

The Wisdom of Solomon, coming from the Hasmonean period, is very insistent upon the acceptance of death, physical and spiritual, as the result of sin coming into God's created world: "For God created man for incorruption, and made him in the image of his own eternity, but through the devil's envy death entered the world, and those who belong to his party experience it" (2:23-24). "Death is an ultimate threat only to the wicked, who assume that death is the end of a meaningful existence."[21]

The Hereafter

At death, in the Israelite's anthropological view, an individual went to the Abode of the Dead, *Sheol,* also called a place of darkness, a pit, and located at the very end of the world. (In the New Testament, this Abode of the Dead is called Hades.)[22] This was a common understanding among other ancient people in the Near East as well — e.g. Canaanites and Akkadians. The word *Sheol* itself is used some 66 times in the Hebrew Bible and is a word found only in the Hebrew language. Other words used to designate this Abode of the Dead, such as the pit, the ditch, or the place of darkness are also found in other Near Eastern cultures of the time.

When an individual died and went to Sheol, all activity ceased. Ecclesiastes tells us "Whatever your hand finds to do, do it with your might; for there is no work or thought or knowledge or wisdom in Sheol, to which you are going" (9:10). Still, death was not considered to be the cessation of all existence because those who actually went to Sheol continued in some sort of shadowy residence there. To be sure, the flesh, *basar,* ended up in the grave, but the person continued a type of existence in Sheol. Job reminds us of the finality of the Abode of the Dead: "Let me alone, that I may find a little comfort before I go whence I shall not return to the land of gloom and the deep darkness. . ." (10:20-21). And again, Ecclesiastes mentions that everyone has the same fate — both the good and evil: "Everything before them is vanity, since one fate comes to all, to the righteous and the wicked, to good and the evil, to the clean and the unclean. . .For the living know that they will die, but the dead know nothing, and they have no more reward; but the memory of them is lost" (9:2, 5).

It is during the latter part of the Old Testament period when the deuterocanonical books (Apocrypha) were written that a distinction about the lot of the dead is found. In 4 Mac 13:17, we read about the "bosom of Abraham" vs the Abode of the Dead: "For if we so die, Abraham and Isaac and Jacob will welcome us, and all the fathers will praise us."[23] In the Gospel, Luke mentions explicitly the bosom of Abraham in 16:22-23: "The poor man died and was buried; and in Hades, being in torment, he lifted up his eyes, and saw Abraham far off and Lazarus in his bosom."

In 2 Mac 7 we find the episode during the reign of Antiochus Epiphanes IV, when the king was persecuting the devout Jews, of a Jewish mother who urged her seven sons not to eat the forbidden swine's flesh which the king had demanded. She urged her children to accept death willingly and, one by one, each of the children was put to death and finally the mother as well. During the course of this celebrated chapter 7, one of the sons says: "One cannot but choose to die at the hands of men and to cherish the hope that God gives of being raised again by him. But for you, there will be no resurrection to life." (7:14). This text speaks clearly about a continuation of life beyond the grave. An even older attestation to life beyond the grave is presented to us in the canonical Daniel which was written during the same historical period, being written during the reign of Antiochus Epiphanes IV (c.165 B.C.).[24] He says: "And many of those who sleep in the dust of the earth shall awake, some to everlasting life, and some to shame and everlasting contempt" (12:2). Regardless of what else can be said about the passage, whether it is speaking of a resurrection of all faithful people or only of the faithful Jews, this is the first passage to "give the first sure teaching of life beyond the grave."[25]

Quality of Life

The Israelites' basic view of humankind was that each individual was an animated body and not some incarnate soul that had to escape at death. Prior to the late period after the year 200 B.C., this present existence was actually the only type of life that the people really understood, at the same time acknowledging some type of shadowy existence beyond the grave. M. Dahood has made a case for an earlier belief in the rewards of the afterlife. He does so based on a philological study of the Psalms. Nevertheless, B. Vawter has presented a successful challenge to the position of M. Dahood.[26]

Prior to the writings following 200 B.C., the emphasis in the Old Testament is not so much upon death, which is to be shunned at all costs, but rather upon the quality of life and the living. Old age was considered to be one of God's greatest blessings. Enoch is said to have walked with God and, after 365 years, God took him (Gn 5:24). To walk with God meant one was close to God, lived according to God's ways, and God took care of that person.

Isaac is said to have been 180 years old at his death when he was gathered to his people "old and full of days" (Gn 35:29). To Abraham, the Lord had promised: "And I will establish my covenant between me and you and your descendants after you throughout their generations for an everlasting covenant, to be God to you and your descendants after you" (Gn 17:7). In both of these citations, we see a relationship of the individual to the group; at death, one went to join the ancestors who had gone on before; what remained was the living covenanted people. The people saw themselves living on in their descendants, and not only direct descendants, but life continued through the successive generations of the family unit. Ezkiel's dry bones coming to life (c.37) concerns the life of the nation which must continue; God's promises made to the patriarchs and kings about the chosen people as a great nation will not be thwarted.

In the earlier passages of the Old Testament, there is an emphasis on parents desiring to have many children; children being seen as a real cause of joy to their parents. For not only did they continue, as it were, to live the life which their parents gave them, but they, too, were fulfilling the promises made by God to their ancestors. The psalmist reminds us that having children is a joyfilled event (Ps 127-128). Yet by the time of the Wisdom of Solomon (c.3), the undefiled barren woman as well as the eunuch who had done no wickedness are said to be among the just and in the hand of God (3:1). "Childlessness with virtue" is rewarded rather than an "unrighteous generation" (4:1). At this late period, the time of Wisdom, death is only to be feared by the wicked (c.2). But the righteous "are in the hand of God" (3:1).

New Testament

The people of the New Testament were the heirs to the Old Testament thought on anthropology, life, and death. For, although they wrote in Greek, they were Semites speaking the living language of the day, Aramaic, a language similar to ancient Hebrew. They wrote Greek, but the Greek had Hebrew/Aramaic meaning. For the people of God redeemed by the blood of Jesus, the quality of life was not limited to present realities, but, continuing in the line of Daniel, Wisdom of Solomon, and 2 and 4 Maccabees, the focus was on the present which would one day issue forth into a glorious future.

The Greek word for immortality, *athanasia,* occurs three times in the New Testament. It is attributable above all to God alone who possesses immortality (1 Tim 6:16). Nevertheless, in speaking to the Corinthians, Paul reminds them that Jesus Christ has vanquished death and that physical death can no longer hold any tyranny over them. In speaking about the resurrection of the body,[27] he can say:

> For this perishable nature must put on the imperishable, but this mortal nature must put on immortality. When the perishable puts on the imperishable, and the mortal puts on immortality, then shall come to pass the saying that is written: "Death is swallowed

up in victory. O death, where is thy victory? O death, where is thy sting?" (1 Cor 15:53-55).

Within the same context of 1 Corinthians (15:45-49), Paul refers back to the biblical account of Genesis 2-3, contrasting humankind's relationship to Adam and dust with its present relationship to Christ and heaven. It would seem that Paul understood death as the result of sin,[28] following in the tradition of the Wisdom of Solomon.[29] Immortality, as Paul used it, would seem to signify human life transformed by the participation in the divine life of Jesus Christ.[30] Throughout 1 Cor 15, the emphasis is upon Christ who through his own death has conquered death, been raised, and given human beings the power "to be made alive" (15:22). The Immortal God has communicated his life to his Son Jesus who in turn gives life to humanity. The life of the believer is founded upon the saving events of the Incarnation, Passion, Death, and Resurrection of Jesus Christ. John tells Christians that an active belief in the person of Jesus Christ, the one lifted up upon the cross, brings the believer to "eternal life" (Jn 3:15). That eternal quality to life begins in time with the historic activity of the redeeming work of Christ on our behalf. It is a quality of life which the believer now possesses and which will continue for all time. The quality far exceeds any type of merely human (unredeemed) life here on earth. Christ's death has vanquished death and sin — his death is understood as an antidote to the sin of Adam.

Paul recounts his own feelings about his death in 2 Corinthians and Philippians. Physical death is not an easy way out from the difficulties of the present.

> So we are always of good courage; we know that while we are at home in the body we are away from the Lord, for we walk by faith, not by sight. We are of good courage, and we would rather be away from the body and at home with the Lord. So whether we are at home or away, we make aim to please him (2 Cor 5:6-9).

Throughout the entire chapter, Paul is making the point that he has work to do for the community. Christ died for everyone and so the individual Christian has work to do here on earth — a work which Paul has found to be a message of reconciliation (5:19).

> For to me to live is Christ, and to die is gain. If it is to be life in the flesh, that means fruitful labor for me. Yet, which I shall choose I cannot tell. I am hard pressed between the two. My desire is to

14

depart and be with Christ, for that is far better. But to remain in the flesh is more necessary on your account (Phil 1:21-24).

Physical death is not the end; a Christian must understand this. Paul himself eagerly looked forward to death so that he might even more fully enjoy that quality of life, already begun in his conversion experience and baptism, in a more complete way.

In giving his last "oration" on the fulfillment of the Old Testament Promises, Stephen, before breathing his last breath while being stoned to death, saw the glory of God coming to him at that moment: "Behold I see the heavens opened, and the Son of man standing at the right hand of God" (Acts 7:56), and then, at the last moment, he cried out "Lord Jesus, receive my spirit" (Acts 7:59).

What the New Testament adds over and above the Old Testament understanding of physical death including that of the Maccabean/Hasmonean period, is that one can look forward to death, not with fear, but with anticipation of the fullness of eternal life. The Christian is to have confidence to enter into the heavenly city of God because, by his blood, Jesus has gone on before in order to open a new and living way (Heb 10:19). The Christian is encouraged to enter into the rest which only God can give (Heb 4:11). It cannot be forgotten that the follower of Jesus is called to lead a life in community. Even now, the faithful on earth are joined, not only to the community of earth, but also to the community which has gone on before (Heb 12:18-24). In Revelation, it is the Living God who causes his people to be sealed so that they not undergo punishment to be visited upon those who have made of God an enemy (Rev 7:2), those who are said to have permanently fixed an abode on earth: "Woe, woe, woe to those who dwell on the earth. . ." (Rev 8:13).

Throughout the New Testament, death is seen as a time for transformation of the faithful individual — a stage in the journey of life. Even though the New Testament writers picked up the Greek vocabulary of body/soul, they, too, still viewed human beings wholistically[31] in the light of the concepts already discussed in this chapter.[32]

The questioning of the legitimacy of capital punishment is not addressed in the New Testament. The identical teaching about murder which is contained in the Old Testament is presupposed and reiterated in the New Testament in the list of the commandments (Mt 19:18; Lk 18:20; Rom 13:9; James 2:11). Murder, which is understood as the killing of an innocent individual who has committed no crime deserving of death, is seen to come deliberately from maliciousness, "from within" (Mk 7:21).

This chapter concludes with one last citation from Sacred Scripture; it is the Gospel of John in which we find the words: "I am the way, and the truth, and the life; no one comes to the Father, but by me" (14:6). Jesus' life, we are reminded, is to be the pattern for our lives; his death too is a pattern for our deaths. As a pilgrim people, we are encouraged to walk in the footsteps of the Lord. We have woven a path through The Book; now, through reflection, we must allow the message to sink into our hearts in order to derive meaning for our lives today.

Summary and Reflection

1. The God of the Bible is a living God who communicates His life to all living things and, above all, to beings made in his image and likeness — humankind. Life, then is a gift from God.

2. As the Living God, He is unique among the various gods of the pagans; He takes care of the human beings He has created. He especially has regard for his covenanted community. There is a communal relationship to God as well as an individual one.

3. Biblical anthropology views the human individual as one whole; it does not follow the bi-partite Greek concepts of body/soul. The New Testament, written in Greek, is nonetheless the heir to the wholistic thought pattern of the Old Testament. There should not be undo emphasis placed upon either the "body" or the "soul", but upon the individual as a whole.

4. In the Old Testament, the quality of a human being's life is measured in terms of God's sustaining influence upon the individual (*ruah*), the breath of life (*nepes*), and the blood (*dam*) in which life resides. The quality of life lived is of great importance.

5. Blood is life; all life belongs to God. For a human being to eat blood is to arrogate to oneself the position of God. The Bible has a great reverence for life. The people of God as a corporate person have the same life blood coursing through their veins. Humankind has an obligation of care and concern toward the individual lives of each of its members. This is especially

true for all people who acknowledge that life ultimately belongs to God.

6. God is the author of life; only He can permit human life to be taken — this is permitted only for specific serious crimes. Murder, the taking of an innocent life, is not permitted.

7. Death occurs when blood has been poured out and when the life breath ceases. Death is an empirical fact.

8. God has intended death as the normal lot for humankind. Superimposed upon this tradition, in the biblical data, is that death is a punishment for sin. Death is part of God's plan; physical death cannot be avoided.

9. There was a gradual development in the belief in an active life beyond the grave; this especially comes to the fore during the Maccabean period and is further developed in the New Testament. The blessings received during life do not terminate with physical death; life becomes richer beyond the grave.

10. The New Testament is insistent that Jesus Christ has transformed death. Death is not the end; it need not be feared unduly. Eternal life, already experienced now, flourishes in the life to come. Having been created by God, baptized into Jesus Christ whose name is confessed, the Christian already enjoys the life of heaven, looks forward to the life which is to flourish after physical death, and continues to live day by day sheltered by the presence of the Lord.

Notes

1. Harris, Stephen L. *Understanding the Bible*. Mayfield Publishing Co. 1980. pp. 3-5.

2. Kallas, James. *Revelation: God and Satan in The Apocalypse*. Augsburg Press 1973. pp. 111-112.

3. All Scripture quotes are from the Revised Standard Version unless otherwise noted. The RSV has been chosen because it is an ecumenical translation; not only have the editors translated the canonical and deuterocanonical books, but also the Books of 3 and 4 Maccabees and Psalm 151 which most Orthodox Churches consider authoritative. cf: *The New Oxford Annotated Bible with the Apocrypha Expanded Edition. Revised Standard Version*. "Introduction to the Apocrypha" p. xiii. Oxford University Press. 1977.

4. Brueggemann, Walter. "Presence of God, Cultic" *Interpreter's Dictionary of the Bible. Supplementary Volume*. 1977. pp. 680-683.

5. Ringgren, Helmer. "Monotheism" *Interpreter's Dictionary of the Bible. Supplementary Volume*. 1977. pp. 602-604.

6. *Ibid*.

7. The Book of Joshua is part of deuteronomic history.

8. Dahood, Mitchell. *Psalms*. Vol. III. *The Anchor Bible*. Doubleday and Co. 1970. p. 46.

9. Underlined English words used for emphasis.

10. McCarthy, Denis, J. "Blood", *Interpreter's Dictionary of the Bible. Supplementary Volume*. 1977. pp. 114-117.

11. Abba, Raymond. "The Origin and Significance of Hebrew Sacrifice," *Biblical Theology Bulletin*. Vol. 7 July 1977. pp. 123-138.

12. DiLella, Alexander. "Conservative and Progressive Theology: Sirach and Wisdom", *Catholic Biblical Quarterly*. Vol. 28 1966. p. 143.

13. *Ibid.* p. 149.

14. Jewett, Robert. "Body" *Interpreter's Dictionary of the Bible. Supplementary Volume*. 1977. pp. 117-118.

15. Abba, Raymond. *op. cit.* p. 135.

16. Hartmann, Louis F. *Encyclopedic Dictionary of the Bible*. Macmillan and Co. 1963. p. 255.

17. Robinson, Wheeler H. *Corporate Personality in Ancient Israel*. Revised Edition. Fortress Press 1980. p. 30.

18. Bailey, Sr., Lloyd R. *Biblical Perspectives on Death*. Fortress Press 1979. pp. 36-38.

19. The Maccabean age encompases c. 175 B.C. - 135 B.C., beginning with the Seleucid oppression of the Jews and ending with the death of the last Maccabee ruler. The Hasmonean age encompases 134 B.C. - 63 B.C., from the reign of the first Hasmonean ruler until the Roman domination of Israel. Among Protestants, this period is linked together with the 100 years previous and is called the *Intertestamental Period*. It is during this time that the deuterocanonical books were written which Catholics consider inspired and pertaining to Old Testament literature.

20. For a discussion of the terms *deuterocanonical* and *Apocrypha* the reader is referred to footnote 1. "Introduction to the Apocrypha," pp. xi-xviii.

21. Bailey, Sr., Lloyd R. *op. cit.* p. 80.

22. Mt 11:23; Acts 2:27; Rev 20:13.

23. cf: footnote 3.

24. *New Oxford Annotated Bible. op. cit.* p. 1067.

25. Hartmann, Louis and DiLella, Alexander. *Book of Daniel. Anchor Bible* Vol. 23. Doubleday and Co. 1978. p. 309.

26. Dahood, Mitchell. *op. cit.* pp. LI-LII responded to by: Vawter, Bruce. "Intimations of Immortality and OT," *Journal of Biblical Literature*. Vol. 91 1972. pp. 158-171.

27. Bailey, Sr., Lloyd R. *op. cit.* p. 93. The author challenges the position advanced by Oscar Cullmann that God gives immortality to the souls of the just. The reader is referred to Oscar Cullmann's essay "Immortality of the Soul or Resurrection of the Dead," *Immortality and Resurrection*. Ed. Krister Stendahl. Macmillan and Co. 1965. pp. 9-53.

28. Rom 6:23.

29. Wis 2:23-24.

30. Norris, Jr., Richard A. "Immortality," *Interpreter's Dictionary of the Bible. Supplementary Volume*. 1977. p. 426.

31. *Psyche* in *Theological Dictionary of the New Testament*. Vol. IX. pp. 645-646. 1971.

32. *nepes, ruah, dam.*

Select Bibliography

Abba, Raymond. "The Origin and Significance of Hebrew Sacrifice," *Biblical Theology Bulletin*. Vol. 7 1977. pp. 123-138.

Bailey, Sr., Lloyd R. *Biblical Perspectives on Death*. Fortress Press. 1979.

DiLella, Alexander. "Conservative and Progressive Theology: Sirach and Wisdom," *Catholic Biblical Quarterly*. Vol. 28 1966. pp. 135-154.

Cullmann, Oscar. *The Christology of the New Testament*. SCM Press Ltd. 1963.

DaHood, Mitchell. *Psalms* Vol. III *The Anchor Bible*. Doubleday. 1970.

Harris, Stephen L. *Understanding the Bible*. Mayfield Publishing Co. 1980.

Hartmann, Louis F. *Encyclopedia Dictionary of the Bible*. McGraw-Hill. 1963.

Hartmann, Louis and DiLella, Alexander. *Book of Daniel, Anchor Bible*. Doubleday. 1978.

Interpreter's Dictionary of the Bible. Supplementary Volume. Abingdon Press. 1976.

Brueggemann, Walter. "Death, Theology of," pp. 219-22.

Brueggemann, Walter. "Presence of God, Cultic," pp. 680-83.

Jewett, Robert. "Body," pp. 117-118.

Jewett, Robert. "Man, nature of, in the NT," pp. 561-563.

McCarthy, Denis J. "Blood," pp. 114-117.

Nickelsburg, Jr., George W. E. "Future Life in Intertestamental Literature," pp. 348-351.

Norris, Jr., Richard A. "Immortality," pp. 426-428.

Ringgren, Helmer. "Monotheism," pp. 602-604.

Kallas, James. *Revelation: God and Satan in The Apocalypse.* Augsburg Pub. Co. 1973.

Leon-Dufour, Xavier. *Dictionary of Biblical Theology.* Seabury Press. Revised English Edition. 1973.

Lyonnet, Stanislas and Sabourin, Leopold. *Sin, Redemption, and Sacrifice.* Pontifical Biblical Institute Press. 1970.

McKenzie, John. *Dictionary of the Bible.* Macmillan and Co. 1965.

Malina, Bruce. "The Individual and the Community: Personality in the Social World of Early Christianity," *Biblical Theology Bulletin.* Vol. 9 1979. pp. 126-128.

Montague, George T. *The Living Thought of St. Paul.* Benzinger Press. 1976.

The New Oxford Annotated Bible with the Apocrypha Expanded Edition. Revised Standard Version. Oxford University Press. 1977.

Robinson, Wheeler H. *Corporate Personality in Ancient Israel.* Revised Edition. Fortress Press. 1980.

Theological Dictionary of the New Testament. 10 Volumes. Editors: Gerhard Kittel and Gerhard Freidrich. Translated by Geoffrey W. Bromiley. W. B. Eerdmans Pub. Co. 1971.

Thompson, Leonard L. *Introducing Biblical Literature.* Prentice-Hall Inc. 1978.

Chapter 2

Consequentialism and the Fifth Commandment

The Reverend Richard R. Roach, S.J., Ph.D.

All ethics are a mixture of prudence and prohibitions. Some choices, even choices that are a matter of life and death, are regulated only by prudential considerations; other choices should be determined by a clear appreciation of what God has prohibited. Manifestly, in the area of medical ethics, where many questions are about matters of life and death, it is essential that practitioners know this distinction between prudence and prohibition. In particular, they should know when that prohibition applies which Catholics know as the Fifth Commandment, although Calvinists number it the sixth, namely, the prohibition, *Do no murder*.

In order to focus our minds on this distinction between a strictly prudential decision and a moral judgment involving the fifth commandment, let us imagine a situation such as the following: a doctor must decide quickly which of two somewhat different procedures to initiate in order to treat a patient; it is a matter of life and death; both procedures are indicated; there are no unequivocal signs which would indicate that one is clearly preferred. His choice, then, will be prudential in the broad sense of the term: his prudence as it has been specialized by training and experience into that art we know as the practice of medicine.

On another occasion, if the doctor has a trained conscience, the choice facing him may give rise to a further consideration of a different kind. He may find himself in a situation facing a dilemma such that he needs to ask himself whether what he contemplates doing or not doing would be murder, and therefore forbidden. Before he can act rightly as his art would dictate, he must settle the question as to whether what he is considering doing or not doing (omitting) is permitted or not, under the fifth commandment. Therefore, we may say that a whole theology of life and death lies hidden in that commandment.

At the heart of that theology is the knowledge that sin, which destroys life and causes death, consists essentially in disobeying God, whereas obedience rendered to God in faith, hope, and love is His redeeming gift which issues in that resurrected life which eventually His true sons and daughters will enjoy everlastingly. The death we all must suffer here because of original and actual sin need not be final. It need not be the death of hell. We may die rendering acts of obedience in faith, hope, and love. Then death leads to everlasting life. But to die obedientially, we must live obedientially. That is to say, at no matter what the cost, we must strive never to perform those acts which deny the kind of creature God made us (i.e., deny our human nature) and which attempt to usurp His sovereignty; or, if we sin, we must repent and seek His forgiveness. Of course, one such act is murder.

Do No Murder

There are two understandings of the prohibition, Do no murder. The first is absolute and the second is either overtly or covertly consequentialist. The Church teaches the first, and rejects the second. No amount of "theological" or other dissent has or can change that. In what follows, I hope the distinction between the two understandings will become clearer.

The Church teaches that this commandment absolutely forbids "intentionally killing the innocent."[1] Anscombe wisely has noted that this notion constitutes the "hard core of the concept of murder," but a simple definition will not do for all possible complicated cases. For example, we would be inclined, and I think rightly, to consider some arsonists as murderers. If an arsonist set fire to a building in which children were sleeping and, as a result of his act, they were burned to death, we would consider the arsonist a murderer. If we tied ourselves too closely to a "simple definition" of murder which designated only the "hard core" of the concept, we would put ourselves in a logical bind. The arsonist might truthfully say that he did not intend to kill the innocent.

I mention this example not only to point out what Anscombe has clearly shown — namely, that a simple definition of murder is helpful, even necessary, but will not do for all cases — but also to obviate the use of normal difficulties in defining this and like concepts by those who want to discredit traditional absolute moral prohibitions. They would have us believe that problems with the "simple definition" are gateways to exceptions, whereas they are really invitations to recall that acts not adequately covered by the "simple definition" also are murderous. In short, murder includes all those acts designated by the simple definition, and a bit more. Nor is this observation weakened by considering those special "hard cases" which men of good will may dispute about, asking whether in truth the simple definition applies. Would I be intentionally killing the innocent if I performed a craniotomy (directly kill a child in the womb so as to facilitate passage through the birth canal)? The Church said that any answer other than yes was not safe.[2] Good men who know that the prohibition is absolute have pondered the issue to see if there might not be a safe way to say no.[3] I am not sure they have been successful, but I am sure that such questioning is not a reason for rejecting absolutes, but a clear sign of how seriously they ought to be taken.

"Intentional," or its synonym, "direct," is perhaps the slipperiest term in the definition, but it is not indefinable. It means simply that I am doing *this* on purpose, and the "this" falls under a specific description which a rational assessment of what I propose to do, am doing, or have done requires. As with all such basic terms, we best understand intentional in contrast with its opposite, unintentional. Unintentional or indirect, in the relevant sense, means something that goes along with what I am doing on purpose, but falls outside a reasonable description of what I am doing on purpose, even when I cannot prevent it from happening along with what I am doing on purpose. For example, I intentionally (directly) brake my car abruptly for very good reason — it is the only way to avoid running over a small child. I foresee that my action will result in another car running into me from behind. I do not intend this to happen, although I foresee it. The wreck is unintentional (*praeter intentionem*) or indirect, although I cause it to happen. ("Unintentional" may also be used of my heart beat or a knee-jerk when the doctor taps the joint, and so forth.)

This review of traditional moral doctrine is intended only to recall to our minds the understanding of that morality with its nuances and casuistry in which a handful of prohibitions are absolute. That is the morality the Church has taught from the beginning, teaches now, and will always teach. She will do so because the morality is true. Furthermore, her faith in God the Creator helps us to see that this morality is true because this morality of absolutes captures accurately our standing as creatures.

Consequentialism

The congeries of theories that contest Church teaching today are all various forms of consequentialism. Consequentialism is a technical term given its best description, in my opinion, by Elizabeth Anscombe in 1958.[4] The salient features of consequentialism are two: the *first* is the claim that no one can prove there are no exceptions to the prohibition, Do no murder, as described thus far. In other words, consequentialists believe that no one can prove the prohibition, Do no murder, is objective, non-tautologous and absolute. The *second* feature is a concession: consequentialism allows that an individual may adopt the prohibition, understood as admitting of no exceptions, as his or her private morality; and such an individual cannot be shown to be wrong any more than the absolute prohibition can be shown never to admit of exceptions.

The concept of "exception" rather than "consequence" is the key to what Anscombe defined as consequentialism, because the use of a consequentialist argument may be hidden even from the arguer and require analysis to expose it, whereas it will be plain that the point of the argument is to justify an exception to what had hitherto been thought of as an exceptionless prohibition. In order to underscore this point, Prof. Anscombe has given me permission, *viva voce*, to refer to what she defined as consequentialism as "exceptionism" when the latter term would be helpful.

In her classic article, Anscombe does not expand on the second feature of her precise definition. Unfortunately, what has happened in our culture since she wrote has made it imperative to add a few words. First, we should note that "consequentialists," while denying that murder as traditionally conceived is absolutely prohibited, have invented another absolute prohibition to take its place: namely, the absolute prohibition against founding public policy on the traditional absolute prohibitions. You may hold to the absolute prohibition against a directly procured abortion, but only if you take that position privately, and in no way seek to shape public policy according to that morality. In other words, the second feature of Anscombe's definition of consequentialism has become an immoral absolute forbidding us to found public policy on the natural law or objective morality as that has been understood from the dawn of Western civilization. What will remain of that civilization as this new morality, consequentialism, works its destructive effects on our society remains to be seen, but I am willing to hazard the prediction that nothing of the public recognition of human freedom and dignity which we have come to cherish will survive.[5]

Meaning of Terms

One of the worst tergiversations consequentialists have begun to engage in is to change the meanings of the ordinary terms used in the traditional moral prohibitions from an objective to a subjective signification, thereby making the prohibitions tautologous. This move is the result of a confusion regarding the meaning of intention which Anscombe has described as follows:

> The reason why people are confused about intention, and why they sometimes think there is no difference between contraceptive intercourse and the use of infertile times to avoid conception, is this: They don't notice the difference between "intention" when it means the intentionalness of the thing you're doing — that you're doing *this* on purpose — and when it means a *further* or *accompanying* intention *with* which you do the thing. For example, I make a table: that's an intentional action because I am doing just *that* on purpose. I have the *further* intention of, say, earning my living, doing my job *by* making the table. Contraceptive intercourse and intercourse using infertile times may be alike in respect of further intention, and these further intentions may be good, justified, excellent. This the Pope (Paul VI in *Humanae Vitae*) has noted. He sketched such a situation and said: "It cannot be denied that in both cases the married couple, for acceptable reasons," (for that's how he imagined the case) "are perfectly clear in their intention to

avoid children and mean to secure that none will be born." This is a comment on two things: contraceptive intercourse on the one hand and intercourse using infertile times on the other, for the sake of the limitation of the family.[6]

In order to bring out the force of Anscombe's point, I shall elaborate on it, bearing in mind that the elaboration expresses my way of thinking about the matter and not necessarily hers. If we assume what I believe is the truth of the matter, namely, that God designed sexual intercourse to be a conjugal act, then what a person is doing when intentionally bringing on an orgasm, or other bodily movements virtually a part of orgasm, is in the first instance right if it is a conjugal act or wrong if it is not. We must add "in the first instance" because the act could qualify as a conjugal act and be vitiated by the further or accompanying intention or circumstances, but if it were not a conjugal act, it would *not* be redeemed by such considerations. It would qualify as a conjugal act if it were intercourse which is apt for procreation engaged in by a man and a woman who are married to each other. Thus, Anscombe continues on from the paragraph quoted above saying:

> But contraceptive intercourse is faulted, not on account of this further intention, but because of the kind of intentional action you are doing. The action is not left by you as the kind of act by which life is transmitted, but is purposely rendered infertile, and so changed to another sort of act altogether.[7]

The basic question is whether sexual intercourse can be normatively described. The answer to this question cuts to the quick where people either see the answer or they do not, where whether one is right or wrong is not a matter of discursive reasoning, but a matter of whether one perceives a fundamental reality or not. Anscombe brings out the point by contrasting a sexual act with eating:

> There is not such a thing as a casual, nonsignificant sexual act; everyone knows this. Contrast sex with eating — you're strolling along a lane, you see a mushroom on a bank as you pass by, you know about mushrooms, you pick it and you eat it quite casually — sex is never like that. That's why virtue in connection with eating is basically a matter only of the *pattern* of one's eating habits. But virtue in sex — chastity — is not *only* a matter of such a pattern, that is of its role in a pair of lives. A single sexual action can be bad even without regard to its context, its further intentions and its motives.[8]

Either a man sees that sex is not like eating or he does not, and if he does not, then I believe that he is wrong and suffers from a singularly impoverished view of reality.[9] But I cannot prove to him that he is wrong by appealing to a more fundamental truth and reasoning to the significance of sex as the conclusion of an argument. Therefore, all the kinds of genital acts we may engage in *except* the conjugal act are rightly judged to be acts that are bad-in-themselves. Once we see this, we understand why fornication or adultery is evaluated differently from going on strike or fighting. I may not fornicate, even if doing so would bring me a better wage; but, I may go on strike for a better wage, other things being equal, if my present wage is unfair. I may not commit adultery in order to protect my country from attack; but I may fight to defend her, other things being equal, if she is unjustly attacked. Again Anscombe has put it all very neatly:

> In considering an action, we need always to judge several things about ourselves. First: is the *sort* of act we contemplate doing something that it's all right to do? Second: are our further or surrounding intentions all right? Third: is the spirit in which we do it all right? Contraceptive intercourse fails on the first count; and to intend such an act is not to intend a marriage act at all, whether or not we're married. An act of ordinary intercourse in marriage at an infertile time, though, is a perfectly ordinary act of married intercourse, and it will be bad, if it is bad, only on the second or third counts.[10]

Going on strike or fighting, like "ordinary intercourse during an infertile time," also fails only on the second or third counts. Fornication and adultery fail on the first. The somewhat distasteful topic of masturbation may serve as the best example of this very important point. A young man may masturbate for the fun of it. A young married couple may engage in a conjugal act for the fun of it. The consequentialist does not analyze correctly the difference between these two acts, because consequentialism excludes the notion of acts that are bad-in-themselves. A consequentialist must adduce something extrinsic to the act in itself in order to reject it.

For example, a somewhat naive consequentialist could argue from a "calculus of pleasures" to a "prohibition" of masturbation. He would then argue that just as the pleasure of listening to Beethoven's Ninth, for example, once you had learned to appreciate it, is more fulfilling, and therefore greater, than the pleasure, if there is any, of listening to punk rock; so solitary sex is not as much fun, in the sense of deep human satisfaction, as sex with a beloved spouse. Therefore, he could further argue that it is preferable to suppress one kind of pleasure in order to cultivate better the other. This kind of argument, of course, provides for exceptions to the prohibition against masturbation which he ostensibly justified. For example, he can hold that it is all right for a young man to masturbate in order to provide a doctor with a sample of his semen if there is, for example, a question of his sterility, because he can claim that, since the masturbatory act was not engaged in for fun, it would not detract from the cultivation of sexual love with a beloved spouse.

The Church's morality implicitly says that this kind of argument simply misses the significance of sex. That significance is such that certain kinds of sexual acts are bad-in-themselves. She teaches that God made sex to signify a conjugal union; any other use fails of its true signification, for the significance of a sexual act is not a consequence of the act, it is immanent in it.

Sexual acts are not the only human acts that have their significance immanent in them, at least a false signification if they are wrong: that is to say, there are some acts which are right or wrong insofar as they meet objective criteria which make them the kinds of acts they are. Murder is, perhaps, the most important of such acts. It is not just killing for a bad reason, it is intentionally killing the innocent for which there can never be a reason good enough. There is never a good enough reason to do any of the kinds of acts that are bad-in-themselves.

Dualism

The alternative to regarding some kinds of bodily acts as inherently significant is to regard all kinds of bodily acts as merely instrumental. That is dualism. It consists in the illusion that what I actually do on purpose cannot determine the meaning of my act morally. For the dualist, the real "me" is my subjectivity, my interiority, my personality, my feelings and the like; and my body is their means of expression.

All dualists are exceptionists or consequentialists with respect to prohibitions against specific bodily acts. So, for them the prohibition against sodomy (standing for all homosexual acts) cannot be absolute as the Church teaches. For example, a consequentialist may choose "love" — of course, it is a dualist's notion of love — as the criterion he uses to discriminate between good and evil bodily acts. He then may reason about engaging in sodomy as follows: If two males love each other, something that is perfectly good in itself, and if at any time for any number of reasons their "love" is accompanied by feelings of attraction, then they may use their sexual organs as instruments to express their love. The fog of wrong-headed analysis has settled. The proper question is whether sodomy is a loving kind of act, and that question is not answered by appealing to subjective testimony about the feelings that accompany engaging in it, or the further intentions with which anyone engages in it. If this kind of analysis were true, then our bodies would be merely tools which our subjectivity (the real "me" inside) can use as it sees fit, as long as it does not hurt anyone else. We are thereby divided in two; we are a subjectivity with a body built around it as a car surrounds its driver.

Anscombe traces this dualism to the work of Descartes. Certainly it has been with us since the Enlightenment. She says the following of the way this dualism works: "According to this psychology (Descartes's), an intention was an interior act of the mind which could be produced at will. Now if intention is all important — as it is — in determining the goodness or badness of an action, then, on this theory of what intention is, a marvellous way offered itself of making any action lawful. You only had to 'direct your intention' in a suitable way. In practice, this means making a little speech to yourself: 'What I mean to be doing is. . . .'"[11] This way lies madness.

The sane or traditional morality says simply that masturbation, for example, is wrong. It is an act that is bad in itself because it is not appropriate for us as God made us. Therefore, it makes no difference whether a man masturbates to produce a semen sample for a doctor or through some mistaken notion of how to relieve sexual tension. From her vast knowledge of God's ways, Holy Mother the Church says rightly and simply that doctor and patient must obtain the sample some other way. No consequentialist can see this, but that is his loss. Let us not make it ours too.

Widespread Consequentialism

A number of observations are immediately in order. We do not have to wait for a formal sociological study to tell us that consequentialism has won almost unanimous acceptance from the educated, or thought-to-be-educated classes of affluent Western Europe and North America, at least since the second World War, although its roots in academia go back almost 150 years before the war. It may well have triumphed during the war as the Allies reworked the definitions of combatant and noncombatant in order to bring their conduct of the war down to the level of Hitler's, as they seem to have thought they had to do in order to win.

A study of the development of the rationalizations behind obliteration bombing, sometimes called carpet bombing, and behind the use of nuclear bombs in Japan is, therefore, a study in the basic formal arguments of consequentialism. Conversely, the formal arguments John Ford, S.J.[12] used in 1944 to condemn obliteration bombing are at depth the same as those he used to defend the teaching of the Church regarding contraception in the 1960s.[13] Both sides have been consistent, although I believe only one side realizes that.

This observation leads me to remind us that the truth of morality is not determined by the majority vote of any group, particularly that of the ruling class in a culture we have good reason to believe is rapidly declining. The observation further leads me to praise the Holy Spirit. If He had not led the Church to define the infallibility of the Pope, it seems most likely that an organization whose clergy and other professionals are drawn in very large number from those classes which I believe are decaying, particularly in Western Europe and North America, and which, as a sign of their decay, succumbed to consequentialism — these clergy and other professionals would have led the whole Church away from authentic morality. Without Peter to stop us, I am confident we would have done so, because I am speaking from experience as one who spent much of his professional life in the darkness of consequentialism. Furthermore, I am a mainline member of a class I am, in this chapter, calling decadent. Our Lord redeems even people like us.

Consequentialism gets its name from the shape its most ordinary arguments take. But, as we have noted, even those who argue differently are consequentialists by definition if they reject moral absolutes as traditionally understood. Consequentialism is exceptionism. Nevertheless, in the most common arguments, we are asked to consider a hard case and then asked to imagine the *consequences* of following the traditional morality. The consequences are imagined to be so horrible that we seem to know at least intuitively, or in some way beyond the reach of logic, that in this case we may make for ourselves an exception to the traditional moral law. So far as I can discover, the pattern was well exemplified in the mind of President Harry Truman when they brought

29

him the proposal to drop the A-Bomb.[14] The A-Bomb both as designed and as targeted, obliterated the distinction between combatant and noncombatant: that is to say, in at least one of the two cases, from the beginning, the plan involved directly killing noncombatants which is murder. But, it was a hard case. If we did not commit murder in Hiroshima and Nagasaki, the war would drag on; we might have to invade Japan, there would be a dreadful loss of American lives, or so we imagined. (Of course, our imaginings were foolishness, as we might have known then, and may know now.) The consequences we imagined if we observed the moral law were so awful, somehow we knew we were permitted to make for ourselves an exception, so we dropped the bombs. You may substitute contraception, abortion, euthanasia, infanticide, lying in a good cause, fornication (now called premarital sex), adultery, sodomy (standing for all homosexual acts), and even treachery, just to mention a few, in the argument in place of nuclear obliteration bombing, and you will find you have the fundamental consequentialist argument for granting exceptions to the prohibitions against each of the items mentioned.

We cannot overemphasize that not all consequentialists follow this pattern openly. Some prefer to re-define traditional moral terms so that absolute prohibitions become tautologies. Thus, the prohibition against masturbation no longer forbids self-abuse, it only forbids abusing yourself when you do not have a justifying reason for doing so. This is to say that the prohibition against masturbation forbids only unjustified masturbation; or it prohibits only what is prohibited, which is a tautology. For these clever consequentialists, their "absolute" prohibition against masturbation does not prohibit all masturbation, but only "wrongful" masturbation, therefore, for them not all masturbation is wrong. These more sophisticated consequentialists would allow that some prohibitions, even a complete list of the traditional prohibitions, are "absolute," *if* they may be allowed to re-define the key terms.

Let us take another example using what some may think of as a more important absolute prohibition, Thou shalt not commit adultery. The sophisticated consequentialist, for example, a representative Roman Catholic "new" moralist, will refer to this commandment as an absolute prohibition. He wants to refer to it as absolute because he knows that is the way it has always been regarded by the Church. But he also wants to allow for exceptions, so he re-defines the prohibition against adultery to forbid all *unjustified* sexual intercourse with someone not one's own spouse, engaged in by persons at least one of whom is married to another. The traditional prohibition has been expanded by only one word, but what a very important word it is. With it, the prohibition does not forbid those cases of adultery the consequentialist feels he can justify. The prohibition against adultery now amounts to saying that unjustified sex is unjustified; it is a tautology. It does not tell us what *kind* of sex is unjustified.

In order to determine when the sin of adultery or murder or any other absolutely forbidden act is "justified," sophisticated "new" moralists (consequentialists) seldom bring a calculation of consequences to the fore. The argument will instead usually appeal first to special circumstances. The widely publicized "situation ethicist," Joseph Fletcher, made a case of this sort notorious.[15] It took place at the end of the Second World War and had to do with a German woman who apparently had no way out of a Russian prison camp except to become pregnant. She was a married woman who believed her family was alive in the West and needed her. With the help of a specially chosen guard, she succeeded in becoming pregnant and was sent back to Allied occupied Germany where she was able to rejoin her husband and family. Fletcher believed that the special circumstances justified the adultery. Although it does not announce itself as an argument from consequences, it is. If we ask ourselves a couple questions, we may see this more clearly.

If before repatriating pregnant women, the Russians had somehow determined whether they were already pregnant before entering the camp, and then repatriated only those who so qualified, the adultery would not have had the desired consequences. Would it then have been "objectively" wrong? Or, if the sexual act required for release from the camp had not been an act of normal intercourse, but instead some expression of sado-masochistic perversion, would we have come up with the "intuition" that justified an exception to the moral law in these special circumstances? The answer to both questions shows that what really counts in the end, whenever anyone enters into this way of think-ing about the moral law, is how one evaluates the supposed conse-quences (and they are always merely supposed before the event takes place, except, of course, in situations where the principle of double effect is legitimately applied). Because, I believe, of Fletcher's notoriety and simplistic arguments, Roman Catholic revisionist ("new") moralists do not follow him directly. Nevertheless, their more sophisticated arguments have the same essence when calling for exceptions to absolute moral prohibitions.

There are also accounts of desperate men choosing cannibalism as the means to survive in dire circumstances. Sometimes, these desperate men murdered those they judged would not survive in order that eating their bodies they, the stronger, might survive. Such stories are less frequently advanced in order to justify consequentialism because they are grisly and far less romantic than an account of adultery.

Medical Consequentialism

In medicine, stories like the following are becoming much more common: A baby is born with spina bifida. He also lacks the normal anal aperture. His mother was recently divorced and has come upon hard times. With corrective surgery, in all probability, he would survive and live to be an adult capable of providing for himself, although disabled. But if the anus is not opened, he cannot be fed and will inevitably die. That will relieve his mother of the burden of raising a crippled child. So, the choice is made *not* to perform corrective surgery, and the baby is fed glucose until he dies. The choice not to operate was made with the intent that, as the direct result of omitting the surgery, the baby might die as easily and quickly as possible. This is murder! The supposed consequences, i.e., an easier life for the baby's mother, do not make the omission anything other than murder.

Consequentialism can also wear another disguise when rationalizing murder in this kind of situation. The catch-phrase, "quality of life," may be employed. For example, Catholics have long known that we do not have to take every possible measure to sustain our lives. If, for example, after I have achieved the age of reason and have exercised that reason to choose to accept God's grace by rejecting mortal sin, I then am faced with the choice of undergoing a difficult operation which may give me six more months of a miserable existence or foregoing it and dying, say, within the next week, I may in good and right conscience forego the operation. (Such a decision could be made for me by a proxy if I were comatose, even though he might not know my state of soul as well as could be desired.) A common sophistical argument takes this truth and says that it is actually a consideration of "quality of life." Then the catch-phrase is transferred to another situation (which actually changes the phrase's meaning) and the consequentialist then concludes that what is justified in the one case is justified in the other. So, if I may forego an operation that prolongs my dying six months (six months of a poor quality of life), then we may forego providing an anal aperture for a baby with spina bifida because he will have to live the life ahead of him handicapped (poor quality) if we operate. It should be evident to all that this is sophistry. The point of living this life is to praise, reverence, and serve God. Sometimes this is done in very mysterious ways, but the baby with spina bifida in our example would have been able to choose to praise, reverence, and serve God in quite ordinary ways. Killing him, therefore, is clearly wrong. On the other hand, in the example I drew around myself, I have had the opportunity to praise, reverence, and serve God. Dragging it out for an extra six months of misery may serve only as an occasion of sin. I cannot rightly to choose to die in order to avoid such occasion of sin, or at all. But, bearing in mind my situation, I can rightly say, "I do not have to undergo this burdensome operation; I choose not to undergo it (even though I know the result will be my death)." Therefore, the decisions in question are not similar, they are not both about quality of life in the same sense; they are in fact quite disparate and must be so treated.

These and other fine distinctions, which the morality the Church teaches requires us to make, are animated by a very specific understanding of the evil of sin. All great and true Catholics, men or women, have shared this understanding, for it comes from the Holy Spirit. Few have expressed it as well as John Henry Cardinal Newman. He said the following about our Holy Mother the Church:

> She regards this world, and all that is in it, as a mere shadow, as dust and ashes, compared with the value of one single soul. She holds that unless she can in her own way, do good to souls, it is no use her doing anything; she holds that it were better for sun and moon to drop from heaven, for the earth to fail, and for all the many millions who are upon it to die of starvation in extremist agony, so far as temporal affliction goes, than that one soul, I will not say, should be lost, but should commit one single venial sin, should tell one wilful untruth, though it harmed no one, or steal one poor farthing without excuse. She considers the action of this world and the action of the soul simply incommensurate, viewed in their respective spheres; she would rather save the soul of one single wild bandit of Calabria, or whining beggar of Palermo, than draw a hundred lines of railroad through the length and breadth of Italy, or carry out a sanitary reform, in its fullest

details, in every city of Sicily, except so far as these great national works tended to some spiritual good beyond them.[16]

We have been obliquely alluding to the fact that consequentialism came out into the open and has become widespread in the Church principally through the work of moralists who rejected the authentic teaching of the Church regarding contraception. The harvest of evil from this rebellion is far from over, but that the harvest is evil can now be seen clearly. Few documents in the history of the Church, and I believe no other document in the 20th century, has been as prophetically accurate as *Humanae Vitae*.

We have also tried to show that the consequentialism used to defend the rejection of the Church's moral doctrine often takes the form of a rejection of the traditional teaching that there are acts which are bad-in-themselves. As we have seen, what this amounts to is the awareness that there are certain kinds of acts that I may know are bad or morally evil simply by knowing that they have been done on purpose (deliberately). For example, if I know the facts about this particular killing, I may know that is was murder if it was done on purpose. I do not have to inquire what the further or accompanying intention was; I do not need to know the spirit in which it was committed in order to know that it was murder. I need know only that it was intended or deliberate. Or, another example, if I know the facts about this particular act of sexual intercourse, I may know that it was adultery, fornication, or sodomy, and thereby know that if it were done on purpose (and, apart from rape, I do not see how else it could be done), then it was bad. I do not have to ask how the participants felt about it in order to determine that it was wrong. The other questions about both the murder and the adultery come into play when trying to understand subjective guilt and when trying to chart a course for pastoral (or psychological, if indicated) guidance. Nevertheless, the first step along that course will be the recognition that the act was bad-in-itself.

This teaching, which I firmly believe is true and is clearly the teaching of the Church, contains at least two hidden benefits: *first*, it makes it possible to assess human acts rationally. Without this teaching ethics must become a guessing game about further and/or accompanying intentions, feelings (psychological states), circumstances, consequences, and the like. The opportunities for delusion in theory and practice become endless. The *second* benefit follows from the first. In order to describe most of the acts that are bad-in-themselves, we must

34

describe bodily realities. This is to say that, although it may be possible to describe blasphemy without reference to bodily realities (and I am not sure that it is possible), it is manifestly impossible to describe adultery or murder without reference to human bodily realities. And this is a real benefit, because this is one very powerful way in which authentic Church teaching keeps us from falling into the great evil of dualism.

We have already described dualism. It is the doctrine that treats all human bodily acts as merely instrumental. The dualist cannot remain consistent with his principles and so describe rape, for example, that it would always and everywhere be morally evil if done on purpose. (I acknowledge, although I believe the possibility is exploited in our day to exonerate evil, that a rapist could be so compelled psychologically that his bodily acts might not be performed "on purpose" in the sense required to make of the act a moral, as opposed to a physical, evil.) The consistent dualist (consequentialist) must allow for the possibility that a rape would be the "lesser of two evils" and therefore the evil which a person ought to do in order to achieve good.

The results of this kind of reasoning are all around us. Consider the moral vacuity, even depravity, in a common dialogue like the following: Jane asks Sue: "Why was it right for you to have an abortion?" Sue replies: "I just knew it was the thing I had to do because of everything that was happening at the time. I hated to do it; it was a tragic thing to have to do, but I just had to do it because of everything!" One of the most dreadful effects of the rebellion against *Humanae Vitae* is that we now find even Catholics rationalizing their sins in dialogues like this.

Acts Bad-In-Themselves

Through the centuries, various thinkers have seen a wide range of good reasons why we may know that there are acts bad-in-themselves or moral absolutes. There are many good thinkers carrying on the work today. In addition to Anscombe, I would recommend the writings of Peter T. Geach and John Finnis, both in England, and Germain Grisez and Joseph Boyle in the United States.

In general, the reasons amount to showing that this is the way God has made us, and in particular that He has made it possible for us to know that there are certain universal values so basic to human life and decent that they are inviolable. They may never be directly attacked. In fact, we may know these values even if we do not know God, so that ignorance about God is no certain excuse for sin. The Biblical exposition of what I am referring to begins in the first chapter of Romans, the sixteenth verse. A superb contemporary exposition may be found in *Natural Law and Natural Rights* by John Finnis.[17]

For example, we may see that God made us to know the truth, and even if we do not know the truth that He created us, we may know that knowledge is a good and from that unshakeable knowledge discover that lying is wrong. Then, once we have properly and quite narrowly defined what it is to lie, we may see that such behavior is absolutely forbidden. Needless to say, there is an elaborate casuistry which allows for some jokes in ordinary living and for some mental reservation in hard cases. These are not lies in the requisite sense.

I mention lying only to recall to our minds the kind of reasoning which enables us to understand what things are absolutely forbidden and why. Members of our culture affected by some form of the prevailing consequentialisms are still slightly better able to see why those acts which directly violate our nature as rational or "spiritual" might be absolutely forbidden or only rarely excepted. What they cannot comprehend are why those acts which violate our rational nature as animal or bodily are forbidden, i.e., why basic values that are more bodily may not be directly attacked. They do not see these bodily acts as only rarely permitted; rather they believe they are frequently allowed, at least for some. Such acts are contraception, fornication, adultery, sodomy and other forms of homosexual behavior, masturbation, and the like. Traditionally, all are absolutely forbidden.

But, we must remember that the modern neo-pagan is a dualist. He does not see the body as God's creation and the first revelation of His will to each creature. He does not see that bodily finalities have an essential place in what is personally, subjectively, "spiritually" chosen. The fact that sex is linked to life through procreation is for the dualist merely an interesting biological detail. It is a fact he must know how to cope with when, for example, he chooses sex for recreational purposes. He must know how to sever the link when he does not want to have to bother with a pregnant partner. Certainly, or so believes the modern dualist, the merely biological fact that sex can lead to pregnancy is not necessarily relevant to distinguishing between good and bad sex. Yet the Church has always said that it is, and the Church is right. I cannot really love as the rational animal I am, and attempt to express love for another sexually while wilfully rejecting (deliberately severing) the link which unites sex to the basic human good of life, namely, procreation.

Through sin, original and actual, sex has become ambivalent, a claim that the history of human lust makes abundantly clear. (I find child pornography the saddest chapter in this history, and it is widespread in the U.S. today.) How and when, then, is sex good? The dualist's answer is when you have the right further or accompanying intention and it is done in the right spirit. For the dualist, what you actually do does not matter a tinker's damn as long as both parties are pleased. But the dualist's answer is, at best, naive. It severs the body from the person and unleashes the tide of lust.

The Church's answer is realistic and therefore true! She teaches that her Lord requires us to respect the bodily link between sex and life. She teaches that when we have sex we certainly must have the right further and accompanying intentions; we must do it in the right spirit, but we also must do only what is right. What we do on purpose must be an act that is open to life, that is, it must be a conjugal act. It is in the context of respect for life that the ambivalence of sex is overcome and it becomes what it was created to be, a good. Outside that context it is in some measure evil. Therefore, when I, a solemnly vowed celibate, sacrificed the great good of marriage for the love of Christ and a particular role of service in His Kingdom, by that sacrifice I gave up sex. There is no good sex outside of marriage. Sex is very good in marriage when it is truly an act of conjugal love. Conjugal love is not merely a matter of the spirit with the body only instrumentally attached; it is rather a human bodily act. Therefore, the way God designed the body must be respected. It should be noted that He designed a woman's body so that most of the time she is infertile. That, too, is part of His design, and spouses may take frequent, happy advantage of the fact without in any way severing sex from life.

I will not attempt here to make the case for the fact that our bodies are normative. It seems manifest to me that they are. Failure to see this, I believe, results in personal and social madness, but I would be the last to deny that our society has become mad. I simply point out again what Pope Paul VI said in effect in *Humanae Vitae*: that is, *the* issue over which one decides whether the body is normative is the contraceptive issue. All the rest follows from it. And look what has followed: widespread movements to persuade us to regard almost all sexual perversions, even sado-masochistic ones, as potential goods, rapidly advancing destruction of the family unit even among Catholics, increases in adultery and

37

fornication, and the attendant loss of faith through loss of purity of heart. Those who rebelled against the Church's teaching were actually rejecting the body as God made it and thereby rejecting the Creator. The rebellion has revived the curses of pagan sex and these drive out the great goods of Christian sex.

My claim that the rejection of the body as normative, if consistently carried out, does involve madness, is not too strong. Since we are bodily, we cannot describe reality without bodily referents either direct or indirect. For us to learn the difference between an elephant and an oak tree is necessarily, at least in part, a bodily activity. Elephants are not oak trees and oak trees are not elephants, and the irreducible difference is unaffected by wish, whim, feeling, or fancy on my part. Furthermore, the difference is not a matter of a trans-rational, non-rational, suprarational, or unrepeatable and ineffable intuition fixed in the unique situation. It is as plain as day, and I can recall the difference perhaps as many times as there are oak trees and elephants in the world, learning something more about it each time. But what I learn will never make the two the same.

For us to learn the difference between good and bad, morally speaking, is very much the same thing, or once again we must concede that it is not a rational matter. For example, we claim to know something about the difference between loving and not loving. We know enough about love to know that rape is not an act of love toward a young girl. We know that every rape is unloving. What we overlook is that the obverse is equally true, no rape is loving. The obverse points out to us bodily creatures that the first step in knowing what love is consists in knowing that there are certain kinds of bodily acts, not one of which is ever an act of love. If we bodily creatures did not have such a boundary separating loving from what is not loving, there would be no way to save ourselves from illusions about love. Anything like love, which is closely associated with wish, whim, feeling, and fancy on my part and seems to hit me on some occasions with the force of an artistic intuition, is the motherlode of delusion, *if* it is not tied by plain, but exact, descriptions to matter of fact things in our everyday world. So, God in His revelation has underscored our common sense and let us know that no masturbation, no fornication, no adultery, no contraception, no sodomy is loving. The full reasons why this is so, He reveals to those who are truly chaste whether wed or unwed, religious, priest, or lay. I think it is time once again that those of us who represent the Church

38

in some professed capacity inform those in our care of this true epistemology of faith. Of course, we must first learn it ourselves.

Murder

Murder lies half-way between lying and contraception in terms of the mix of the rational and the bodily in those acts which are bad-in-themselves. What actually counts as a lie in hard cases can involve complicated reasoning and amount to next to nothing in bodily terms. A young man carrying a bible into Russia to help a brother in Christ will probably engage in complicated reasoning about what he can say in his customs declaration which will result in an almost imperceptible difference in his spoken or written word from what another person would call lying. A man contemplating contraception may engage in some complicated reasoning, but not because the act he contemplates is subtle. The difference between putting on a condom or not putting on a condom is not subtle like the difference between what is a lie and what is not when you are trying to withhold information from the agents of a tyranny. Determining whether this act is or is not murder is a bit of both.

In hard cases, determining whether this contemplated act or omission would or would not constitute murder may require all the complicated reasoning of a mental reservation and the lack of subtlety of contraception. But note, neither the young man smuggling the bible into Russia nor the doctor contemplating removing the still useful kidneys from what may or may not be a corpse would have to engage in any complicated reasoning at all if each were not serious about observing the moral law. I assure you that as God is our judge, He asks only that when doing this kind of reasoning, we do our best *modo humano*, as the theologians used to say, and that will be good enough for Him. He has given us these difficult cases to test our mettle.

From that fuller knowledge of reality which faith provides, this testing of our mettle should not surprise us. All of life is such a testing, or if you prefer, such an invitation to enter more deeply into His love, which in this life, tainted by sin as it is, always includes overcoming evil.

From the third chapter of Genesis to the last word recorded as Holy Scripture we discover that sin consists in disobeying God. It is irony itself that what motivated the first sin, namely, the desire to determine the difference between good and bad for ourselves, which the lying serpent promised would make us gods, is proposed today as the morality of the mature Christian. I would say it is the Christian gone to pot. Therefore, the way back to God from sin consists in special and tested obedience, an obedience which, when it is mature, becomes love itself. The difficulties we encounter in taking His commands seriously are opportunities for progress in the school of love.

From this perspective, we can see how the effort to dissolve real laws which prohibit specific things always and everywhere has the effect of trivializing our spiritual lives. There would be no sins, only mistakes. God would not then be someone whom we must obey. Rather, He would then be a wise and avuncular counselor whose advice we ought to take into consideration.

Then, what He really meant when He commanded us not to murder would be the wise counsel that it is better not to kill the innocent intentionally or directly except when it would be "kind" or when it is "necessary" to do so. The prohibition against adultery would have been intended really as the wise counsel not to cheat on your wife unless you had justifying cause. David's sin with Bathsheba would, thereby, have consisted in a failure to have a very good reason for adultery; his murderous order which brought about Uriah's death would have been a sin because it was not really the "kind" thing to have done. And, of course, the paradigm of consequentialism given in the Scriptures, which is Caiaphas's reasoning about why they should have Jesus killed, would be reduced either to a mistake in identifying Jesus as a threat to the people or to a mistake in calculating the effects in killing him. St. John recorded the scene: "One of them, Caiaphas, the high priest that year, said, 'You don't seem to have grasped the situation at all; you fail to see that it is better for one man to die for the people, than for the whole nation to be destroyed.'"[18]

Sin

This reduction of sin to a mistake makes an absurdity out of that understanding of reality which faith provides. If sin were just a mistake, then there is no explanation for what we suffer as a consequence of its entrance into the world. If our sins are just mistakes, then how did we ever have Auchswitz, how do we understand a Gulag Archipelago, whence comes a Cambodia? If sin is just a mistake, what is the sense of Hell?

40

But if sin consists in disobeying God, then we can make some sense of the rest. Sin is such a catastrophe, such an offense, it is only natural that its effects should include turning mere human beings into Hitler's, Stalin's and Pol Pot's. There is a proportion between the effect or consequence of sin and the cause which is the sin itself. Perhaps that is why God allows these things, so we can see what sin is. Perhaps that is why He chose to save us by that sacrifice which is Our Lord's cross. I believe that these and like reflections can lead us to the truth about sin.

For sin to be disobedience rather than a failure to take wise advice or simply to make a human mistake, God must command and we must know what He commands. God could command us all individually, one to one, as it were, by direct inspiration. I believe He has commanded some few in this way regarding fundamental matters: for example, Abraham. And, I believe He has commanded a much larger number regarding a choice between relative goods: for example, He has asked some chosen souls to accept a special vocation, as was the case with the apostles and the rich young man in the gospels. But to claim that He has left fundamental matters, as whether to kill or not, to personal inspiration is madness. He governs by general law. That law specifies acts we may not perform. There may be honest doubt as to whether this or that medical procedure qualifies as such an act under these circumstances — for example, whether removing these kidneys for transplant is intentionally killing the innocent or making legitimate and respectful use of a corpse. Such doubts about specifics, no matter how frequent, do not add up to a doubt about the general law or its absolute character. Rather, knowledge of the general law and its absolute character is our starting point for resolving the specific questions, since what we want to do above all is obey God. In short, God commands by general law binding on all and admitting of no exceptions.

These laws are limited to exercising the appropriate authority over his voluntary creatures. That is to say, He rules us by the nature of things and not by arbitrary whim. After all, He is the wise and benevolent Creator of all. Reflection on this point helps us understand why the traditional morality contains so few absolute prohibitions and what they have in common.

As Genesis informs us, we stand to irrational creation in a way not unlike the way God stands towards us. That is to say, I have a kind of sovereign authority over the farm animals, albeit as part of a stewardship which I must account for, which is different from the authority I exer-

41

cise over my own life and the lives of other men. I do not have to prove a pig guilty in order to execute him; I do not have to respect the stallion's preference in mares when it comes to breeding; and I may put my pet dog out of his misery long before he dies a natural death. There are no commandments forbidding murder or adultery with respect to farm animals. We are sovereign.

God exercises a much greater sovereignty over us. He determines the difference between right and wrong, not arbitrarily, but reasonably, according to the way He has created and redeemed us. Nonetheless, we know that sovereignty in a special and immediate way when we contemplate an act that is bad-in-itself. Our choices at times like that are the choices that set the fundamental meaning of our lives. One choice determines whether we are chaste or unchaste, a murderer or not, a liar or truthful, and so forth. In these matters there is never any question of what benefits may or may not be gained for me or for anyone else. The only consequence I calculate is whether I am courting damnation. If we have sinned in these ways or have led others to sin, as I believe I did when I taught consequentialism, then our only hope is in the forgiving mercy of Our Lord and Savior Jesus Christ. Fortunately, He abounds in such mercy, not in a way that makes grace cheap, but in a way that makes conversion real.

Conclusion

I said at the beginning that the fifth commandment contains a whole theology of life and death. I hope we now see better that it does. It is, therefore, only as obedient sons and daughters of God that we may rightly solve the hard cases that trouble us. Pope Pius XII expected this understanding of each of us when He addressed the question of the Prolongation of Life in 1957.[19] His work, what preceded it, and what has followed, presuppose that we all ask ourselves whether the act we contemplate doing or omitting constitutes intentionally killing the innocent, not whether under these circumstances we are justified in killing. Therefore, we want to know whether in fact the acts we contemplate performing or omitting are directly lethal or not; or whether in fact the body we are dealing with is living or dead. By God's mercy I know as well as Pope Pius XII did that such matters of fact are beyond the competence of moral theology.[20] What the moral theologian may and must say about these matters to the health professional and to himself, is "Be sure you solve the question in fact and not just with some

42

mental intention produced at will before you proceed, or you may commit murder." And that, I take it, will be the center of our concern whenever we do moral theology about life and death.

Notes

1. I am in debt in this discussion to the work of Miss Elisabeth Anscombe, particularly to a talk, as yet unpublished, which she delivered at St. Thomas College in St. Paul, MN, during the Spring of 1980. For this definition, see the unpublished manuscript of that talk, p. 3.

2. John Connery, S.J., *Abortion: The Development of the Roman Catholic Perspective* (Chicago: The Loyola University Press, 1977), pp. 225-303.

3. Cf., Germain Grisez, *Abortion: The Myths, the Realities, and the Arguments* (New York: Corpus Books, 2nd printing, 1972) pp. 267-346; Joseph M. Boyle, Jr., "Double-Effect and a Certain Type of Embryotomy," in *The Irish Theological Quarterly,* Vol. 44, No. 4 (1977), pp. 303-318.

4. G.E.M. (Elisabeth) Anscombe, "Modern Moral Philosophy," in *Philosophy: The Journal of the Royal Institute of Philosophy,* Vol. XXXIII, No. 124 (January, 1958), pp. 1-19; the definition is given on pp. 9-10.

5. C. S. Lewis, *That Hideous Strength* (New York: Macmillan Publishing Co., 17th printing, 1976).

6. Anscombe, *Contraception and Chastity* (London: The Catholic Truth Society, 1979 — reprinted from *The Human World,* issue 7), pp. 17-18.

7. *Ibid.,* p. 18.

8. *Ibid.,* p. 22.

9. Cf. 1 Cor. 6.

10. Anscombe, *Contraception and Chastity,* p. 18.

11. Anscombe, "War and Murder," in *Nuclear Weapons and Christian Conscience;* ed. by Walter Stein (London: The Merlin Press, 1961, reprinted 1965), p. 58.

12. John C. Ford, S.J., "The Morality of Obliteration Bombing," in *Theological Studies,* Vol. 5, No. 3 (September, 1944), pp. 261-309.

13. John C. Ford, S.J. and Germain Grisez, "Contraception and Infallibility," in *Theological Studies,* Vol. 39, No. 2 (June, 1978), pp. 258-312.

14. Cf., Robert C. Batchelder, *The Irreversible Decision: 1939-1950* (New York: The Macmillan Company, 1961).

15. *Situation Ethics: The New Morality* (Philadelphia: The Westminster Press, 1966), pp. 164-5.

16. *Certain Difficulties Felt by Anglicans in Catholic Teaching Considered;* Vol. I (rpt.; Westminster, MD: Christian Classics, 1969), pp. 239-40 (Part II, Lecture VIII, section 4).

17. Oxford University Press, 1980.

18. John 11: 49-50.

19. Pope Pius XII, "The Prolongation of Life," in *The Pope Speaks,* Vol. 4, No. 4 (Spring, 1958), pp. 393-398.

20. *Ibid.,* p. 396 and p. 398.

Chapter 3

The Medical Approach to the Determination of Death

Kenneth R. Smith, Jr., M.D.

Now that physicians have the ability to maintain heartbeat and circulation and respiration in a human body which has no functioning brain, it is necessary for physicians to determine when the brain is completely, totally, and irreversibly without function, so that the remainder of the body is not kept functioning for days or even weeks after the organ which is responsible for human life is dead. This paper will review the current medical approach to determination of brain death.

In the autumn of 1980 the Institutional Review Board of Saint Louis University published its *"Position on Declaration and/or Definition of Death"* as agreed to by the Executive Faculty of the Saint Louis University School of Medicine. It states:

> *The following discussion and criteria outline the clinical definition*
> *of death for individuals for whom vital functions are maintained by*

cardiopulmonary support systems. These criteria may be used in declaring death in hospitals of, associated with, or affiliated with, Saint Louis University. These seven criteria may have a generally useful function for the faculty and administrative staff of the above hospitals, and are acceptable to the Institutional Review Board when applied with the following stipulations:

A registered Missouri physician who believes an individual is dead, requests confirmation via consultation from a physician faculty member of the Saint Louis University who is currently a specialist or is currently eligible to be a specialist in Neurology and/or Neurological Surgery. That faculty member discusses the situation with the physician, learns the basis of his decision and applies his own judgment, is guided by the criteria, noted below, and states his concurrence or non-concurrence with the opinion of the physician originally seeking consultation.

Organ donation involving death declaration and needing IRB approval will receive such approval when concurrence and affirmation of death have followed the outline provided and are documented and signed by the two individuals concerned, neither one of whom may be part of the organ transplant team referred to at the beginning of this statement.

A statement to the IRB from the organ donation program requiring approval of the IRB should declare, e.g.

"The Death of _____ *(name) was pronounced on* _____ *(date) at* _____ *(time) at* _____ *(place) on the basis of an initial examination and study (1) by Dr.* _____ *and confirmed (2) by Dr.* _____ *both following the guidelines for such declaration of death including the prerequisites and criteria as needed.*

Signature (1) _____

Physician of Patient

Signature (2) _____

Consultant Physician

The seven criteria that follow must be met, but also must have been preceded by the following prerequisites:

PREREQUISITES:
1. *All appropriate diagnostic and therapeutic procedures have been performed.*
2. *The potential donor is over the age of 3 years.*

3. The inhibition of reflex or respiratory activity must not be on the basis of any drug administration or central nervous system infection or abnormalities in acid-base balance.
4. The body temperature is above 32.2° C (90° F).

CRITERIA: All must be present for at least six hours.
1. There are no spontaneous movements except spinal reflexes.
2. There are no responses to painful stimuli except spinal reflexes.
3. There is coma and cerebral unresponsiveness.
4. There is irreversible apnea.
5. There are fixed and dilated pupils.
6. The cephalic and brain stem reflexes are absent.
7. One of the two following procedures must be done and shown to be negative, and the same procedure repeated at least six hours later:
   a) There is electrocerebral silence, with an absence of electrical potentials of cerebral origin over 2 microvolts from symmetrically placed electrode pairs over 10 centimeters apart and with an electrode impedance between 100 and 10000 ohms. This flat electroencephalogram remains isoelectric when retested at least six hours later, or
   b) The cerebral circulation is at a standstill as witnessed by 1) angiogram, or 2) the use of a radioisotopic arterial bolus, or 3) standstill of the blood in the retinal vessels.
   c) Either of criteria 7 (a) or 7 (b) should be reconfirmed at least six hours after the initial observation.

These seven criteria apply in the absence of an irreparable intracranial lesion such as massive gun shot wound, cerebral hemorrhage, etc., associated with absent brainstem reflexes, no spontaneous movement, and irreversible apnea. These conditions must continue for at least six hours. When such severe lesions occur, as described in the last paragraph, alternatively, a declaration of death may be provided by two physicians as required, earlier, without the collection of evidence of electrocerebral silence or absence of cerebral circulation. Where no such evidence of an irreparable intracranial lesion and its sequela exist, then the requirements listed under Prerequisites and Criteria will apply.

Why is this long document necessary when for the past several years physicians at St. Louis University have pronounced patients dead without formal criteria or prerequisites? One of the most compelling reasons is that, according to several lawyers who give legal advice to the University and its physicians, the law of the State of Missouri concern-

46

ing the definition of death probably is contained in Black's Law Dictionary[1] which defines death as "the cessation of life; the ceasing to exist; defined by physicians as a total stoppage of the circulation of the blood and a cessation of the animal and vital functions consequent thereon, such as respiration, pulsation, etc." Two other law dictionaries define death as "a cessation of life."[2,3] Certainly, all physicians would have no problem with this latter definition of death, but the Black's Law Dictionary is clearly wrong, because physicians today do *not* define death as a total stoppage of circulation of the blood and a cessation of animal vital functions consequent thereon, such as respiration, etc.

In the last 20 years, we have devised respirators, artificial hearts, and many other technological advances which enable physicians to take a dead human being and force oxygenated blood through his organs and can keep most of the body functioning except for the neurons of the brain. Therefore, a cadaver can be "alive" for days and sometimes even weeks. This leads to many problems, such as needless mental anguish of relatives and loved ones who falsely hope, hour after hour, and day after day, that the patient may recover. There is certainly anguish and despair on the part of all medical and paramedical personnel caring for the patient. There is needless financial expense and utilization of scarce medical resources which could benefit other patients, if the cadaver were not kept on the machines. Therefore, the concept of brain death has evolved and, in a recent survey of some 60 neurologists and neurosurgeons in the St. Louis Society for Neurological Sciences, 100% agreed that, when a patient's brain is dead, the patient is dead, and 100% agreed that medical/clinical criteria are available to make this determination. How did these criteria evolve?

One of the first recognitions of brain death was published in 1959 by French workers who observed patients who had resuscitation after cardiac arrest.[4] These patients' brains were partially or totally destroyed by the period of anoxia and they never awakened from a state of coma. This state was called *"coma dépassé."* In 1968, the well-known Harvard criteria for defining irreversible coma were proposed by an ad hoc committee of the Harvard Medical School to examine the definition of brain death.*[5] This group of neurological and medical experts tried to

---

*The authors of the Harvard criteria for brain death originally used the term "irreversible coma." The word coma has many different meanings to different people. In the original Harvard paper "irreversible coma" meant the same as "brain death." Because of the confusion about the meaning of the word coma, the consensus today is to use the words "brain death" rather than "irreversible coma."

determine the characteristics of a permanently non-functioning brain. They felt that the condition could be satisfactorily diagnosed by: 1) unreceptivity and unresponsivity; 2) no movements or breathing; 3) no reflexes; and 4) of great confirmatory value is the flat or isoelectric electroencephalogram. All four of these criteria should be repeated at least 24 hours later with no change. The validity of this data as indications of irreversible cerebral damage depends on the exclusion of two conditions: 1) hypothermia and 2) central nervous system depressants. Four years later, these criteria were appraised by the Task Force on Death and Dying of the Institute of Society, Ethics, and Life Sciences, a group of eminent physicians, philosophers, theologians, attorneys and sociologists.[6] Their conclusion was, "nevertheless, we can see no medical, logical or moral objection to the criteria as set forth in the Harvard Committee Report. The criteria and procedures seem to provide the needed guidelines for the physician. If adopted, they will greatly diminish the present complexity about the status of some 'patients' and will thus put an end to needless, useless, costly, time consuming, and upsetting ministrations on the parts of physicians and relatives."

Since 1968, five other widely quoted papers defining criteria for cerebral death have been published: 1) the Minnesota criteria in the Journal of Neurosurgery, 1971,[7] 2) the Swedish criteria published in 1972,[8] 3) the Japanese criteria presented at the Fifth International Congress of Neurological Surgery, Tokyo, 1973,[9] 4) the Conference of Royal Colleges and Faculties of the United Kingdom, 1976,[10] and 5) the collaborative study of cerebral death of the National Institutes of Health, 1977.[11]

The question of whether to continue extraordinary measures (such as respirators) in patients who have irreversible brain damage, and have hopelessly severe deficits which prevent them from living any sort of useful human existence, arises occasionally in patients who have some functioning brain tissue remaining. As Pope Pius XII has stated, it is not obligatory to continue to use extraordinary means indefinitely in hopeless cases, but normally one is held to use only ordinary means, that is to say, means that do not involve any grave burden for oneself or another.[5] It is much more difficult to make a determination that a patient has hopeless, irreversible, brain damage and that extraordinary life-support mechanisms should be removed, than it is for a physician to determine that the brain is dead and that the patient should be pronounced dead. The complicated medical, moral, ethical, and religious

48

question of what measures to use in patients with severe brain damage (but not total, irreversible loss of all brain function) is not being considered in this essay.

Many hundreds of patients have been studied by eminent physicians of many specialties, ranging from electroencephalography to electronmicroscopy, in almost every country in the world, and there is universal agreement that physicians, in 1980, can set down certain criteria which, when rigidly met, can make a definition of brain death with absolute certainty, and no patient who is declared brain dead has any chance of recovering and living so that there need be no fear that doctors are declaring patients dead when they really are only in some reversible unconscious condition. Hundreds of autopsies with careful study of the brain have shown that, when the criteria of brain death are met, the brain is dead and cannot recover. Hundreds of patients who have met the criteria for brain death have been kept on respirators and all other artificial supportive measures for days and (rarely) weeks, and no patient has recovered brain function.

There are a few anecdotes published in newspapers and letters to editors making some claims about patients who have been declared dead, but have recovered to normal life and mentation. However, when these are examined, each one has been found to have failed to meet one or more of these important criteria. The Saint Louis University criteria, stated at the outset, are a distillation of the essential features of all these many studies, and represent the state of the art in 1980. Certainly, in the future, changes will occur in these criteria, but they will be relatively minor, and the criteria will apply to only a tiny fracture of 1% of all the patients who are declared dead in the United States in the next 10 to 20 years. These criteria are only used on patients in very special circumstances, mostly in intensive care units where elaborate resuscitative and supportive equipment is available. The criteria are only considered for use when the patient is determined to have irreversible, hopeless brain damage. Any time there is any chance of recovery from hypothermia, from drug intoxication, from metabolic states, from anoxic or hypoxic conditions after cardiac arrest or drowning, all modern (almost miraculous) techniques which we have at our disposal today are used. Miraculous recoveries do occur in patients who are seemingly dead when they arrive in the emergency room, or who seemingly die and are brought back to life in the cardiovascular units, after heart attacks and strokes which certainly would have been fatal a few years ago.

The criteria for death used today meet the definition of "good criteria" as published by the Task Force on Death and Dying.[6] 1) They are clear and distinct and the tests performed yield vivid and unambiguous results. 2) The tests are simple, easily performed and interpreted by an ordinary physician or nurse and depend as little as possible on the use of elaborate equipment and machinery. 3) The procedures include an evaluation of the permanence and irreversible absence of functions and the determination of the absence of other conditions that may be mistaken for death. 4) The determination of death does not rely exclusively on a single criterion or on the assessment of a single function. 5) The criteria do not undermine, but are compatible with, the continued use of the traditional criteria (cessation of spontaneous heartbeat and respiration) in the vast majority of cases where artificial maintenance of vital function has been in use. The revised criteria provide an alternative means for recognizing the same phenomenon of death. 6) The alternative criteria, when they are used, should determine the physician's actions the same way as the traditional criteria: that is, all individuals who fulfill either set of criteria should be declared dead by the physician as soon as he discerns that they have been fulfilled. 7) The criteria and procedures are easily communicable both to relatives and other laymen as well as to physicians. They are uniformly acceptable by the medical profession as a basis for uniform practice. The criteria and procedures are accepted as appropriate by the general public. 8) The reasonableness and adequacy of the criteria and procedures have been vindicated by experience in their use, and by autopsy findings.

The Task Force went on to state that:

There are ample reasons both necessary and sufficient, and independent of the needs of potential transplant recipients, of the patient's family and of society, for clarifying and refining the criteria and procedures for pronouncing a man dead. It is the opinion of the Task Force that widespread adoption and use of . . . clearly defined criteria will in fact allay public fears of possible arbitrary or mischievous practices on the part of some physicians. We also believe that if the criteria of determining death are set wholly independently of the need for organs, there need be no reticence or embarrassment in making use of any organs which may actually become more readily available if the criteria are clarified (provided, of course, that other requirements of ethical medical practice are met). While we cannot deny the fact that the growth of the practice of transplantation with cadaveric organs provided a powerful stimulus to reassess the criteria for determining death, the members of this Task Force are in full agreement that the need for organs *is* not and *should* not be a reason for changing these criteria, and especially for selecting any given criterion or procedure. Choice of the criteria for pronouncing a man dead ought to be completely independent of whether or not he is a potential donor of organs. The procedures, criteria and the actual judgment in determining the death of one human being must not be contaminated with the needs of others, no matter how legitimate those needs may be. The medical profession cannot retain trust if it does otherwise, or if the public suspects (even wrongly) that it does otherwise.

The Colorado Supreme Court concluded on October 15, 1979, that the brain death concept for determining death was appropriate and adopted that standard in the absence of any legislative action to define death.[12] The American Medical Association and American Bar Association support this definition. The Chairman of President Carter's Commission for the Study of Ethical Problems in Medicine and Biomedical and Behavioral Research, Maurice Adam, predicts that the drafting of a uniform definition based on brain death, without criteria attached, would post no major problems.[13]

So the legal, medical, religious and sociological professions are united behind the concept that, when a human being's brain is dead, then the human being is dead. I have shown that the medical profession has reached a consensus concerning criteria for determining brain death. There will be constant efforts to refine these criteria and make them more precise and accurate. There will be quibbles about semantics such as the difference between "definition" and "determination," between "irreversible coma" and "death," between "permanent cessation of function" and "destruction," between "total brain function (without an s)" and "brain functions (with an s)."

The quibbles will not change the basic fact that doctors can and do each day declare patients dead because they have decided on unassailable scientific evidence that the patients' brains are dead.

Notes

1. Black's Law Dictionary, Fourth Edition 1951, p. 48, St. Paul, West Publishing Company 1968.

2. Bouvier's Law Dictionary (Rawle's Edition) p. 775, Vernon Law Book Company, Kansas City, MO., together with West Publishing Company, St. Paul, Minn. 1914.

3. Cyclopedic Law Dictionary, p. 285, Publisher, Callaghan, Chicago, Ill. 1922.

4. Mollaret, P. and Goulon, M.: *Le coma dépassé*. Rev. Neurol. 101: 3-15, 1959.

5. Beecher, H. K. *et al*, A Definition of Irreversible Coma; report of the ad hoc committee of the Harvard Medical School to examine the definition of brain death, J.A.M.A. 205: 337-340, 1968.

6. Cassell, E. and Kass, L. *et al*, Refinements and Criteria for the Determination of Death: an appraisal, J.A.M.A. 221: 48-53, 1972.

7. Mohandas, A. and Chou, S., Brain Death, A Clinical and Pathological Study, Journal of Neurosurgery 35: 211-218, 1971.

8. Ingvar, I. and Widen, L.: *Hjärndod-Sannmanfattning av ett symposium,* Lakartidningen 69: 3404-3814, 1972.

9. Uek, K., Takevchi, K. and Katsurada, K., Clinical Study of Brain Death. Presentation No. 286, Fifth International Congress of Neurological Surgery, Tokyo, 1973.

10. Conference of Royal Colleges and Faculties of the United Kingdom, Diagnosis of Brain Death, Lancet 2: 1069-1070, 1976.

11. Walker, A. *et al*, An appraisal of the criteria of cerebral death, a summary statement, J.A.M.A. 237: 982-986, 1977.

12. *Lovato vs State of Colorado*, 1979.

13. Sun, M., Panel asks "When is a person dead?", Science 209: 669-670, 1980.

Dr. Smith was invited to prepare the above essay on the medical approach to the determination of death for his presentation at the Institute on "Moral Responsibility in Prolonging Life Decisions," sponsored by the Pope John Center and the Catholic Health Association September 19-21, 1980. Dr. Paul A. Byrne, with two other authors, has published an article in the *Journal of the American Medical Association* on November 2, 1979, which is severely critical of efforts to determine irreversible cessation of brain functions and pronounce death without evidence of the destruction of the brain. Dr. Byrne offered to respond to Dr. Smith's presentation. We have included his response in this chapter. — *Ed. Note*.

Response

Paul A. Byrne M. D.

My purpose is to clarify some aspects of death, especially from the medical viewpoint, regarding the use of brain-related criteria for the determination of death. I am not proposing that a ventilator may not be removed until putrefraction or gangrene has occurred. Furthermore, even though I am opposed to removing a vital organ from someone who is not yet dead, in principle, I am not opposed to organ transplantation, thus, that topic need not be confused with this issue.

The subject of death can be broached from the disciplines of theology, philosophy, medicine, and the law. Needless to say, there is not agreement from the aspect of the first three disciplines. While accord has not been reached, legal acceptance has been propelled by a movement to legitimize that which has been incompletely formulated, and which, in my opinion, is morally wrong and is based on data that is not scientifically valid. Presently, twenty-six states have laws accepting cessation of brain function as indicating death, and the Uniform Law Commissioners are urging passage in the other twenty-four states of the Uniform Determination of Death Act.

Life on earth for an individual is a continuum from conception until death. An individual is still alive, even when dying. One cannot be dead until and unless life on earth has ended.

A human person is the entire living human being in one single, though composite, organism. The function of an organism depends on an adequate structure and an appropriate environment. Hostile environmental factors, such as lack of oxygen, the presence of drugs or chemicals, or the accumulation of toxic wastes like lactic acid, result in dysfunction, or nonfunction. These same or similar factors may result in altered structure, or even destruction. A return, then, to a more normal environment may result in a return of function or activity. However, this return is dependent on adequate structure. A cessation of function without altered structure does not indicate anything regarding the return of function. Hence, in a determination of death, there must be evidence of destruction, over and above cessation of function.

The proponents of brain-related criteria propose that the brain is the critical organ, whose function is necessary for human life. Furthermore, they indicate that the brain is the radical human structure. But actually within the human organism there exists an asymmetric inter-dependence of organs.

The brain itself has multiple parts that have anatomical proximity and are functionally inter-related. However, no part is in complete control of the other. The cortex is recognized as that part which has control over voluntary motor activity, for example, running. But, should the individual trip, while running, the mid-brain activity reflexly supersedes the cortical activity, keeping the individual from falling.

The brain-related criteria revolve around testing for absent function. If a set of functions is absent for a period of time, then the neurologist concludes that the individual has brain death. Furthermore, if all "tested" functions of the brain have ceased, then, whatever the term "total brain function" may designate, this also has ceased.

The Harvard Criteria, published in the journal the *American Medical Association* in 1968, listed the characteristics of irreversible coma.[1] Subsequently, there have been at least thirty sets of criteria which have grown out of at least five separate studies. One set of criteria, commonly known, in medical circles, as the Minnesota Criteria, was published in the *Journal of Neurosurgery*, in 1971.[2] This study involved only twenty-five patients, nine of whom had the electroencephalogram evaluated. Two of these nine showed "low voltage, fast activity at the time of brain death." It was then concluded that it was not necessary for the neurosurgeon to include the EEG in the evaluation. Dr. A. E. Walker stated "if the EEG is omitted, 8% of the cerebrally dead would have biologic activity on the EEG, ... representing an anomalous and undesirable situation."[3]

Another well-recognized study, known as the Collaborative Study, was undertaken by the National Institute of Neurological Diseases and Stroke.[4] Eight hundred and forty-four patients were entered into the study. They then reported on five hundred and three of these. Of these, four hundred and thirty-eight (87%) died within three months. Sixty-five (13%) survived. Nineteen (4%) fulfilled the Harvard Criteria, but all of these died within three months. Autopsies were performed on two hundred and twenty-six, of which 10% had a grossly normal brain. Forty percent had findings consistent with "Respirator Brain." Dr. Molinari[5] stated that this was "one of the major and most disturbing findings."

54

The Collaborative Study then used the same subjects, but with a more strict set of criteria which included apnea, electrocerebral silence, and cerebral unresponsiveness. There were one hundred and eighty-seven of these patients of which one hundred and eighty-five did die within three months; however, forty-four of these had non-dilated pupils, another fifteen had unequal pupils. Seventy-one of these had stretch reflexes. At the conclusion of this report, it was stated, "these criteria are recommended for a larger clinical trial." Thus far, such a trial has not been published.

An article published in *Neurology* in 1978, entitled *Duration of Apnea to Confirm Brain Death*, included the following: "In ten apparently brain-dead subjects, we measured arterial gases for up to ten minutes." There were seven who remained apneic, and three patients in whom respirations began during unassisted oxygenation. Thus, three of these patients who were "apparently brain-dead," did not have irreversible cessation of brain function.[6]

Dr. Fost in the *Journal of Pediatrics*, in January, 1980, wrote there is "deep disagreement . . . . whether brain death is synonymous with death." "Brain-death . . . . is a valid indication for discontinuing some medical care . . . . reason is not because patient is dead, but because patient no longer has interest in being maintained." Brain-death ". . . . might simply be another on a long list of medical care problems from the patient and family's perspective." "Death of the brain is not the same as death in a traditional sense."[7]

The new criteria confound the loss of function with destruction. We have written on this aspect in the *Journal of the American Medical Association* on November 2, 1979, entitled *Brain Death, an Opposing Viewpoint*.[8] So long as we are dealing with cessation of function, we are dealing with a living patient. If he happens to be dying, he is not yet dead. The cessation of brain function does not imply destruction of the brain, or death of the patient; however, the converse is true. Death of the person includes destruction of the brain, and at this time, there is cessation of brain function which is irreversible. Doctor Safar, in *Critical Care Medicine*, reported on forty patients who were treated with barbiturates.[9] Twenty-two of these had an arrest time lasting between five and twenty-two minutes. The expected neurological recovery would be less than 10%. However, fourteen of the twenty-two (64%) made complete neurologic recovery. The reason that recovery is possible is because there was cessation of brain function and *not* destruction.

The ABA definition of death was introduced into the Missouri Legislature in 1978. It read, "for all legal purposes, a human body, with irreversible cessation of total brain function, according to usual and customary standards of medical practice, shall be considered dead." This was not acceptable to the legislators of the state of Missouri. Many of those that supported passage of the ABA definition of death switched allegiance to support of the passage of the Uniform Brain Death Act, which has subsequently been replaced by the Uniform Determination of Death Act, which says that, "An individual who has sustained either: (1) irreversible cessation of circulatory and respiratory functions, or (2) irreversible cessation of all functions of the entire brain, including the brain stem, is dead. A determination of death must be made in accordance with accepted medical standards."

This is not acceptable for many reasons, including the following: cessation of function is not acceptable as a criterion. The Uniform Determination of Death Act accepts two separate, distinct clinical situations, both of which can be manifest in the same individual. Both situations are clearly distinct to a physician and to many others. The same individual is dead only one time.

Those that accept "irreversible cessation of brain function or functions" as a determinant of death, after making such a determination, indicate that there is now a cadaver. The "cadaver" is then treated "as alive," i.e. the ventilator is continued, postural drainage is used to prevent pneumonia, turning is done to prevent bed-sores, until the time is convenient to remove the vital organs. Who has heard of a cadaver developing pneumonia or a bed sore? A body undamaged, except for destruction of the brain, is a mortally wounded human person, who, however, is not yet dead. While transplantation and the advancement of science are, in general, commendable and often highly emotional issues, it is not acceptable to remove a vital organ from someone, who, if he is not yet dead, will be killed by the excision of the vital organ.

In conclusion, an individual exists on earth from conception until death, and still exists when dying. A cessation of brain function, no matter what adjectives are used to modify the cessation, is not acceptable. Codification into law does not make it morally acceptable.

I would propose repeal of those laws that have been passed, and, to prevent further abuse, would suggest "no one shall be declared dead unless there is destruction of the circulatory, respiratory, and central nervous systems."

56

Notes

1. Ad Hoc Committee of the Harvard Medical School to Examine the Definition of Brain Death, A Definition of Irreversible Coma, J.A.M.A. 205. 337, 1968.

2. Mohandas, A. and Chow, S. Brain Death: A Clinical and Pathological Study, J. Neurosurg., 35: 211, 215, 1971.

3. Walker, A. S., "Cerebral Death," in Tower, O. B., Chase, T. N. (eds): *The Nervous System: The Clinical Neurosciences*, (New York, Raven Press, 1975), Vol. 2, p. 87.

4. An Appraisal of the Criteria of Cerebral Death: A summary statement, a collaborative study. J.A.M.A. 237: 982-986, 1977.

5. Molinari, G. F., Medical Criteria of Brain Death: Clinical Criteria, N.Y.A.S. 62-69, 1978.

6. Schafer, J. A. and Caronna, J. J.: Duration of Apnea to Confirm Brain Death. Neurology, 28: 661-666, July, 1978.

7. Fost, N., Research on Brain Death, J. of Peds., 96: 54-56, 1956.

8. Byrne, P. A., O'Reilly, S. and Quay, P. M., Brain Death — An Opposing Viewpoint, J.A.M.A. 242: 1985-1990, 1979.

9. Breivik, H., Safar, P., Sands, P.: Clinical Feasability Trials of Barbiturate Therapy after Cardiac Arrest, Crit. Care Med. 6: 228-244, 1978.

Chapter 4

Determination of Death:
A Medical-Legal Consensus

Dennis J. Horan, J. D.

In the past ten years twenty-seven state legislatures have passed statutes "defining death."[1] In addition, three state supreme courts and several trial courts have adopted brain death definitions.[2] This flurry of legal activity has been precipitated by much scholarly legal, medical and ethical writing addressing this topic which has been loosely described as definition of death legislation.[3] That description is somewhat imprecise since what really is at issue is not a definition of death but a decision as to whether an additional criterion for determining death may be made legal. The phrase "brain death" is likewise inartful and somewhat confusing. Death is diagnosed when you are dead. The phrase "brain death" is merely a descriptive, short-hand way of referring to the debate as to whether this additional method of diagnosing death may be used by physicians when circumstances so warrant.

Obviously, the issue is not an additional definition of death since what has been true remains true: you are dead when you are dead. One does not suddenly redefine the fact that you are dead unless someone intends to define that as dead which is not dead. Such intended definitions have been part of the problem surrounding this issue as we shall discuss later.

Historical Background

Death is a diagnosis. Physicians have diagnosed death without the aid of statutes for ages. Why then in the last ten years has it become necessary for state legislatures and courts to embark on a sea of legislative controversy to do for the medical profession what it heretofore has been capable of doing for itself? Why, indeed, did the medical profession itself see a necessity for promoting legislative determination of brain death?

Part of the answer lies in the problems created by technology. As resuscitative technology became more and more sophisticated, its use became more and more common. That use created a problem. People were maintained on machinery after a resuscitative crisis but they never regained consciousness. Physicians soon realized that that state of unconsciousness had become irreversible and that the brain was no longer functioning. The machinery was maintaining heart and pulse rate but was it maintaining the life of a person? A conceptual problem became obvious at this point.

In the past, the diagnosis of death had always been based on the customary standards of medicine for making such a diagnosis: absence of circulatory and respiratory functions. Even the law accepted this standard although its inquiry into the problem had been practically non-existent.[4] In the current problem, however, circulatory and respiratory functions were present because a machine was causing them to be present. On what basis, then, could a person whose circulatory and respiratory functions were being maintained by machinery be declared dead?

A little common sense reflection at this point would have solved the problem and headed off much of the unnecessary great debate which followed. Someone should have realized that circulatory and respiratory functions ceased when the brain ceased functioning and thereby caused the circulatory and respiratory systems to stop. In short, you were dead when your brain was dead.[5]

Instead, several movements began at this time among certain circles which caused even greater confusion. Let me explain. The brain is composed of several parts which include the medulla, cerebellum, midbrain and cerebrum. Cognitive function is thought to be a product of the cerebrum. One group of commentators proposed to society that once the cognitive function was lost, then that person should no longer be considered a person and should be defined as dead. Cognition, they said, makes you human. Your thoughts are your humanum and, when the power to think is gone, the humanum is gone. That is to say, death of the cerebrum alone, they argued, was the equivalent of death of the person.[6] In the brain death debate, this position presents the greatest danger to a value system which rejects euthanasia.

Two more groups of physicians added to the confusion. Fear of litigation made one group hesitant to arrive at the very common sense notion that you are dead when your brain is dead. Since circulation and respiration were being maintained, albeit artificially, they wondered if declaring such a person dead might lead to malpractice suits or criminal prosecution. This fear rendered them unable to act.[7]

Another group of physicians were interested in developing the medical art of transplanting organs from one person to another. In recent years, organ transplantation had become possible and advances in technology were speeding its use. Organ transplantation, however, had to take place as soon as possible after death in order that the donor organs would be optimally viable to facilitate successful transplants. Delays in diagnosing death, it was said, make organ transplantation difficult, if not impossible. This group of physicians saw brain death as a possible acceptable social means for curing what they considered an important problem stalling medical progress.[8]

A movement began to resolve the impasse. The medical profession was split on the issue but enough physicians feared the growing momentum of litigation to feel it necessary to seek legislative help in an area that should have been solved by the common sense use of customary medical practice.

State Statutes

The impasse was broken by the passage of the first brain death statute in Kansas in 1970. Since that time twenty-six other states have passed similar statutes.[9] Basically, what these statutes do, or attempt to do, is to retain the traditional standards for diagnosing death (absence of respiration and circulation) while adding another standard (brain death).

The statutes generally follow one of four different types.[10]

1) One type is modeled after the *Kansas* law, which provides for alternative definitions of death — one based on brain death, the other based on absence of spontaneous respiratory and cardiac functions. The "brain death" alternative is as follows:

> A person will be considered medically and legally dead if, in the opinion of a physician, based on ordinary standards of medical practice, there is the absence of spontaneous brain function; and if based on ordinary standards of medical practice, during reasonable attempts to either maintain or restore spontaneous circulatory or respiratory function in the absence of aforesaid brain function, it appears that further attempts at resuscitation or supportive maintenance will not succeed, death will have occurred at the time when these conditions first coincide. Death is to be pronounced before artificial means of supporting respiratory and circulatory function are terminated and before any vital organ is removed for purposes of transplantation.

Maryland, New Mexico and *Virginia* have enacted statutes virtually identical with the Kansas enactment, except that the Virginia statute requires the opinion of a consulting physician who is "a specialist in the field of neurology, neurosurgery, or electroencephalography" in addition to the opinion of the attending physician that there is an absence of spontaneous brain function. Commentators have criticized this alternative definition approach on the basis that in reality there are not two different ways of dying as the statute seems to imply.[11]

2) A second type of statute provides a determination of death based on absence of brain function, to be used only when the heart and lungs are artificially maintained. This approach is illustrated by the *Michigan* provision:

> A person will be considered dead if in the announced opinion of a physician, based on ordinary standards of medical practice in the community, there is the irreversible cessation of spontaneous respiratory and circulatory function. If artificial means of support preclude a determination that these functions have ceased, a person will be considered dead if in the announced opinion of a physician, based on ordinary standards of medical practice in the community, there is the irreversible cessation of spontaneous brain function. Death will have occurred at the time when the relevant functions ceased.

Statutes in *Alaska, Hawaii, Iowa, Louisiana* and *West Virginia* are substantially similar except that the *Iowa* and *Hawaii* statutes require the opinion of a consulting physician as well as the attending physician.

3) The Tennessee statute is an example of a third type of statute which follows the American Bar Association model and which reads:

> For all legal purposes, a human body, with irreversible cessation of total brain function, according to the usual and customary standards of medical practice, shall be considered dead.

This type differs in that there is no explicit provision made for determination of death based on respiratory and cardiac cessation although such is implied since brain death is a clinical diagnosis and it was not intended by the ABA that traditional means of determining death were to be superseded by the statute. This approach is also followed in *California, Idaho, Illinois, Montana* and *Oklahoma*. California and Idaho require independent confirmation of death by a second physician.

4) A fourth type of statute provides that a person *may be* pronounced dead if he has suffered irreversible cessation of spontaneous brain function. Unlike the Tennessee statute, this type of statute permits, but does not require, a physician to pronounce a person dead if brain function cessation has occurred. The *Georgia* statute is of this type, stating:

> A person may be pronounced dead if it is determined that the person has suffered an irreversible cessation of brain function. There shall be independent confirmation of the death by another physician.

Similarly, the *Oregon* statute provides:

> In addition to criteria customarily used by a person to determine death, when a physician licensed to practice medicine under ORS Chapter 677 acts to determine that a person is dead, he may make such a determination if irreversible cessation of spontaneous brain function exists.

A number of states make provision within their statutes for organ donation. The *California, Hawaii* and *Louisiana* statutes provide that a physician who makes a determination of brain death may not participate in the removal or transplantation of any organs of the deceased. Most ethical commentators see such a provision as necessary in order to remove potential conflicts of interest for the physician making the determination of brain death.[12]

Court Action

Several courts have had the opportunity to deal with the brain death problem. Their basic approach has been to accept the testimony of the neurological experts on this issue. That testimony generally is provided so that instructions can be drafted which will indicate to the court and jury an intelligible meaning and definition of brain death. In *Tucker v Lower*, for example, which was one of the earliest cases to present the question of definition of death in the context of organ transplantation, the court instructed the jury that death occurs at a precise time, and that it is defined as the cessation of life; the ceasing to exist; a total stoppage of the circulation of the blood and a cessation of the animal and vital functions consequent thereto such as respiration and pulsation. This court initially refused to employ a medical concept of neurological or brain death in establishing a rule of law. In its charge to the jurors, however, the court did allow all possible causes of death to be considered by them including brain death. Unfortunately, the case was never appealed and there is no reported precedent. In addition, the instructions are somewhat confusing.[13]

The Massachusetts Supreme Court accepted the concept of brain death in the case of *Commonwealth v Golston*.[14] The court instructed the jury that brain death occurs "when in the opinion of a licensed physician based on ordinary and accepted standards of medical practice, there has been a total and irreversible cessation of spontaneous brain functions and further attempts at resuscitation or continuous support of maintenance would not be successful in restoring such functions." In *New York City Health and Hospitals Corporation v Sulsona*,[15] a New York trial court in a declaratory judgment suit construed the definition of death in the context of the anatomical gift statute. The court held that the word "death" implies a definition consistent with generally accepted medical practice. Doctors are qualified to testify as to what the general standards are and a general standard of death based upon the diagnosis of brain death was found acceptable by the court.

Recently, the Supreme Courts of Arizona and Colorado have accepted brain death. The Colorado opinion is illustrative.[16] A seventeen-month-old child was discovered to have breathing difficulty and was unresponsive. He was taken to a hospital where it was determined that he had been grossly abused and was not breathing. He was placed on a respirator. Subsequently, the mother was arrested for child abuse and custody of the child was taken from her and placed with the Department of Social Services. The child's attending physician and consulting neurologist as well as the court-appointed neurologist testified that the child had suffered total brain death caused by extensive brain damage resulting from head trauma. The child had sustained multiple bruises, was completely comatose, was not breathing spontaneously and his respiration was maintained entirely by artificial means. He had no spontaneous muscular movements, no reflexes, including stretch or tendon reflexes, and no response to even the most intense pain or other stimuli. Corneal reflexes were absent, his pupils were dilated and fixed, electroencephalograms were flat. The unanimous opinion of the physicians was that the respirator and any other artificial mechanisms supporting the vital functions of the child's body should be discontinued since the child had suffered brain death.

The court viewed the case as one involving the definition of death in Colorado. Conceivably, it said the common law might be interpreted broadly enough to include permanent cessation of brain functions as one of the definitions of death since one of the common law definitions of death was "cessation of life". The court rejected this definition as applicable to the circumstances here where respiration and circulation were being artificially maintained.

The court then proceeded to discuss modern scientific views, judicial decisions and comparatively recent legislation in other states as well as model legislation offered by the American Bar Association, the American Medical Association and the National Conference of Commissioners on Uniform State Laws. As the rule of this case, the court adopted the provisions of the Uniform Brain Death Act which was created by the National Conference of Commissioners on Uniform State Laws.

The Colorado and Arizona cases illustrate our courts' willingness to act in instances where legislative activity have not provided a solution. Of significance is the Colorado Supreme Court's view that:

> Under the circumstances of this case we are not only entitled to resolve the question, but have a duty to do so. To act otherwise, would be to close our eyes to the scientific and medical advances made worldwide in the past two or three decades.[17]

In *State v Fierro*,[18] the Arizona Supreme Court was faced with the issue of brain death when the defendant argued that the victim's death was not caused by the bullets he fired but rather by the physicians who,

64

after declaring the victim brain dead, removed his life support systems. The court rejected this view stating that, when supported by expert testimony, either the Harvard criteria or the standard created by the National Commissioners was appropriate.

Recommended Models

The American Bar Association, The American Medical Association and the National Conference of Commissioners on Uniform State Laws each adopted a recommended brain death statute. In each case, the wording varied slightly but the substance was the same. Each required irreversible cessation of all brain function which can be determined in accordance with reasonable medical standards. The AMA version added legal immunity for the physician.

The version adopted by the National Conference of Commissioners of Uniform State Laws reads:

> For legal and medical purposes, an individual with irreversible cessation of all functioning of the brain, including the brain stem, is dead. Determination of death under this act shall be made in accordance with reasonable medical standards.[19]

This definition is very similar to the definition adopted by the American Bar Association in 1975 which stated as follows:

> For all legal purposes, a human body with irreversible cessation of total brain function, according to the usual and customary standards of medical practice, shall be considered dead.

The determination of death provision in the American Medical Association model bill was as follows:

> A physician, in the exercise of his professional judgment, may declare an individual dead in accordance with accepted medical standards. Such declaration may be based solely on an irreversible cessation of brain function.

Conclusion

Fortunately, it was early recognized that the use of cerebral or cortical death alone as an equivalent for brain death was unacceptable to medicine and society and constituted the introduction of euthanasia into our society.[20] Consequently, all of the brain death statutes require total brain death, or its equivalent, as an acceptable standard. That standard is usually expressed as irreversible cessation of total brain function or equivalent language.

Recently, a full day meeting was held in Chicago which was attended by the Chairman of the Medicine and Law Committee of the ABA, two attorneys from the American Medical Association, the Executive Director of the NCCUSL and three of its board members, as well as the Executive Director of the President's Commission for the study of Ethical Problems in Medicine and Biomedical and Behavorial Research. As a result of that day long meeting, an agreement was reached by the participants as to language for a model statute concerning death. That model statute reads as follows:

UNIFORM DETERMINATION OF DEATH ACT

An individual who has sustained either (1) irreversible cessation of circulatory and respiratory functions, or (2) irreversible cessation of all functions of the entire brain, including the brain stem, is dead. A determination of death must be made in accordance with accepted medical standards.

Each participant returned to his respective association and began the process whereby each association would determine whether they would adopt the proposed definition. Eventually, the AMA, the ABA, and the NCCUSL adopted the Uniform Determination of Death Act as their policy position on this issue. In addition, the President's Commission on BioEthical Issues has urged the passage by Congress of the same Determination of Death Act so as to create a national standard on the issue.

The brain death statutes constitute a legislative determination which is really no different than the common sense insight that should have been made by the physicians ten to fifteen years ago. When the brain has irreversibly ceased to function, then the person is dead in spite of the fact that respiration and circulation are artificially maintained.

This is not to say that determining when the brain has irreversibly ceased to function is an easy diagnosis to make or that it is made easier by the existence of legislation supporting it.[21] What these statutes and cases are simply saying is that when your brain has irreversibly ceased all of its functions you are dead. When your total brain is dead, you are dead. We should not confuse that acceptable medical fact with the also acceptable medical fact that, in any given case, it may be difficult to prove that the brain has irreversibly ceased all of its functions.

66

Irreversibility, of course, is the key. The diagnosis of brain death as irreversible is made with caution in the cases of children or drug induced coma states. Experience has shown the difficulty of making the diagnosis in these instances.[22] That difficulty, however, is no greater than the difficulty medical practitioners experience in making many diagnoses and should not deter entry into the area of diagnosing brain death. The customary concern and caution of physicians, including even transplant physicians, will deter hasty diagnoses and will protect patients. The history of the slow development of brain death and its cautious use by the medical profession are proof of the profession's concern for the well-being of the patient, even dying patients.

Another key is the universally accepted criterion that brain death must be total. All brain centers must be dead. Death of the cortex alone has been correctly rejected by state legislatures and ethical commentators as the introduction of euthanasia which is contrary to our law. Karen Quinlan is in deep coma; she is not dead nor is she brain dead.

Some have argued that brain death is an acceptable criterion for death only if the words "brain death" were merely other words for saying the complete destruction of the entire brain.[23] If by destruction is meant the irreversible cessation of all neuronal activity, then understanding the issue in that fashion presents no insurmountable problems.[24] However, it seems that some understand that word "destruction" in its anatomical sense, thus arguing that brain death is only acceptable when it involves the anatomical destruction of brain tissue. We do not ordinarily wait for anatomical destruction of tissue before determining that death has occurred, having almost universally accepted permanent and irreversible loss of function as the standard.[25]

A more significant problem in my judgment is what direction the law would take in the absence of the currently existing statutes.

All of the currently existing statutes require total brain death. Thus, the fear of introduction of euthanasia through brain death is, as I have argued elsewhere, obviated.[26] Without such legislation, the avenue is left open for courts through judicial pronouncement to accept other, but lesser, standards of brain death if supported by competent neurological testimony. If that testimony supports only cerebral brain death as death, only a judge very sophisticated in these medico-legal problems would understand and be able to overcome the thrust of such ideologically oriented expert testimony.

The important problem is that without brain death legislation requiring total brain death, courts may unwittingly accept a much lesser standard and create even greater problems for society. Thus, legislation limiting the concept of brain death to the irreversible cessation of total function of the brain including the brain stem is beneficial and does not undermine any of the values we seek to support. Indeed, total-brain-death legislation enhances those values by prohibiting euthanasia and allowing only those to be declared dead who are really dead. The definition also serves a teaching function by clearly delineating the distinction between the living, the dead, and the "virtually" dead, a problem which has confused and plagued the definition of death issue for many years.[27] Medical treatment is terminated for the dead because one does not treat a dead patient. Medical treatment may be terminated for the virtually dead but not because they are dead. Rather, it is terminated in those cases because it has become useless, offering no hope of benefit for the patient and only serving to unduly prolong the dying state. The distinction, however, is vital, and, if not understood, causes great confusion.

In addition, it is interesting to note that the emerging medical-legal consensus on the acceptance of brain death as an additional diagnosis for the determination of death may represent one of the first on new bio-ethical issues in the United States.

Notes

1. Ala. Act. 165, 1979; Alaska Stat. §09.65.120; Ark. Stat. Ann. §82-537; Cal. Health & Safety Code §1780; Conn. Public Act 79-556; Ga. Code §88-1715.1; Haw. Rev. Stat. §327 C-1; Idaho Code §54-1819; Ill. Rev. Stat. Ch. 110 1/2, §302; Iowa Code §702.8; Kan. Stat. §77-202; La. Civ. Code Ann. Art. 9-111; Md. Ann. Code Art. 43, §54F; Mich. Comp. Laws §14.228(2); Mont. Rev. Codes Ann. §50-22-101; Nev. Stats. Ch. 451 (S.B. No. 5, Ch. 162, Sixtieth Sess., 1979); N.M. Stat. Ann. §1-2-2.2; N.C. Gen. Stat. §90-322; Okla. Stat. Tit. 63 §1-301; Or. Rev. Stat. §146.087; Tenn. Code Ann. 53-459; 1979 Tex. Sess. Law Serv., p. 368; Va. Code §54-325.7; W. Va. Code §16-19-1; and Wyo. Stat. §35-19-101; Fla. B 293; Colorado.

2. *Lovato, et al v. District Court et.al.*, Supreme Court of Colorado, No. 79 SA 407 Dec. 10-15-79; *Commonwealth v. Golston*, 373 Mass. 249, 366 N.E.2d 744 (1977) cert. den. 434 U.S. 1039, 98 S. Ct. 777, 54 L.Ed 2d 788 (1978) (Court adopts brain death as alternative definition of death); *Arizona v Fierro* (Ariz. Sup.Ct.) 124 Ariz. 182, 603 P.2d 74.

See also: *State v. Shaffer*, 223 Kan. 244, 574 P.2d 205 (1977) (upholding constitutionality of Kansas brain death statute); *Cranmore v. State*, 85 Wis.2d 722, 271 N.W.2d 402 (1978) (error not to instruct jury on what constitutes death); *State v. Brown*, 8 Oreg. App. 72 (1971) (gunshot wound rather than termination of life supports was cause of death); *Tucker v Lower*, No. 2381 Richmond, Virginia, L&Eq. Ct., May 23, 1972 (jury instructed that it can consider brain death as an alternative definition of death); *People v Lyons*, 15 Criminal Law Reporter 2240, Cal. Super Ct. (1974) (court instructed jury that victim legally dead from gunshot wound because of brain death before respirator turned off); *New York City Health and Hospitals Corp. v Sulsona*, 367 N.Y.S.2d 686 (1975) (court declares brain death as an alternative definition of death).

3. See e.g.: *Euthanasia and Brain Death: Ethical and Legal Considerations;* Horan, D. J., Annuals of the New York Academy of Sciences Vol. 315 pp. 363-375, Nov. 17, 1978; (this entire volume is devoted to the issue of brain death); Conway, *Medical and Legal Views of Death: Confrontation and Reconciliation,* 19 *St. Louis U.L.J.* 1972 (1974); Arent, *The Criteria for Determining Death in Vital Organ Transplants — A Medical-Legal Dilemma,* 38 Mo. L. Rev. 220 (1973); Biorck, *When is Death?,* 1968 *Wis. L. Rev.* 484; Black, *Brain Death, Part I,* 299 *N. Eng. J. Med.* 338 (1978); Black, *Brain Death, Part II,* 299 N. Eng. J. Med 393 (1978); Cantor, *Quinlan, Privacy, and the Handling of Incompetent Dying Patients* 30 Rutgers L. Rev. 243 (1977); Collestar, Jr., *Death, Dying and the Law: A Prosecutorial View of the Quinlan Case,* 30 Rutgers L. Rev. 304 (1977); Frederick II, *Medical Jurisprudence — Determining the Time of Death of the Heart Transplant Donor,* 51 N.C.L. Rev. 1972 (1972); Friloux, Jr., *Death, When Does it Occur?,* 27 Baylor L. Rev. 10 (1975); Hirsh, *Brain Death,* 1975 Med. Trial Tech. Q. 377; Hoffman and Van Cura, *Death — The Five Brain Criteria,* 1978 Med. Trial Tech. Q. 377; Note, *The Tragic Choice: Termination of Care for Patients in a Permanent State,* 51 N.Y.U.L. Rev. 285 (1976); Wasmuth, Jr., *The Concept of Death,* 30 *Ohio St. L. Rev.* 32 (1969); *Refinements in Criteria for the Determination of Death: An Appraisal.* 221 J.A.M.A. 48 (1972); *An Appraisal of the Criteria of Cerebral Death, A Summary Statement,* 237 J.A.M.A. 982 (1977); Capron and Kass, *A Statutory Definition of the Standards for Determining Human Death: An Appraisal and a Proposal.* 121 U. Penn. L. Rev. 87 (1972).

For an excellent review of this subject see: Van Till, A. *Diagnosis of Death in Comatose Patients under Resuscitation Treatment: A Critical Review of the Harvard Report,* American Journal of Law and Medicine 2, 1-40 (1976). See also Veith, F. et al. *Brain Death,* 238 J.A.M.A. 1651-1655 (1977) and 238 J.A.M.A. 1744-1748 (1977); *Brain Death — An Opposing Viewpoint,* Byrne et al. 242 J.A.M.A. 1985-1990 (1979); *Editorial,* 242 J.A.M.A. 2001, 2002 (1979); Horan and Mall, *Death, Dying, and Euthanasia,* University Publications of America, Inc. Washington, D.C., 1977.

4. Under the common law a person was considered dead when there was "total stoppage of the circulation of the blood, and a cessation of the animal and vital functions consequent thereon, such as respiration, pulsation, etc." *Black's Law Dictionary* (4th Ed. 1951), p. 488.

5. The common law can be interpreted broadly enough to include permanent cessation of brain functions as one of the definitions of death. One of the common law definitions of death was "cessation of life," *Bouvier's Law Dictionary* (Rawle's Ed.) p. 775 (1914); *Cyclopedic Law Dictionary,* p. 285 (1922).

6. Olinger, S. D. *Medical Death,* Baylor Law Rev. 22-26 (1975) (the entire issue of this law review is devoted to the issue of euthanasia).

7. See, e.g., Editorial of J.A.M.A., Nov. 2, 1979, Vol. 242, No. 18, p. 2001, 2002 where Robert M. Veatch Ph.D. says: "But the historical evolution has slowed. While approximately 20 states have adopted legal changes in the years after the Harvard report, the rate of change has recently decreased. Physicians are, or should be, bound by law. Where the definition of death has not been changed, newer criteria for death pronouncement based on brain function should not be used."

8. See the discussion in: Paul Ramsey, *The Patient as Person* (New Haven & London: Yale University Press, 1979).

9. Op. Cit. ft. 1.

10. For these classifications, I am grateful to the Jan. 1979 memo of the legislative department of the Public Affairs Division of the AMA.

11. Capron & Kass, op. cit. ft. 3 at pp. 108-11.

12. Ramsey op. cit. ft. 8 at p. 101.

13. Op. Cit. ft. 2.

14. 366 N.E. 2d 744 (Sup Ct. Mass, 1977).

15. 376 N.Y.S.2d 686 (1975).

16. *Lovato, et al. v. District Court, et al.,* Supreme Court of Colorado, N. 79 SA 407 dec. 10-15-79. Slip Opinion.

17. Ibid p. 20.

18. *Arizona v Fierro* 124 Ariz. 182, 603 P2d 74.

19. Uniform Brain Death Act drafted by the National Conference of Commissioners on Uniform State Laws, approved at its annual conference July 28 - August 4, 1978.

20. Horan, D. J. *Euthanasia and Brain Death: Ethical and Legal Considerations,* 315 Annals of the New York Academy of Sciences, 363-375 (1978).

21. That the diagnosis may be medically difficult to make is made clear by Volume 315 of the Annals of the New York Academy of Sciences, the entire volume of which is devoted to the subject of brain death on a medical, scientific, legal and moral basis.

22. *An Appraisal of the Criteria of Cerebral Death,* 237 J.A.M.A. 982-986 (1977).

23. Byrne, et al. *Brain Death — An Opposing Viewpoint,* 242 J.A.M.A. 1985-1990 (1979).

24. See, Van Till, op. cit. ft. 3 at p. 8-12. In his rebuttal editorial to the Byrne article, Veatch praises the Byrne article as a challenge to be more precise in specifying what it is whose irreversible loss signals death of the person.

25. Robert M. Veatch, 242 J.A.M.A., 2001, 2002 (1979).

26. Horan, *Euthanasia and Brain Death: Ethical and Legal Considerations,* 315 Annals of the New York Academy of Sciences, 363-375 (1978).

27. Paul Ramsey, *Statement on Matters Related to the Definition of Death,* Testimony submitted to the President's Commission for the Study of Ethical Problems in Medicine and Biomedical and Behavioral Research, July 11, 1980.

Part II

Prolonging Life Decisions

Introduction

These eight chapters view moral responsibility in prolonging life decisions through the insights of three theologians, a physician, a philosopher, a historian of theology, a lawyer, and a sociologist. In chapter 5, Dr. Oscar B. Hunter, Jr., looks briefly at medical treatments and procedures which prolong human life, without pretending to offer an exhaustive catalogue. In chapter 6, philosopher Joseph M. Boyle, Jr., opens up the central theme of moral responsibility by arguing that both patients and physicians, at least in the teaching of the Church, share responsibility toward the personal good of health so that their relationship cannot be reduced simply to that of purchaser and purveyor of a commodity.

71

Gary M. Atkinson Ph.D., of the philosophy department of the College of St. Thomas in St. Paul, MN, prepared chapter 7 as a historical introduction to the theological development of the parameters of moral responsibility in prolonging life decisions. He focuses on key theologians from Thomas Aquinas in the 13th century to Gerald Kelly, S.J., and Bishop Daniel Cronin in the 20th.

Chapters 8 and 9 contain the central ethical and theological reflections of this entire resource volume. In chapter 8, Father Benedict M. Ashley, O.P., professor of moral theology at the Aquinas Institute, now located in St. Louis, MO, describes simply and directly four moral principles which function in the Judeo-Christian stewardship of life tradition. Father John R. Connery, S.J., a professor at Loyola University in Chicago, devotes chapter 9 to a detailed and sometimes difficult analysis of the implications of Father Ashley's second principle, the obligation to do whatever is required for the healthy functioning of one's own body. He distinguishes the question of useful and useless means of prolonging life (useless means are clearly not obligatory), from the more problematic discussion of burdensome means. From this latter discussion originated the ethical distinction of ordinary and extraordinary means of prolonging life. A careful study of chapter 9 will fortify the reader for practical decision-making in the complex and confusing situations which arise.

Father Lawrence T. Reilly presents, in chapter 10, a readable and helpful approach to conscience formation in decisions about prolonging life. He emphasizes that everyone involved in prolonging life decisions, not only health care providers, but patients, families, and advisors, all are challenged to form their consciences according to objective moral norms as applicable to individual situations.

In chapter 11, Dennis J. Horan, author of chapter 4, returns to contribute a magnificent legal analysis of legislative statutes and judicial decisions in the United States relevant to prolonging life decisions. His critical argument for the dubious relevance of the constitutional right of privacy to refusal of treatment questions adds additional importance to this outstanding chapter. Professor William J. Monahan, of St. Louis University, concludes Part II with a sobering look at a steadily increasing acceptance of mercy killing, and, *a fortiori*, the omission of ethically ordinary medical treatment, by popular opinion in the United States population.

Chapter 5

Prolonging Human Life in Medical Practice

Oscar B. Hunter, Jr., M.D.

Introduction

From the earliest days of medicine as a profession, physicians have followed a code of ethics which embodied the principle of prolonging life by prevention or treatment of disease, and of never taking life. The Oath of Hippocrates is still adhered to today, although in some schools of medicine, modifications, such as approval of abortion, have crept in. These principles of prolonging life and not using poisonous potions or abortifacients constitute ethical principles completely compatible with Christian teaching and are elevated by faith to the theological status of following God's will as taught by Christ.

Using this principle in the practice of medicine has given patients the confidence to seek the assistance of the physician who would impart only sound treatment and cause no harm.

The decision, therefore, of seeking a physician to treat an illness and prolong life is first of all the patient's. By requesting a physician for treatment, a contract is made by which the physician is authorized by the patient to relieve him of symptoms and/or cure the disease and thus to prolong his life. Under dire circumstances, the decision to seek medical help is taken over by family members if the patient is unable to make such decisions rationally. Thus the responsibility of prolonging life follows a precise sequence — patient to physician or patient's family to physician. The only way such responsibility can be countermanded is by the patient or the patient's family withdrawing this permission and thus breaching the contract. The physician, however, must make the decision as to what means or methods are to be used to prolong life and must follow his conscience in pursuing therapy as long as he concludes that it is for the patient's best interest — and that interest is both physical and spiritual. When the therapy becomes worse than the disease, prolongation of life by artificial means can hardly be justified. Most physicians, however, will make the decision to discontinue further therapy only with the full knowledge and consent of the patient or, if that is not possible, of the family.

Using this principle as the basis of practice, we can explore various life-prolonging treatments according to the principal stages of human life, followed by a discussion of pain management and trends for the future.

Intrauterine Life

Physicians generally regard life as beginning with conception. In the first trimester of pregnancy, signs of early miscarriage may be evident by a bloody vaginal discharge associated with uterine cramps. Bed rest, sedation, and hormones are generally used to prevent the miscarriage and prolong the life of the fetus to the time of delivery. If placental slough occurs, death of the fetus is inevitable and the use of further therapy is of no value. Preservation of the mother's health and life then become the most important considerations.

In the second trimester, the child is usually non-viable if delivered before the sixth month; but if it does survive, the child does so only with aggressive supportive measures. A threatened miscarriage is usually evident from the same signs and symptoms evident in the first trimester. The therapy is generally the same. However, late in the second trimester, the question arises as to whether the fetus is mature enough to survive if delivered. This may be determined under proper circumstances by amniocentesis, and determining the creatinine or the lecithin sphingomyelin ratio in the amniotic fluid.[1] In addition, the degree of severity of certain fetal diseases may be determined such as erythro blastosis or diabetes.[2] Corrective measures can be taken and, in some instances, early delivery be effected by induction of labor or Cesarean section.

The latter problems are usually seen in the third trimester along with the threats of post maturity syndrome and fetal effects of maternal alcoholism and/or malnutrition. For the latter, corrective therapy is best done before delivery while in the post maturity state.[3] Early delivery is most important.

Newborn Life

The newborn child may suffer from a host of ailments, such as those seen as a result of difficult labor, cranial injury or damage because of malfunctions. In today's world, the careful obstetrician is usually aware of the problem before birth, and, where necessary, will perform a Cesarean section which is associated with a low morbidity and mortality.

Decisions must occasionally be made as to whether or not it is truly of benefit to the child to expend life-preserving measures on newborns who have suffered severe cranial damage or have life-threatening malfunctions.

Such medical decisions today are made by a neonatologist. As a rule, most such afflicted infants are given a trial period on life-support systems to determine their viability. Such systems include a respirator with intermittent positive pressure and an individual venous catheter for feeding or blood sampling. The latter is most important since control of the electrolytes and blood gasses is extremely important to the control of all bodily functions. If the trial period proves satisfactory, continuation of the support is warranted. If, on the other hand, the child is doing poorly and death appears inevitable, continuation of heroic support exposes the child and parents to needless pain and anguish as well as the tying up of six people per day at a cost not only of time, but also of $2,000 - $3,000 per day. The same holds true for deformed babies where the malfunction is so extreme that death is inevitable. Use of heroic measures under these conditions is not only not wise, but also wasteful.

Babies suffering from neonatal illnesses today can often benefit

75

from very helpful therapeutic treatment. Those suffering from erythro-blastosis due to blood incompatibility can be treated with exchange transfusions and relieved of their anemia and threats of cerebral damage due to jaundice.

A frequent complication of premature babies is pulmonary disease —such as Hyaline membrane disease.[4] Treatment with respirators and careful control of electrolytes and blood gasses past 96 hours usually will allow the child to survive.

With any of these problems, neonatal intensive care units can frequently control all of the necessary life-support systems. This is done by the respirator with intermittent positive pressure, electrodes continually to monitor cardiac function and a catheter in the umbilical vein for feeding and blood sampling. All of this is done with constant monitoring by the pathology laboratory and maintenance of a warm moist environment in an incubator.

Childhood and Adulthood

Life-threatening situations arise in childhood and adulthood as a result usually of seven major disease areas or conditions:
1) Malnutrition
2) Toxic substances or radiation
3) Cancer
4) Cerebral disease
5) Heart disease
6) Arteriosclerosis and the aging process
7) Trauma

Medicine's role enters the picture when one of these life-threatening situations arises or its effects are seen in the patient. To prolong the life of the patient is, first of all, a decision-making process which may be simple or most complex. For example, an accident victim may arrive in the emergency room with an avulsion of the scalp, depressed fracture of the skull, and fragments of brain extruding from the skull while cardiac and respiratory function persist. The patient is inevitably going to die, and thus therapy is fruitless. On the other hand, with the patient having a less severe injury, yet admitted in a coma with skull fractures, all measures for support and relief should be initiated until such time as it becomes evident that the patient is indeed "brain dead."

A recent case in Washington occurred in a local hospital with a nine-year-old boy accidentally poisoned by phencyclidine (PCP). The child was maintained on life-support systems. EEG waves were absent but he still had some spinal reflexes. The father refused to give permission to turn off the machines but the courts ultimately gave permission after medical consultation found gangrene of the extremities and other evidence of tissue death.

What are these life-support systems and how do they work?[5] All of the tissues of the body need circulation of oxygen and nutriment to sustain life. Self-sustained life does this by the brain instructing the heart and blood vessels to circulate blood and instructing the respiratory muscles to fill and empty the lungs with O_2 and CO_2. Without these stimuli from the brain medulla, these activities cease. Introduce a cardiac pacemaker and vasopressor drugs, and the heart and vascular system can be maintained. A respirator supplying O_2 and abstracting CO_2 will maintain lung function.[6] All other organs can then be maintained. To assist the physician, electrodes are connected from the body to an ECG machine and monitors to register pulse and blood pressure continuously. Catheters in the vena cava give central venous pressure to monitor for early signs of shock. Also blood gasses and electrolytes can be continually monitored by the laboratory. Hyperalimentation can be dripped through the catheter in the interim. To treat cardiac fibrillation, a defibrillator with its shock paddles are left by the bedside. The patient can then be maintained for prolonged periods even when there is no evidence of brain waves.

Patients receiving life-support, as well as others critically ill, may experience cardiac arrest. Normally, a "code blue" alert is called. Such alerts are called in response to apparent deaths. A team of doctors and nurses move rapidly to the patient's bedside with resuscitation gear, oxygen, and drugs. The respirator is initiated and cardiac compression is applied to the chest. Under favorable conditions the patients will respond, while under others all attempts at resuscitation prove fruitless.

"No code blue" may be ordered by the physician properly when the patient is in a dying state, where death is near at hand and there is no moral obligation to institute such measures. To die in dignity without the code blue procedure is, under those circumstances, a blessing.

Intractable Pain and Prolonging Life

Pain and suffering are the lot in life for humankind. None of us will go through life without this inheritance from Adam and Eve.

Some pain and suffering purifies the spirit and individuals become stronger by overcoming their effects, but, for the physician seeing a patient these are symptoms of a disease to be treated and, where possible, relieved or cured.

Pain is both physiological and psychological. Many people will have pain which they can disregard. The body senses the pain but the psyche rejects it and continues without heeding it. Usually persistent, severe pain will destroy the patient's ability to cope with life and many times drive him to desperate measures.

Intractable pain due to an invasive malignancy is not infrequently a terminal problem for some patients. Medicine today has many adjuncts with which to cope with pain. A few are:

— Local and general anesthesia
— Narcotics and sedatives
— Intravenous alcohol drips
— Hypnosis and psychologic suggestions including acupuncture
— Biofeedback — using low level pain stimuli to reduce more severe pain and finally surgery using either neurectomy or cordotomy.

All of these procedures may be used individually or in various combinations to obtain relief. Under most circumstances, modern care can satisfy the problem without keeping the patient in an unconscious state.

The degree of therapy, of course, must be measured in conjunction with the severity of the pain and the state of the primary pathology. Terminal cancer patients should be given relief but consideration of the spirit is of primary importance as the patient approaches death and should be given its proper place in the decision. Deliberate overdoses with medication are not only wrong, but unnecessary with the tools available today.

The Future

What will life be like 20 years from now in the year 2000? We cannot evade the fact that medicine, with all of the new technologies developed from the space program, is yearly becoming more and more able to prolong life and to do so with a more rewarding type of living.

Nutrition and immunology are proving to be quite helpful in preserving life. Arteriosclerosis can be relieved and many of the diseases associated with premature aging can be, in part, prevented.

Surgical procedures to relieve sclerotic vessels and even to replace organs are becoming more commonplace. Replacement of diseased vessels has given years of happy living to many who would have otherwise died of heart attacks.

But of all the new knowledge, the science of immunology will, perhaps, make the most significant discoveries to identify the causes and relief of the aging process whereby tissues become worn out by stress and the interaction of antigen-antibody complexes. The endocrine world is finding ways to relieve the body's reaction to outside antigens which cause more rapid deterioration of the body tissues.

Life will not be eternal youth, but the quality of life, if cared for properly and not abused, will be more rewarding in the future.

Notes

1. Aubrey, R. H. et al. The Lecithin Sphingomyelin Ratio in a High Risk Obstetric Population. Ob. & Gyn., 47:21, 1976.

2. Henry, J. B. Clinical Diagnosis by Laboratory Methods. Evaluation of Placental Function. Sanders, 1979, p. 880.

3. Morrison, J. C. et al. Amniotic Fluid Test for Fetal Maturity, Ob. & Gyn., 49:20, 1976.

4. Forman, D. T. Biochemical Basis of Hyaline Membrane Disease. American Clinical Laboratory Science, 3:242, 1973.

5. Lawn, B. et al. The Coronary Care Unit, New Perspectives and Directions. JAMA, 199:188, 1967.

6. Beal, J. M. & Eckerdoff, J. E. Intensive and Recovery Room Care, McMillan Company, 1971.

7. Goodman, M.D., J. M. and Heck, M.D., L. L. Brain Death. JAMA, pp. 966-968, 1977.

8. Collins, V. J. Managing Pain and Prolonging Life, *New Technologies of Birth and Death*, Proceedings of Pope John XXIII Center Workshop, St. Louis, MO, 1980.

Chapter 6

The Patient/
Physician Relationship

Joseph M. Boyle Jr., Ph.D.

The relationship between the patient and the physician is an essential part of the context within which life-prolonging decisions are made. Many of the moral and legal obligations of those involved in such decisions are based upon or shaped by this relationship. Thus, it is important — but by no means sufficient — for dealing with the issues addressed in this volume that the patient/physician relationship be understood. In particular, it is necessary that this relationship be understood in a normative way — that is, we should know not only how this relationship does, in fact, work, but how it should work. It is from this latter, normative conception of the relationship that light will be shed on the proper procedures and content of life-prolonging decisions.

The patient/physician relationship is, as we shall see, very different in cases in which the patient is a legally competent adult and in cases in which the patient is a child or a non-competent person. Many of the most difficult life-prolonging decisions concern those who are non-competent. However, the relationship between a competent adult and his or her physician provides the central, paradigm case of the patient/ physician relationship. It is by understanding the relationship in this context that its morally and legally essential features emerge. And it is by contrasting the relationship of a non-competent person and his or her physician to this standard that the special difficulties of making decisions for non-competents come to light.

For this reason, this chapter is divided into two parts; the first deals with the relationship between a competent patient and his or her physician. The second with the relationship between a physician and the non-competent patient. Because of its centrality, the first part is more extensive — consisting of a review of the legal status of the patient/ physician relationship, a survey of Church teaching on this relationship and a brief theological/philosophical reflection.

1) The Competent Patient and His or Her Physician

The patient and his or her physician are related to one another — in the simplest case at least — insofar as they together pursue the patient's health. Some dimension of health is always at stake in the patient/ physician relationship, but in some experimental and public health contexts it is not the patient's health which is directly and centrally the goal. These special contexts will not be discussed here. The common pursuit by patient and physician of the patient's health most often takes place when the patient is ill or in pain and the services of the physician are sought and provided to cure or arrest the illness or to alleviate the pain. Thus, the relationship between patient and physician is a union in cooperative activity for the sake of the patient's health. Of course, the performances of the patient and the physician are quite different. The patient initially seeks the help of the physician, accepts the physician's advice and submits to the physician's regimen or treatment. The physician diagnoses, prescribes and treats. Yet, these different performances do not prevent the activity of the patient and the physician from having an underlying unity, any more than the different functions of the members of a team prevent them from being joined in the common activity of playing a game.

Of course, the physician/patient relationship is frequently not experienced or understood as a common action. One reason for this is that the patient must often submit to treatment by the physician — as in the extreme case of surgery. It appears that the patient endures or undergoes not only the pain and debilitation of illness but also the treatment of the physician. Thus, it may seem that the actions are those of the physician, and that the patient is no more than a voluntary recipient of the physician's action. Nevertheless, the relationship between patient and physician is a unity in common action, and, paradoxically, it is the patient, and not the physician, who is the primary decision-maker. The physician serves as the agent or helper of the patient in the common pursuit of the latter's health.

A. The Law on Patient Intangibility and Informed Consent.

Anglo-American law takes for granted that as a rule every competent adult is at liberty to seek medical treatment and not to seek it, and to give or to refuse consent to any treatment which is proposed. No police officer takes one to the doctor; one chooses to go. If one is negligent about one's own health, one cannot be charged with any offense or sued for damages by anyone else. If one does not like the treatment which physicians propose, one can dismiss them and find other physicians or one can refuse to follow directions, not take one's medicine, reject the suggestion that one go to the hospital, refuse to sign forms consenting to surgery — in general, be an uncooperative patient. The physician has no choice but to put up with one's uncooperativeness or to withdraw from the case.

In a 1914 New York case, Judge (later Justice) Cardozo stated this proposition clearly:

> Every human being of adult years and sound mind has a right to determine what shall be done with his own body; and a surgeon who performs an operation without his patient's consent commits an assault, for which he is liable in damages.[1]

The underlying concept is that a person has a basic right to bodily integrity and intangibility — that is, nobody can cut a person or even so much as touch a person who is not willing to be cut or touched without violating that person's rights and providing him or her with a legal claim to compensation for the violation. In principle, this claim is no less against a physician who treats a person without consent than it is against someone who attacks another in anger or with premeditated malice, for although the latter might be guilty of a crime of which the physician would be innocent, the personal offense is the same.

82

In effect, the law intends to enclose everyone in an invisible shield and to give to each person the right to decide when to lower the shield and when to keep it in place. The underlying theory, which surely is sound, is that bodily contact can be repugnant — if not harmful, distasteful — and that each person is the best judge of what contact is acceptable.

In the medical context, the mere fact that one puts oneself into the hands of physicians does not mean that they can proceed as they see fit. They have a duty to explain what sort of treatment they propose and why, and to point out any significant risks or reasonable alternatives. They also have a legal duty to limit treatment to that to which one has consented. If they go beyond the boundaries, even for the patient's good and with good results, physicians violate the patient's rights.[2]

The extent and nature of the right of a competent adult to refuse treatment are revealed in those cases in which patients have sued physicians for malpractice because of treatment for which there was not proper consent and in those cases in which courts have been asked to override the patient's right to refuse treatment.

Most of the actions in the former category are civil cases in which the physician's action was judged to be a battery. "In most general terms, a battery is committed when there is an intentional contact with the plaintiff's body, and that contact neither has been consented to nor is legally privileged."[3] A battery is essentially an affront to personal dignity; injury or financial loss is not essential.[4]

Courts have overridden the right of a competent adult to refuse medical treatment on a number of distinct grounds. Overriding the right of a competent adult to refuse treatment is distinct from the important and common exception to the requirement of informed consent — namely, the emergency situation in which the patient can neither give nor refuse consent. In such cases, consent is presumed. The physician may proceed provided the treatment supplied is medically appropriate and such that a reasonable person normally would consent to it, and provided the physician has no knowledge that the particular patient would not consent. In other words, when a patient cannot decide about treatment, the law establishes a reasonable assumption that the ordinary person who needs care would want the treatment a normally competent physician can give. Were this assumption not made, the intangibility of those few who would refuse treatment if they could do so would be held paramount to the actual desires as well as to the well-being of most people.

In several of the cases in which the right of a competent person to refuse treatment is overridden, the court's overriding the right to refuse treatment is well grounded and obviously legitimate. In other cases, the reasoning of the court is tendentious and doubtful, going against the trend of the law and in effect rendering empty the right to refuse treatment.

Medical treatment, even against the patient's explicit wishes, can be legally required when demanded by the clear interest of public health and safety. For example, the United States Supreme Court ruled that the interest of the state in protecting its members from smallpox overrides the right to refuse treatment — in this case vaccination — whether this right is based on the right of free exercise of religion or bodily intangibility.[5]

Courts have also overridden the right to refuse treatment on the grounds that this refusal would lead — by the patient's death or incapacitation — to a failure to care for minor children. The application of this line of reasoning to various cases can be questioned;[6] but the *parens patriae* authority of the state is unquestioned and this limitation of the right to refuse treatment is clearly justifiable.[7]

In other cases, the right to refuse treatment by a competent adult has been overridden on the grounds that the individual had become incompetent by the time of adjudication or on the grounds that there was suspicion that the individual actually desired the refused treatment. These opinions are widely disputed.[8] Likewise, the rulings which override the patient right to refuse treatment on the grounds that honoring this refusal would infringe on the rights of physicians or hospitals are agreed to be unsound.[9] Such reasons would render the right to refuse treatment nugatory and would amount to a medical paternalism contrary to the direction of the law.

Finally, there are several cases in which the right to refuse treatment was overridden because this refusal would predictably lead to death and, thus, the refusal was held to be tantamount to attempted suicide.[10] However, the common law definition of suicide includes the person's purposefully setting in motion the death-producing agent. Thus, these decisions adopt a non-legal definition of suicide because the refusal of treatment does not involve setting in motion the death-causing agent. These decisions also involve imputing to the patient intentions the patient almost certainly did not have. For these reasons, these decisions go against the direction of the law.[11]

These cases must be distinguished from cases in which treatment is given to a person who has attempted suicide and whose refusal of treatment is pursuant to the suicidal act. In these cases, overriding the refusal to accept medical treatment is clearly justified by the state's undeniable interest in preventing suicide.[12]

The important point here, however, is that refusal of medical treatment by a competent adult is *not* justifiably overridden *simply because the refusal predictably leads to death*. The grounds for this right of refusal are the right to bodily intangibility and, in many cases, the right to free exercise of religion. In several recent cases, there is appeal to the right to privacy and the right to die.[13] These appeals are unnecessary since the right to bodily intangibility is well established as is the right to free exercise of religion, and these are sufficient to justify the right to refuse treatment. The exact import of the right to privacy — to the extent that it is not simply equivalent to the right to bodily intangibility and to free exercise of religion — is not clear. The "right to die" seems to include the right to commit suicide or at least to treat a person's death as a socially protected good. By substitute consent, this "benefit" might be extended to many who are not legally competent. Since the right to refuse treatment — even when the refusal predictably leads to death — should be understood as based on the right to bodily intangibility and free exercise of religion, the broad extent of this right should be understood not as based on any public interest in a person's death or on the legitimacy of a person's desire to die; it should be understood as based on the importance of these rights in a society committed to individual freedom and dignity.[14]

The legal status of the right of a competent adult to refuse medical treatment certainly supports the primacy of patient choice in the patient/physician relationship; it clearly rejects medical paternalism which, however widespread in practice, has little legal foundation. The state of the law, however, does not *by itself* provide a full, normative account of the patient/physician relationship. For the law allows a view of the relationship as a buyer/seller relationship in which the patient voluntarily seeks and the physician voluntarily provides certain services or commodities. This view of the relationship requires patient consent and in principle rejects medical paternalism: after all, the consumer should be properly informed and should not be forced to buy what he or she does not want. But this understanding of the patient/physician relationship obscures the patient's moral responsibility for his or her health, misconstrues health as an object which can be purchased, and reduces the physician's role to that of a technician or expert purveyor of a commodity. By considering the teaching of the Church on the patient/physician relationship, a more adequate understanding of this relationship will emerge.

B. The Teaching of the Church on the Patient/Physician Relationship.

On several occasions, Pope Pius XII affirms that the physician has no rights over the patient except those which have been given him by the patient.

> First of all, one must suppose that the doctor, as a private person, cannot take any measure or try any intervention without the consent of the patient. The doctor has only that power over the patient which the latter gives him, be it explicitly, or implicitly and tacitly. The patient, for his part, cannot confer rights which he does not possess.[15]

In his famous discussion of ordinary and extraordinary means, Pope Pius says much the same thing:

> The rights and duties of the doctor are correlative to those of the patient. The doctor, in fact, has no separate or independent right where the patient is concerned. In general he can take action only if the patient explicitly or implicitly, directly or indirectly, gives him permission.[16]

Pope Pius' position seems very close to that of the Anglo-American legal tradition, and one might claim to find in his statements support for a consumer model of the patient/physician relationship in which patient desires are basic. However, Pope Pius rejects any such understanding of the patient/physician relationship: the physician's duties and rights are correlative to the patient's *duties* and *rights* — not to the patient's desires and wants. Thus, the patient too has certain obligations bearing upon his or her health: "As far as the patient himself is concerned, he is not absolute master of himself, of his body, or of his soul. He cannot, therefore, freely dispose of himself as he pleases. Even the motive for which he acts is not by itself sufficient or determining."[17]

Pope Pius immediately draws the implication that there are some things which a physician may not do to a patient even if the patient consents, because these things are wrong and patient consent cannot justify them.[18] So, the Pope's statements undercut one mistaken implication of the primacy of patient choice — namely, the proposition that patient *wants* are normative. Moreover, since the consumer model almost certainly reduces the physician's role to that of a highly expert technician, this model is inconsistent with the Pope's affirmation of the dignity of the medical profession:

> Spirit and dust compounded to form an image of the Infinite; living in time and space, yet headed towards a goal that lies beyond both; part of the created universe, yet destined to share the glory and joy of the Creator, that man who places himself in the care of a doctor is something more than nerves and tissue, blood and organs. And though the doctor is called in directly to heal the body, he must often give advice, make decisions, formulate principles that affect the spirit of man and his eternal destiny. It is, after all, the man who is to be treated: a man made up of soul and body, who has not only temporal interests but also eternal and as his temporal interests and responsibility to family and society may not be sacrificed to fitful fancies or desperate desires of passion, so his eternal interests and responsibility to God may never be subordinated to any temporal advantage.[19]

The recent teaching of the Church, therefore, rejects the consumer model of the patient/physician relationship, while, nevertheless, affirming the primacy of patient choice and consent in this relationship.

C. Theological/Philosophical Reflections

Reflection on the nature of health and on the role of health within the personal vocation of each person makes it clear that the patient/physician relation must be understood as a unity in common action in which the patient is the primary decision-maker and the physician is his or her agent or helper.

Leon Kass, following Aristotle, defines health as "the well working of the organism as a whole."[20] According to this definition, health is the perfection of a certain dimension of the human person — namely, that dimension in which human beings are living bodies or organisms.[21] Health, then, is a value in two senses: first, it is the standard for evaluating activities, disabilities, and so on, as healthy or unhealthy.

Second, health is a basic personal good — an aspect of the good of human life — since it perfects one dimension of human existence. Thus, health has a place among the basic principles of practical reasoning and generates moral obligations.

Since health is a personal good, it is not something that can be *objectified* and given to people as if it were a commodity. Health is not something one has, it is part of the way a person exists, thus, a person's health is effectively promoted only when the person himself is actively involved in its promotion. This personal involvement differs greatly according to the age, condition and responsibility of the person in question; there can be little doubt, however, that for people capable of responsible choice, health will be effectively promoted only through the choices and commitments of the person himself.[22] In this respect, health and other human goods are like the virtues; individual initiative is essential for their effective realization.

Even more importantly, personal initiative is absolutely required if the realization of such goods as health is to be a morally significant part of a person's life. One can be lucky enough to be healthy; but this is not by itself morally significant. The commitment to health on the part of a person who seeks to integate this concern reasonably into his or her life is morally significant even if the person is unlucky enough to be unhealthy in spite of his or her best efforts. The importance of the individual's exercise of choice is one of the grounds for the principle of subsidiarity — a basic principle of Catholic social teaching. According to this principle, "one should not withdraw from individuals and commit to the community what they can accomplish by their own enterprise and industry."[23] After discussing this principle in *Mater et Magistra*, Pope John XXIII brings it to bear on the multiplication of social relationships in modern society. One area in which there is growing intervention by public authorities into the intimate aspects of personal life is the area of health care. Pope John sees this trend as a great help to people but also as a genuine danger.

> But as these various forms of association are multiplied and daily extended, it also happens that in many areas of activity, rules and laws controlling and determining relationships of citizens are multiplied. As a consequence, opportunity for free action by individuals is restricted within narrower limits. Methods are often used, procedures are adopted, and such an atmosphere develops wherein it becomes difficult for one to make decisions indepen-

dently of outside influences, to do anything on his own initiative, to carry out in a fitting way his rights and duties, and to fully develop and perfect his personality. Will men perhaps, then become automatons, and cease to be personally responsible, as these social relationships multiply more and more?[24]

It seems to me that the concern of Pope John applies not only to the public and legal dimension of health care but also to the patient/physician relationship itself. Here, too, the initiative and responsibility of each person for his or her own health must be protected and encouraged. Thus, we have at last a ground for primacy of patient decision in the patient/physician relationship which does not reduce the relationship to that of buyer and seller, or reduce the physician's role to that of a servant of the patient's whims.

The nature of the moral obligations imposed by the personal good of health also provides a reason for the primacy of patient choice in the patient/physician relationship. Health, like other goods, is the basis for a number of distinct obligations.[25] First of all, one should not choose against this good or choose its appearances when these prevent its full realization. One should also take care not to neglect one's health and to integrate the pursuit of health with one's entire vocation. Thus, it is wrong never to think of health except when one is sick and then to give it a priority inconsistent with the set of commitments which form one's personal vocation.

Health, like life itself, is a great good but it is not the only good and one's pursuit of health — including its minimal realization in staying alive — must fit into one's vocation. How the pursuit of health fits into one's vocation is determined by one's choices; health, therefore, has no definite priority vis-a-vis the other goods in a person's life. What priority it has can only be determined by the person himself. The physician is in no special position to determine the role health has or should have within the commitments and duties of a person's unique life. In fact, many saints have lived lives which, by the standards of modern medicine, were decidedly unhealthy. No physician can rightly decide that a person should forgo unhealthy practices of asceticism, missionary activity in unhealthy climates and so on. The same applies with respect to the more mundane lives of most people.

To sum up: the primacy of patient choice and responsibility in the patient/physician relationship is not based on the primacy of patient *wants* or on an understanding of the relationship as a kind of commercial transaction. Rather, this primacy is based on two related considerations: first, that health is a personal good which is effectively realized only by the activity of the individual, and second, that the priority of this good in each person's life can be settled only by the person's unique vocation and obligations.

Before turning to the relationship between the physician and the non-competent patient, two objections to my view of the nature of the patient/physician relationship must be considered.

One might object that the emphasis on the primacy of patient choice is inefficient. This emphasis requires an inefficient use of the physician's time in deliberating with the patient, informing the patient, and perhaps persuading the patient. Furthermore, patients aware of their own active responsibility are less likely to cooperate, more likely to demand a wider range of options and, in general, to act so as to make health care delivery more cumbersome and to make the over-all quality of health decline.

In response, I concede that my understanding of the patient/physician relation makes the physician's role a difficult one, and that this understanding might make certain procedures less efficient technically. However, it is by no means clear that the overall good of health will be realized less fully if the responsibility for health is placed on the individual.[26] Moreover, the actual realization of good health is not the only nor even the primary value that is at stake. The goods of human persons are also realized in the very commitments of the persons who choose them. Whether these goods are actually realized is less existentially important than that the person's choices towards them are the right ones. But again, the goods are more likely to be actually realized when persons are properly committed to them.

A second objection is that my view of the patient/physician relationship does not do justice to the nobility of the medical profession — that it removes the moral judgment altogether from the physician. In response, it seems to me to be false to suppose that medicine is not a moral enterprise unless the moral judgments of the physician are determinative of the patient's actual care. Of course, the physician should not do things he or she thinks immoral. Moreover, the physician is legally free to refuse to provide what he or she regards as substandard care; such a refusal is morally defensible — at least where the professional standard of medical care is not unreasonably set up, and where lesser standards are not arbitrarily precluded.

It is worth noting that the honoring of a competent patient's refusal of treatment is not either of these things. To honor such a decision, even when one is convinced that it is mistaken or immoral, is not to choose the evil involved but to respect the established right which, as we saw above, is morally well founded even if sometimes abused.[27]

Furthermore, the physician who sees his role as helping the patient in the patient's pursuit of health will have a clear moral role. He or she will not simply take it for granted that the level of health established as the object of good medical care and wanted by the patient is normatively established and beyond question; rather the physician will participate in the patient's deliberation by clarifying options and articulating values. This role, it seems to me, is not that of a mere technician but of one who truly treats the whole person without the paternalistic assumption that all of a person's life is an organic object for medical expertise or that medical values are the only relevant ones in medical decisions.

Furthermore, the physician is morally obliged to give good medical care and to seek to provide that care in accord with the patient's consent. If the patient does not consent to treatment which corresponds to the medical profession's standard for good medical care, the physician should still seek to provide good medical care consistent with the patient's consent. One who refuses chemotherapy, for example, ought still to be provided with pain killers and other ordinary treatments.

Finally, the emphasis on the primacy of patient responsibility does not mean that the obligations are all on the side of the physician. The patient has obligations to his physician, and to other potential users of health care services, to cooperate, to follow orders, and so on. Most important, the patient cannot morally ask a physician to do what the physician regards as immoral.

2) The Physician and the Non-Competent Patient

The misunderstanding of the patient/physician relationship in the case of competent adult patients has the effect of giving people treatments they do not choose. Here the tendency of medical paternalism is towards overtreatment and a diminishing of individual responsibility for health. The problem which arises in dealing with non-competent patients is very often a different one; the main danger for non-competent persons is that their basic rights will be neglected and that they will be denied treatment they morally ought to be given. This problem — the problem of passive euthanasia and neglect of the elderly and of "passive infanticide" for severely deformed babies — is one of the great challenges to the justice of our society and to the fairness and humanity of our health care institutions. The understanding or the misunderstanding of the relationship between a physician and his or her non-competent patient contributes to this problem but it is by no means the only or the primary factor. The anti-life attitudes of many parents and adult children, the unclarity about the roles of patient, family, and the courts in these decisions, and the often radical disagreements about principles and their applications all contribute to the problem.

When his patient is not a competent adult, the physician — although committed to the health and welfare of his patient — is not acting as the patient's agent since the patient cannot be presumed to be a responsible decision-maker. The physician is, nevertheless, the agent of those who bear primary responsibility for the patient. The responsible decision-makers are thus most often the parents or guardians of a dependent child or a non-competent adult. Sometimes the responsible party is a designated person in a public institution or even the court when treatment is judicially mandated. These persons are rightly presumed to have a deep concern for the patient's best interests and to be in a position to know the patient's mind and will so as to be most able to construct consent for the patient — that is, to choose responsibly on the patient's behalf. In the case of court-ordered treatment, the grounds for the responsibility lie in the court's authority to protect the basic rights and interests of children and non-competent adults. The physician, as such, lacks this authority and lacks an intimate relationship to the patient. So, in the case of the treatment of non-competent patients as well as in the case of the treatment of competent patients, the physician acts as the agent of other parties.

The moral situation of the physician in such cases is different than in cases in which the patient is competent, because here the person whose health the physician is promoting is distinct from those who authorize the treatment. The moral difference arises because the physician's judgment as to what is medically or morally or legally required may be quite different from the judgment of those who authorize treatment — in particular, a physician may feel that a treatment is required for the good of his patient which those who bear responsibility for the treatment have refused. Since the patient is a person who has not, in fact, refused the treatment, the appeal to patient autonomy cannot settle the issue as it does in the case of a competent patient. Moreover, those who are in a position to authorize or to refuse to authorize treatment are not literally exercising the patient's own autonomy. Thus, their constructed consent cannot be merely what they want for the patient or would want for themselves if they were in the patient's position, but what is morally and perhaps legally required of them on the patient's behalf.[28] Since most people want treatment up to the standard of good medical care and since there is no evidence that non-competent persons would want or are entitled to anything less than this, the physician — who is in the best position to know what this standard is — is rightly concerned if care up to this standard is denied to his non-competent patient. The physician would be morally remiss if he failed to do what he could to see that treatment up to this standard is carried out. To do less is to fail in his duty to his patient.

Of course, as a private person, the physician cannot initiate treatment without authorization, but the physician can seek to persuade those authorized to consent, and, in the extreme case of a violation of the patient's basic rights, can appeal for a court order or make use of other mechanisms to insure that the patient's basic rights are not violated.[29] This activity by physicians and hospitals is common enough; for example, courts have routinely ordered blood transfusions for children of Jehovah's Witnesses over their parents' objections.[30]

Thus, the complication of the physician/patient relationship in cases where the patient is not a competent adult imposes a special moral obligation on the physician to provide for the health of his patient. This obligation exists even in the face of the refusal of treatment by those who have the responsibility to authorize treatment. Although the physician operates as their agent, he acts for the good of his patient and must do what is possible to promote this good and protect his patient's rights.

Notes

1. *Schloendorff v. Society of New York Hospital,* 211 N.Y. 125, 105 N.E. 92 (1914) at 93.

2. Angela Roddey Holder, *Medical Malpractice Law* (New York, London, Sydney, Toronto: John Wiley & Sons, 1975), pp. 225-234; Norman L. Cantor, "A Patient's Decision to Decline Life-Saving Medical Treatment: Bodily Integrity Versus the Preservation of Life," *Rutgers Law Review,* 26 (1973) pp. 236-237. The preceeding paragraphs follow closely the analysis in Germain Grisez and Joseph M. Boyle Jr. *Life and Death with Liberty and Justice,* 'A Contribution to the Euthanasia Debate,' (Notre Dame: The University of Notre Dame Press, 1979) pp. 87-88.

3. Charles Fried, *Medical Experimentation: Personal Integrity and Social Policy* (New York: Elsevier North-Holland, Inc., 1974), p. 14.

4. *Ibid.*, pp. 15-16.

5. *Jacobson v. Massachusetts,* 197 US II (1905).

6. See Robert M. Byrn, "Compulsory Lifesaving Treatment for the Competent Adult," *Fordham Law Review,* 44 (1975) pp. 33-35. I am indebted to this important article in the legal summary which comprises this section.

7. *Ibid.;* see also John C. Ford, S.J. "Refusal of Blood Transfusions by Jehovah's Witnesses," *Catholic Lawyer,* 10 (1964), pp. 216-219. Fr. Ford's article is limited to the difficulties arising from the refusal of blood transfusions by Jehovah's Witnesses. He articulates the principles of law and Catholic morality relevant to this entire discussion.

8. See Byrn, *op. cit.* pp. 24-26; Grisez and Boyle, *op. cit.,* p. 94 and the literature cited there.

9. See Byrn, *op. cit.,* pp. 29-33; Grisez and Boyle, *op. cit.,* pp. 95-96.

10. See Byrn, *op. cit.,* pp. 16-24; Grisez and Boyle, *op. cit.,* pp. 94-95.

11. See Byrn, *op. cit.,* pp. 17-19.

12. See Byrn, *op. cit.,* p. 17; Grisez and Boyle, *op. cit.,* p. 95.

13. See *In re Yetter;* 62 Pa. D & C 2nd 619 (C. P., Northampton County Ct. 1973). Byrn discusses this case, pp. 3-10.

14. See Grisez and Boyle, pp. 96-99.

15. Pope Pius XII, "Allocution to the First International Congress of Histopathology," September 13, 1952; this translation is from *Papal Teachings: The Human Body,* Selected and Arranged by the Monks of Solesmes, (Boston, St. Paul Editions, 1960) p. 198. See also, "Allocution to Military Surgeons," October 19, 1953 in *Human Body,* p. 281.

16. Pope Pius XII, "Allocution to Gregor Mendel Genetic Institute," November 24, 1957: *AAS,* 1957, pp. 1027-1033. The translation is from *The Pope Speaks,* 4 (1957-1958), p. 397.

17. Pope Pius XII, Allocution of September 13, 1952, cited in note 15; translation from *Human Body* pp. 198-199.

18. See *ibid., Human Body* p. 199; and Allocution of October 19, 1953, cited in note 15, *Human Body* pp. 281-282.

19. Pope Pius XII, "Allocution to Doctors of Allied Countries," January 30, 1945; *Human Body,* p. 66.

20. Leon Kass, "Regarding the End of Medicine and the Pursuit of Health," *The Public Interest,* 40 (1975) p. 19. See also Aristotle, *Categories* 9A 21-24.

21. For a fuller defense of a narrow, biological definition of health see my "The Concept of Health and the Right to Health Care," *Social Thought* 3 (1977) pp. 7-12.

22. See Kass, *op. cit.,* pp. 29-38.

23. This principle is enunciated in Pope Leo XIII's *Rerum Novarum* and cited in Pope John XXIII's *Mater et Magistra* #53.

24. *Mater et Magistra* #62; the translation is from the Paulist Press edition, (New York: 1961), p. 26.

25. For a discussion of the way human goods ground various types of moral obligations, see Grisez and Boyle *op. cit.,* pp. 361-371.

26. See Kass, *loc. cit.*

27. See Ford, *op. cit.,* pp. 214-217.

28. See Pope Pius XII, Allocution of November 24, 1957 cited above in note 16; *The Pope Speaks loc. cit.;* on the abuse of substitute consent, see Grisez and Boyle, *op. cit.,* pp. 175-176, and on how to forestall such abuse, pp. 289-297.

29. The decision of the Supreme Court of New Jersey in the Karen Quinlan case establishes a mechanism within hospitals that avoids use of the courts. For a critique of this decision, see Grisez and Boyle, *op. cit.,* pp. 283-287.

30. See Ford, *op. cit.,* pp. 216-218. The classic decision is that of the United States Supreme Court, *Prince v. Massachusetts* 321 U.S. 1944.

Chapter 7

Theological History of Catholic Teaching on Prolonging Life

Gary M. Atkinson, Ph.D

Introduction

On November 24, 1957, Pope Pius XII delivered to an international congress of anesthesiologists an address known as "The Prolongation of Life".[1] That address, in a sense, represents a culmination of the theological development of the Church's official teaching regarding the prolongation of life, and at the same time provides an indispensable basis for understanding the contemporary situation. The purpose of this chapter is to present a brief description of the historical development of theologians' answers to questions regarding the duty to preserve life.

In looking at the historical development of an idea or concept, one is frequently faced with the difficulty of deciding just how far back to trace that development. Concerning the question of the prolongation of life, one is inclined to say that any starting point is bound to be somewhat arbitrary. But there are at least two reasons for beginning here with the writings of the Angelic Doctor. First, his assimilation of human reason and divine revelation is held to be without parallel, and the impact of his thinking on his successors down to the present day has been immense. Second, as a practical matter, the history of the development of the idea from Aquinas to the present is a topic of manageable proportions for a chapter of this length.

St. Thomas Aquinas (1224-1274)

Aquinas sees life as a gift from God, so that a person who takes his own life sins against God and violates God's mastery over life and death. Thus, we have a negative duty owed God not to kill ourselves. But do we possess a corresponding *positive* duty to take steps to keep ourselves alive? Aquinas answers this question in the affirmative. In his lectures on the Epistles of St. Paul, Aquinas writes:

> A man has the obligation to sustain his body, otherwise he would be a killer of himself . . . by precept, therefore, he is bound to nourish his body and likewise we are bound to all the other items without which the body can not live.[2]

Now it would seem reasonable to draw from this quotation the inference that Aquinas believes we have an absolutely binding obligation to take every step necessary for the preservation of one's life. But there is a basis within the *Summa* for denying such an inference. In the *Secunda Secundae*, Aquinas takes up a discussion of fearlessness, and his first question is whether fearlessness ought to be considered a sin. Aquinas' answer is that it can be:

> It is inbred for a man to love his own life and those things which contribute to it, but in due measure (*tamen debito proprio*); that is, to love things of this kind not as though his goal were set in them, but inasmuch as they are to be used for his final end. So if a man falls below the due measure of love of temporal goods this is against the basic tendency of his nature and consequently a sin . . . .

> So it is possible for someone to fear death and other temporal evils less than he should, because he loves life and its goods less than he should . . . .[3]

Temporal goods ought to be despised in so far as they hinder us from love and fear of God. And in this sense they ought not to be a cause of fear; so *Ecclesiasticus* says (34:16), *He who fears God will not tremble.* But temporal goods are not to be despised in so far as they are helpful means of attaining things which promote fear and love of God.[4]

It is important here to note two things: *first*, that by man's "final end" Aquinas means here the happiness of eternal life with God and, *second*, that by "temporal goods" Aquinas means to include life on this earth. Thus, Aquinas is saying that there are temporal goods and evils and that they ought to be sought or avoided, but in *due measure* as this pursuit or avoidance is conducive or appropriate to the person's final end who is God. To seek a temporal good or avoid a temporal evil, *not* in due measure, is to act in such a way that God, the final end, is lost sight of. Now Aquinas in this article is concerned with a lack in seeking temporal goods (*aliquis deficiat a debito modo*). But one can also conceive the possibility of an *excess*, of too much of a love for temporal goods. Just as one can sin by a lack of love for one's life, so one can sin by an excess of such love. In either case, the test is whether the pursuit or avoidance is useful in serving to obtain the final end of knowing, loving, and serving God (*secundum quod eis utendum est propter ultimum finem*).

Francisco De Vitoria (1486-1546)

Aquinas set the parameters for the discussion regarding the prolongation of life: (1) suicide is ruled out, (2) as is the intended killing of the innocent; (3) mutilation is recognized as a legitimate means of saving life; (4) an obligation to preserve life is admitted, but (5) this obligation is seen to be somewhat circumscribed by considerations relating to the proper pursuit of one's final end.[5] The task of the successors of Aquinas became that of elaborating on and specifying the implications of these basic points.

The moral theologians who immediately succeeded Aquinas were content to restate his arguments opposing suicide, and we find in them little discussion regarding the obligation to preserve one's life. This neglect is abruptly altered by the great sixteenth century Dominican moralist, Vitoria. In his *Relectiones Theologicae* he discusses the virtue of temperance and the eating of food. It is in connection with food, and its usefulness in preserving life, that Vitoria raises some points of special interest.

Following Aquinas, Vitoria argues that a person has an obligation to preserve his life, based on the natural inclination toward self-preservation. Furthermore, the malice of suicide would arise from the non-preservation of oneself. But if this is so, then it would seem that a sick person who does not eat because of some disgust of food would be guilty of a sin equivalent to suicide. Vitoria denies this inference, and, in response, makes eight important points:

(1) A sick person is required to take food *if* there exists some hope of life (*cum aliqua spe vitae*).

(2) But, if the patient is so depressed or has lost his appetite so that it is only with the greatest effort that he can eat food, this right away ought to reckoned as creating a kind of impossibility and the patient is excused (*jam reputatur quaedam impossibilitas et ideo excusatur*), at least from mortal sin, especially if there is little or no hope of life.

(3) Furthermore, the obligation to take drugs is even less serious. This is because food is *"per se* a means ordered to the life of the animal" (*per se medium ordinatum ad vitam animalis*) and is natural, whereas drugs are not. A person is not obliged to employ every possible means of preserving his life, but only those that are *per se* intended for that purpose (*media per se ad hoc ordinata*).

(4) Nevertheless, if one had a moral certitude that the use of a drug would return him to health, and that he would die otherwise, then the use of the drug would be obligatory. If he did not give the drug to a sick neighbor, he would sin mortally, so it seems he would have the same responsibility to save his life. Medicine is also *per se* intended by nature for health (*medicina per se etiam ordinata est ad salutem a natura*).

(5) On the other hand, it is rarely certain that drugs will have this effect, so it is not mortally sinful to declare abstinence from all drugs, though this is not a praiseworthy attitude to take since God has created medicine because of its usefulness.[6]

(6) It is one thing not to protect or prolong life; it is quite another thing to destroy it. A person is not always held to the first.

(7) To fulfill the obligation to protect life, it is sufficient that a person perform "that by which regularly a man can live" (*satis est, quod det operam, per quam homo regulariter potest vivere*). Again, if a person "uses foods which men commonly use and in the quantity which customarily suffices for the conservation of strength" (*quibus homines communiter utuntur et in quantitate*), then the person does not sin even if his life is notably shortened thereby, and this is recognized.

(8) Thus, a sick person would not be required to use a drug he could not obtain except by giving over his whole means of subsistence.[7] Nor would an individual be required to use the best, most delicate, most expensive foods, even though they be the most healthful. Indeed, the use of such foods would be "blameworthy" (reprehensibile). Nor would one be obliged to live in the most healthful location.[8] In another work (Comentarios a la Secunda Secundae de Santo Tomás), Vitoria cites as examples of "delicate foods" hens and chickens. He says that if the doctor were to advise the person to eat chickens and partridges, the individual could still choose to eat eggs and other common items instead, even though he knew for certain he could live another twenty years by eating such special foods.[9]

In a later Relectio on the question of homicide, Vitoria summarizes his position as follows: "One is not held, as I said, to employ all the means to conserve his life, but it is sufficient to employ the means which are of themselves intended for this purpose and congruent" (ad hoc de se ordinata et congruentia).[10] This makes clear the point also made by Aquinas: that one is not obliged to use any and every means for the preservation of life.

Furthermore, Vitoria is inclined to view the obligation to use certain means not in the abstract but in the concrete. As the second point on the above list shows, what produces a "kind of impossibility" (and no one is obliged to do the impossible) need not be the means themselves but the impact of their use on the individual patient. Thus, the obligation to preserve life is neither absolute nor invariant, but rather can depend on the peculiar circumstances of the individual.

Vitoria raises the question of the relevance of the distinction between natural means (e.g., foods and drink) versus artificial means (e.g., drugs). It should not be surprising that Vitoria himself displays some ambivalence on the subject. On the one hand, (Point 3), the obligation to use drugs is less stringent than the obligation to use food because food is a means per se ordered to the life of the animal, and is natural, whereas drugs are neither. But on the other hand, (Point 4), medicine is also intended by nature for health. It would seem, then, that medicine is also natural.

Daniel Cronin offers the following as a possible explanation for Vitoria's distinction between artificial and natural means:

> Food is primarily intended by nature for the basic sustenance of animal life. Food for man is basically and fundamentally necessary

from the very beginning of his temporal existence. It is basically required by his human life and nature intends food for this purpose. That is why man has the right to grow food and kill animals. Furthermore, because it is a law of nature that man sustain himself by food, it is a duty for man to nourish himself by food. In the case of drugs and medicines, the same is not true. Drugs and medicines are intended per se by nature to help man conserve his life. However, this is by way of exception. Drugs and medicines are not the basic way by which man is to nourish his life. They are intended by nature to aid man in the conservation of his life when he is sick or in pain or unable to sustain himself by natural means. These artificial means are not natural means but they are intended by nature to help man protect, sustain, and conserve his life. If man were never to be sick, he would never need medicines. If he is sick, however, it is quite *natural* for him to make use of *artificial* means of *conserving* life.[11]

Thus, natural means are intended by nature for the preservation of life, whereas artificial means are likewise intended, but only as means supplementing the natural, when this becomes necessary. Such a distinction may be able to explain some moral difference regarding the obligation to employ them, but it would also seem to permit calling artificial means obligatory under certain conditions.

Juan Cardinal De Lugo (1583-1660)

A period of a hundred years stretches between the work of Vitoria and de Lugo. During this time a number of prominent theologians were writing on the topic of obligatory means of preserving life: Soto, Molina, Sayrus, Banez, Sanchez, Suarez. These are important writers, but their work did not advance much beyond Vitoria. This is not to say that their work is inconsequential or insignificant, for it does serve to demonstrate a rough consensus with only the relatively minor details to be worked out. By and large, we find few new basic principles being enunciated. The writers seem mostly content to elaborate on old themes.

By paying special attention to de Lugo, then, we may convey the false impression that his ideas are radically new. In fact, many of the topics discussed by de Lugo were thoroughly covered by his predecessors. Both Aquinas and Vitoria admit that there are restrictions on the duty to preserve life, that there can be conditions under which one is not morally obliged to preserve life. It must follow, then, that there are conditions under which not-saving is morally different from killing. De Lugo follows his predecessors in this. What he has to say is not always new, but some of the examples he employs are historically important.

De Lugo deals with one topic not yet discussed in any great detail but of great interest for his predecessors and contemporaries, the question of mutilation. Agreeing with Aquinas, de Lugo held that, just as a person does not possess full dominion over his own life, so he does not possess complete dominion over the parts of his body. Thus, arguing as Aquinas had argued, mutilations of the body are wrong if they are not necessary for the body's health.

The question at issue here is whether certain mutilations can become *obligatory*, as being necessary for life or health. De Lugo holds that such a mutilation is obligatory, *provided* that it can be accomplished without intense pain:

> He must permit this cure when the doctors judge it necessary, and when it can happen without intense pain; not, if it is accompanied by very bitter pain; because a man is not bound to employ extraordinary and difficult means to conserve his life (*media extraordinaria et difficillima*).[12]

Vitoria had insisted, (see the seventh point in summary above), that in most cases one is obliged to use only those means that are regularly (*regulariter*) and customarily (*communiter*) employed for the preservation of life. Here de Lugo seems to be making basically the same point, but he chooses to phrase his position in the negative, that one is not obliged to employ extraordinary or out-of-the-ordinary means for the preservation of life. Thus, de Lugo is saying that the difference between not-saving and overt killing is morally important if the means being refused are either difficult to employ or out of the ordinary. He uses, as an example of means difficult to employ, a mutilation causing intense or bitter pain (*intenso acerbissimo dolore*). Indeed, a means may be out of the ordinary precisely *because* it is painful to employ.

Nevertheless, it is important to recognize that there may be a number of reasons why a means may be out of the ordinary, other than that it is difficult to employ. Thus de Lugo considers many of the examples of optional means earlier mentioned by Vitoria: the use of choice and costly medicine, or even the drinking of or abstaining from wine.[13] Indeed, one senses in de Lugo a striking attempt to be most liberal in judging a means to be optional. Any reason that would make

101

a means out of the ordinary suffices for de Lugo as a justification for calling it optional. And he is quite willing to relativize this element of the extraordinary (as Vitoria was with the element of the burdensome) to the particular circumstances of the individual. Thus de Lugo argues that a novice in a religious order is not bound to return to the secular world in order to eat better food to preserve his life, since such food, even though ordinary and common for the secular world, is not ordinary for those in the religious life.

De Lugo holds that the failure to employ available means necessary for preserving one's life or the failure to avoid a potentially death-dealing natural cause can be morally equivalent to the positive taking of one's own life. But this is true only where the means are ordinarily employed and not difficult to use, or where the death-dealing natural cause can easily be avoided.

In the previous discussion the opinion of Vitoria argued that a sick person is required to take food to preserve his life, at least if the food can be employed without great difficulty. But Vitoria adds a further qualification: for the taking of food to be obligatory, there must exist "some hope of life." The implication there is that a person is not obliged to employ means if there is no hope of their being useful in preserving life.

De Lugo is in agreement with Vitoria on this point and employs an example which will be discussed by later moralists and will be seen to have considerable theoretical and practical significance for the present day. De Lugo considers the case of a man facing certain death in a burning building. The man notices that he has water to extinguish part of the fire, but not all of it, and that he can only delay his death by the water's use. Is the man under an obligation to use the water? De Lugo answers in the negative, "because the obligation of conserving life by ordinary means is not an obligation of using means for such a brief conservation — which is morally considered nothing at all" (*quae moraliter pro nihilo reputatur*).[14]

On the other hand, de Lugo holds that if the person could put out the fire completely, he would be obliged to use it. In this latter case, the use of water would be analogous to eating ordinary foods. Certainly the use of water is an ordinary means of putting out a fire (and so saving a life). And, in the example, the means can be easily employed. Thus, de Lugo wished to admit the possibility that an ordinary means need not be obligatory because the benefit to the person is too slight to carry moral weight.

Alphonsus Liguori (1696-1787)

The next author in this survey, St. Alphonsus Liguori, lived about a hundred years after Cardinal de Lugo. Alphonsus adds little to the work of his predecessor. His *Theologia Moralis* has been of great historical importance, but he covers no new ground in his treatment of the duty to preserve life, being content to make a number of well-covered points: (1) that there is no obligation to use costly or uncommon medicines; (2) that one need not move to a more healthful climate; (3) that one is not required to use difficult or extraordinary means of preserving life, such as the amputation of a leg; (4) that one might have an obligation to use ordinary medication if there were good hope for recovery.

Alphonsus does raise a point not yet discussed, though it is not new with him, that a person's subjective repugnance toward the use of a means might make that means nonobligatory for that individual. Alphonsus mentions the case of a woman (particularly a maiden) who might find examination by a male physician greatly abhorrent. This element of subjectivity in the assessment of the obligatoriness of means is firmly in the tradition of Vitoria and de Lugo.

Danial Cronin, whose work on the history of the ordinary/extraordinary distinction is the most thorough to date, sees little of novelty in the writers of this period. He finds moralists using the very same phrases and examples already well-worn by their predecessors. Cronin offers as one hypothesis for this lack of originality the fact that

> progress in the medical field had not actually reached such a degree as to initiate any speculation on whether a particular remedy should be considered obligatory or not. Evidently an amputation, at this period in history, was the perfect example of a terrible torture which no one ordinarily could be held to undergo. . . . Had doctors and other scientists created doubts or difficulties by advancing new and secure methods of health and cure, no doubt these very moralists would have settled them, as they did in so many other instances. The absence of speculation therefore seems due to the fact that difficulties in the matter were not presented to the moralists, rather than any want of appreciation of the problem itself.[15]

Alphonsus' *Theologia Moralis* shares this general lack of originality. Furthermore, the writers between the time of Alphonsus and the twentieth century have little new to say. To be sure, there are differences in emphases and disagreements on some points. For example, Vincent Patuzzi, an eighteenth century theologian, takes issue with de Lugo, and maintains that a maiden does possess an obligation to accept treatment from a male physician even at the cost of great embarrassment and shame.[16] But it is the *scarcity* of such differences that is the most striking feature of this period. Daniel Cronin writes:

> After St. Alphonsus and in the nineteenth century, the characteristics of the treatments given this problem of the ordinary and extraordinary means of conserving life were fairly well standardized. St. Alphonsus had emerged as a recognized authority and leader in the field of Moral Theology. What he had learned from the previous theologians was now to be passed down by the authors who followed him. This is particularly true regarding the problem of the ordinary and extraordinary means of conserving life. Here and there different speculation is discovered, but for the most part, the authors are content to paraphrase Alphonsus.[17]

And since there is little new in Alphonsus himself, the basic positions can be traced back to de Lugo, Vitoria and Aquinas.

One last point will be noted before closing this section. In their work Vitoria and de Lugo insisted that in assessing the obligatoriness of a given means, the issue must be relativized to take into account the particular condition of the patient. Thus, if the eating of food produces intense repugnance, that means could become non-obligatory for *that* patient even though the means would remain obligatory for most patients. But one may turn the question around and ask whether there are some *non-obligatory* means that remain optional *regardless* of the condition of the patient? A surprising number of theologians in the nineteenth and twentieth centuries answer this question in the affirmative. Noldin and Schmitt hold that not even a rich person would be required to seek the services of very skilled doctors or to leave home for a more healthful climate. What is required of the sick is only what can be required of any one else: the use of means ordinarily employed.[18] This judgment is echoed by Genicot and Salsmans[19] and by Herbert Jone and Urban Adelman.[20] Edwin Healy goes further in his work *Moral Guidance*. In that work, published in 1942, Healy sets as an *absolute* norm the sum of $2,000 beyond which *no one* is obliged to go

104

in saving his life.[21] This position would hold that although the judgment of a means as ordinary and therefore obligatory must *always* be made *relative* to the condition of the individual patient, the judgment of *some* means as extraordinary and optional can be made *absolutely* and independently of the patient's particular circumstances.

Gerald Kelly (1902-1964)

Kelly is an important figure for this study. As a moral theologian he was intrigued by the history of the concept of ordinary and extraordinary means. He published two key articles in *Theological Studies*, "The Duty of Using Artificial Means of Preserving Life" (1950, hereafter "Artificial")[22] and "The Duty to Preserve Life" (1951, hereafter "Preserve").[23] The earlier article, "Artificial," is the lengthier of the two. In it Kelly presented a resumé of the traditional position and requested help from his readers in resolving a few of the more difficult questions raised. The shorter, "Preserve," appeared eighteen months later and contains Kelly's further reflections on the topic in response to suggestions from his readers.

In the first article, Kelly summarized a descriptive approach to the distinction of ordinary and extraordinary means of prolonging life:

> Speaking of the means of preserving life and of preventing or curing disease, moralists commonly distinguish between *ordinary* and *extraordinary* means. They do not always define these terms, but a careful examination of their words and examples reveals substantial agreement on the concepts. By *ordinary* they mean such things as can be obtained and used without great difficulty. By *extraordinary* they mean everything which involves excessive difficulty by reason of physical pain, repugnance, expense, and so forth. In other words, an extraordinary means is one which prudent men would consider at least morally impossible with reference to the duty of preserving one's life.[24]

Kelly also notes the uncertain status of major operations in these days of anesthesia and antibiotics. He finds a tendency among modern authors to consider most operations today as ordinary means, though there is also a common willingness to admit the possibility that a strong subjective repugnance on the part of the patient could render those operations extraordinary means for some people.

Kelly raises the question of whether the concept of the "extraordinary" should be treated as relative or absolute, a question raised already in this chapter. Kelly writes that his "general impression" is that "there is common agreement that a relative estimate *suffices*. In other words, if any individual would experience the inconvenience sufficient to constitute a moral impossibility in the use of any means, that means would be extraordinary for him."[25] On the other hand, Kelly cites a number of authors who believe that there is an absolute standard of an extraordinary means beyond which no one, regardless of his condition, need go.

Kelly makes two other points that should be mentioned here. First, he notes that the standard moralists he has consulted are concerned solely with the responsibility of the individual patient and say nothing about the duties of the family or of the medical profession. Second, Kelly points out that the moralists are in agreement that although a patient is *per se* not obliged to use extraordinary means in preserving his life, the use of such means is permissible and usually admirable. Furthermore, a patient *per accidens* may even be obliged to use extraordinary means "if the preservation of his life is required for some greater good such as his own spiritual welfare or the common good." As traditionally cited examples, one might consider the obligation of a person to take extraordinary steps to preserve his life until he can receive the sacraments, or the obligation of a government leader to keep himself alive if his leadership is necessary for the welfare of the community.

The foregoing is relatively unproblematical, at least on a theoretical level. But Kelly continues in a way that will produce terminological difficulty. This occurs when Kelly raises the question whether a patient can be obliged to employ *useless ordinary* means. Kelly cites several authors, including Alphonsus, Ballerini-Palmieri and Noldin-Schmitt, as seeming to espouse the view

> that no *remedy* is obligatory unless it offers a reasonable hope of checking or curing a disease. I would not call this a common opinion because many authors do not refer to it, but I know of no one who opposes it, and it seems to have intrinsic merit as an application of the axiom, *nemo ad inutile tenetur* [i.e., No one can be obliged to do what is useless]. Moreover, it squares with the rule commonly applied to the analogous case of helping one's neighbor: one is not obliged to offer help unless there is a reasonable assurance that it will be efficacious.[26]

Kelly is thus willing in "Artificial" to countenance the possibility of some means being ordinary and yet optional and non-obligatory. At the close of that article, Kelly admitted that many of the points he had raised call for further discussion. Two in particular, he said, were of "special import," and one of these was the possibility "that even ordinary, artificial means are not obligatory when relatively useless." His original article can be seen, then, as a call for further discussion on certain controversial issues.

In his second article, Kelly presents some of the reactions his earlier paper had elicited from theologians and offers further reflections of his own. He writes in "Preserve":

> Theologians have responded favorably to the suggestion that even an ordinary artificial means need not be considered obligatory for a patient when it is relatively useless. It was proposed, however, — and I agree with this — that, to avoid complications, it would be well to include the notion of usefulness in the definitions of ordinary and extraordinary means. This would mean that, in terms of the patient's duty to submit to various kinds of therapeutic measures, ordinary and extraordinary means would be defined as follows:
>
> *Ordinary* means are all medicines, treatments, and operations, which offer a reasonable hope of benefit and which can be obtained and used without excessive expense, pain, or other inconvenience.
>
> *Extraordinary* means are all medicines, treatments, and operations, which cannot be obtained and used without excessive expense, pain, or other inconvenience, or which, if used, would not offer a reasonable hope of benefit.
>
> With these definitions in mind, we could say without qualification that the patient is always obliged to use ordinary means. On the other hand, insofar as the precept of caring for his health is concerned, he is never obliged to use extraordinary means; but he might have an extrinsic obligation to use such means, e.g., when his life is necessary for the common good or when a prolongation of life is necessary for eternal salvation.[27]

It will be helpful to compare these definitions of ordinary and extraordinary means with the descriptions cited from the first article above. There we see the term *ordinary* as encompassing only those means "as can be obtained and used without great difficulty." The new definition of *ordinary* is changed in two ways, one obvious and other more subtle. First, Kelly quite obviously adds the concept of usefulness to the definition of *ordinary*. But, secondly, there is a more radical change in the way in which the term *ordinary* is treated. In the earlier definition, the term is treated as *descriptive* term, as simply referring to how easily the means may be obtained and employed. In the latter definition, and the quotation makes this clear, Kelly treats the term as an *essentially normative or evaluative one*. It is no longer used simply to *describe* ease of use; it is now used to make a judgment regarding *obligatoriness* of use. For the earlier definition, it made quite good sense to suggest as a theoretical possibility that some ordinary means might not be obligatory. But in the second definition, it makes no sense (at least in Kelly's mind) to suggest an ordinary means (as newly defined) might not be obligatory: "without qualification the patient is always obliged to use ordinary means." In other words, to call a means non-obligatory one *must*, using Kelly's new definitions, call the means extraordinary. *Ordinary = obligatory, extraordinary = per se optional*, and these two equations are justified by reducing the obligatoriness of means to their being easily obtained and employed *and* their offering reasonable hope of benefit.

Kelly's two articles mark, as it were, a kind of watershed between the descriptive and normative senses of *ordinary* and *extraordinary*. Writing in his first article and surveying the past history, Kelly could provide a *descriptive* analysis of *ordinary*. Writing in his second, in response to suggestions, he provides a *normative* analysis. Of course, this descriptive/normative distinction can be pushed too far, for even in the first definition the feature of "without great difficulty" has normative elements. And in the second, the elements of being without excessive burden and offering reasonable hope of benefit are somewhat descriptive. Nevertheless, the differences between the two definitions are sufficiently great to warrant calling them definitions of *different types* of concepts. Thus, the possibility of serious confusion is created when the same word is used to bear such fundamentally different meanings.

In his first article, in discussing the case of a dying patient whose life can be extended for a few weeks by intravenous feeding, Kelly holds that the issue comes down to the usefulness of the means. "To me, the mere prolonging of life in the given circumstances seems to be relatively useless, and I see no sound reason for saying that the patient is obliged to submit to it."[28] A conscious patient should be allowed to decide for himself. If unconscious, Kelly still says, "I see no reason why even the most delicate professional standard should call for their use. In fact, it seems to me that, apart from very special circumstances, the artificial means not only need not, but should not, be used, once the coma is reasonably diagnosed as terminal."[29]

Kelly cites the positions of two earlier commentators on the case. The original commentator, Joseph P. Donovan, had held that the IV feeding itself involves no moral impossibility and hence should be considered an ordinary means. Stopping IV would, according to Donovan, be a form of mercy killing.[30] On the other hand, Joseph V. Sullivan had held the position that extraordinary means are relative to the patient's condition, and, because IV feeding is an artificial means of prolonging life, one may be more liberal in application of principle.[31] Therefore, Sullivan considers the means to be extraordinary and the physician to be justified in discontinuing the IV.

Kelly's position is to offer a distinction. He is in agreement with Donovan in calling IV an ordinary means, but he says that "one may not immediately conclude that it is obligatory." Rather, Kelly wishes to consider such means ordinary, but useless, artificial means of preserving life and so optional. Thus, Kelly is in practical agreement with Sullivan over the discontinuance of the means, but sides with Donovan on designating the means as ordinary. The strong impression conveyed is that both Sullivan and Donovan are using the concept of *ordinary* which Kelly *later* adopted in his second article. Under his revised conception, Kelly would have agreed with Sullivan *in toto*, calling the means useless, and therefore extraordinary, and therefore optional.

Kelly says that using oxygen or IV feeding merely to sustain life for a while in "hopeless" cases can be called *remedies* "only in the very wide sense that they delay the hour of death." Because they sustain life, they in a sense offer a hope of success. But their expense quickly can mount up. For a combination of reasons, then, the use of artificial means of preserving life for a few days or weeks is optional.

Kelly notes that his principles embody a great deal of imprecision:

> There are degrees of "success." It is one thing to use oxygen to bring a person through a crisis; it is another thing to use it merely to prolong life when hope of recovery is practically negligible. There are also degrees of "hope," even when it concerns complete recovery. For example, in one case the use of oxygen to bring a

patient through a pneumonia crisis may offer very high hope, whereas in another case the physical condition of the patient may be such that there is only a slim chance of bringing him through the crisis. Finally, there are degrees of difficulty in obtaining and using ordinary means. Some are inexpensive and very easy to obtain and use; others may involve much more difficulty, though not moral impossibility.[32]

All of these features add considerably to the practical difficulties encountered in deciding about concrete cases. But they do not necessarily create theoretical problems of understanding.

Daniel A. Cronin (1927-   )

The most complete work on the history of the ordinary/extraordinary means distinction is Daniel A. Cronin's doctoral dissertation (1958) from the Gregorian Pontifical University in Rome: *The Moral Law in Regard to the Ordinary and Extraordinary Means of Conserving Life*. The author, now the Most Reverend Daniel A. Cronin, S.T.D., Bishop of Fall River, Massachusetts, presents a study of the views of fifty or more moral theologians from Thomas Acquinas to the early 1950's, followed by his own recommendations. His position is presented here in two sections.

A. THE ORDINARY/EXTRAORDINARY MEANS DISTINCTION

Following his discussion of the views of individual authors, Cronin attempts to summarize and categorize their positions by listing various features commonly cited as grounding the distinction between obligatory and optional means.[33] None of these features is employed by every author Cronin cites, but each of the features is employed by enough of the authors to justify calling it an important aspect of the distinction as it has been drawn historically.

Concerning the concept of *ordinary* (obligatory) means, Cronin mentions four commonly cited features:

(1) *hope of a beneficial result (spes salutis)*: even natural means, such as the taking of food or drink, can become optional if this element is not present. Cronin sees this feature as relative to the condition of the patient, so that no means can be said to be absolutely obligatory regardless of the patient's own status;

(2) *commonly used (media communia)*: Cronin sees this notion of what is in common use as basic. "For the moralists, the duty of conserving one's life does not demand a diligence or a solicitude that exceeds the usual care that most men normally give their lives."[34]

(3) *comparison with one's social position (secundum proportionem status)*: This feature serves to emphasize even further the relative feature of what is obligatory. Cronin sees this idea as connected with the idea of commonly used means and also with the feature of cost;

(4) *not difficult to obtain and employ (medicina non difficilia)*: this feature is alternatively phrased positively as "convenient" means, though Cronin notes that most moralists prefer using the negative expression. The difficulty in question must be *excessive*, and, once again, this can be determined only as relative to the patient's own condition.

In addition to characterizing ordinary means, the moralists have also used terms to refer to means held to be extraordinary and therefore as optional. Cronin lists five of these commonly used phrases:

(1) *impossibility (quaedam impossibilitas)*: this feature refers to the element of *moral* as opposed to *physical* impossibility. We may characterize the morally impossible as what one cannot be reasonably expected to do. Again, this feature is relative to the condition of the patient;

(2) *great effort (summus labor, media nimis dura)*: such a quality can encompass even the taking of food;

(3) *pain (quidam cruciatus, ingens dolor)*: Cronin maintains that this should also be understood as relative to the patient's condition;

(4) *expense (sumptus extraordinarius, media pretiosa, media exquisita)*: again, relative to the condition of the patient, though some authors, as we have noted, would permit some appeal to an absolute standard of expense beyond which no one need go;

(5) *intense emotion (vehemens horror):* fear and repugnance are the two emotions commonly appealed to. This feature is closely related to the first as creating a moral impossibility, and, like the first, is also a relative norm.

Turning from the more historical dimensions of his study, Cronin examines the views of Gerald Kelly. Cronin is generally favorable toward Kelly's definitions of *ordinary* and *extraordinary* quoted above.

Cronin's definitions may be understood simply as clarifications of Kelly's:

> *Ordinary means of conserving life* are those means commonly used in given circumstances, which this individual in his present physical, psychological and economic condition can reasonably employ with definite hope of proportionate benefit.

> *Extraordinary means of conserving life* are those means not commonly used in given circumstances, or those means in common use which this individual in his present physical, psychological condition cannot reasonably employ, or if he can, will not give him definite hope of proportionate benefit.[35]

Cronin's definitions provide *two* standards, one absolute and one relative. If a means is not ordinarily or customarily used, then *no one* has an obligation to employ it (in the absence of exceptional features). This is an absolute standard. The relative standard enters when a means is customarily employed, but would be unreasonable for that particular patient. Cronin's definitions are unclear, though, about the extent to which the individual's own (social or economic) status determines what is to be considered to be customary or ordinary.

It also should be pointed out that, at least with regard to the relative standard, the burden of the definition is carried by the term *reasonably*. Also, Cronin's definitions are like Kelly's second pair of definitions in being *normative* or *evaluative* rather than primarily *descriptive*. To call a means "ordinary" in Cronin's sense is not simply to describe how frequently it is used, but is also to call that means obligatory. This is also true of Cronin's definition of *extraordinary*: to characterize a means as extraordinary is also (special circumstances apart) to regard it as morally optional.

B. SPECIAL OBLIGATIONS OF PHYSICIANS

With regard to the special obligations of physicians, Cronin maintains that the physician has the obligation of using ordinary means of conserving life when treating the patient, and that, if the patient chooses to employ extraordinary means, the doctor has no choice but to follow his wishes. "In the last analysis, it is the patient who has the right to say whether or not he intends to use the extraordinary means of conserving life."[36] This position, like Kelly's, skirts the question

112

of what the physician ought to do if the patient refuses ordinary (morally obligatory) means.

Cronin discusses a number of specific cases which permit him to illustrate principles regarding the special responsibilities of the physician. Cronin's views are consistently patient-centered. A few of the rules he proposes as guides for the physician are:

(1) if it is unknown what means a patient would wish employed, the doctor's duty does not extend to the use of extraordinary means, even if these would benefit the patient. "We are not bound in charity to force a neighbor to save his life by means which he, personally, is not bound to use to save his own life."[37]

(2) if the patient's actual wishes cannot be ascertained, the physician should make a reasonable effort to determine what the patient *would* wish, *were* he able to respond;

(3) if relatives are present when the patient's wishes cannot be ascertained, then they should try to make the decision for the patient and the doctor should follow their wishes;

(4) if no relatives or friends or guardians are present, then the doctor should decide on the basis of what he believes to be the greater good of the patient;

(5) the physician's prime duty is to the patient and not the medical profession. The doctor should never judge that an unconscious or mentally incompetent patient or a patient receiving charity should be given extraordinary means merely for the advancement of scientific knowledge or because he believes that the professional ideal requires fighting death to the bitter end. Surreptitious experimentation carried on without informed consent by the use of extraordinary means is wrong. If the common good does not oblige the patient to use extraordinary means, that good cannot oblige the physician either.[38]

Cronin writes:

In practice, therefore, a doctor should take his norm from the obligation of the patient himself. The doctor must employ the ordinary means of conserving life and then those extraordinary means which, *per accidens*, are obligatory for the patient or which the patient wants to use. He must never practice euthanasia and he must conscientiously strive never to give the impression of using euthanasia. Furthermore, he must strive to find a remedy for the disease. However, when the time comes that he can conserve his patient's life only by extraordinary means, he must consider the patient's wishes, expressed or reasonably interpreted, and abide by them. If the patient is incurable and even ordinary means, according to the *general norm*, have become extraordinary for this patient, again the wishes of the patient expressed or reasonably interpreted must be considered and obeyed.[39]

The foregoing represents not only a summary of Cronin's views but a remarkable recapitulation of the ideas that derive from a study of the historical development of the concept of obligatory and optional means of preserving life. That development, given its history of some five hundred years, is surprisingly consistent.[40] There are indeed differing emphases, and individual authors may disagree on specific points. But the overall appearance is one of uniformity and at times almost one of tedious repetition. No doubt changing circumstances require applications in novel areas, but the basic principles have been firmly laid in a coherent development stretching back at least to the time of Aquinas.

Notes

1. *The Pope Speaks*, 4 (1958), 393-98.
2. St. Thomas Aquinas, *Super Epistolas S. Pauli* (Taurini-Romæ, Marietti, 1953), II Thess., Lec. II, n. 77. Translation in: Cronin, Daniel, *The Moral Law in Regard to the Ordinary and Extraordinary Means of Conserving Life*, (Dissertatio ad Lauream in Facultate Theologica Pontificiae Universitatis Gregorianae, Romæ, 1958) p. 48.
3. *Summa Theologica*, Blackfriars Translation, Anthony Ross, O.P., and P. G. Walsh. (New York, McGraw-Hill Book Co., 1966), II, II, q. 126, a. 1.
4. *ibid.* ad. 3.
5. For example, for the teaching of Thomas Aquinas on suicide, see II,II, q. 64, a. 5; for his teaching on killing the innocent: II,II, q. 64, a. 6; on self-defense: II,II, q. 64, a. 7 and 8; on mutilation: II,II, q. 65, a. 1.
6. F. Vitoria, *Relectiones Theologicae*, (Lugduni, 1587), Relectio IX, de Temp. n. 1, (Transl. as in Cronin, *op. cit.*, pp. 48-49).
7. *ibid.*, n. 9 (Cronin, p. 49).
8. *ibid.*, n. 12 (Cronin, p. 49).
9. F. Vitoria, *Comentarios a la Secunda Secundae de Santo Tomás* (Salamanca, ed. de Heredia, O.P., 1952) in II,II, q. 147, a. 1 (Transl. as in Cronin, p. 50).
10. F. Vitoria, *Relectiones*, Relectio X, de Homicidio, n. 35, (Transl. as in Cronin, p. 50).
11. Cronin, *op. cit.*, p. 90.
12. J. de Lugo, *Disputationes Scholasticae et Morales* (ed. nova, Parisiis, Vivès, 1868-69), Vol. VI, *De Iustitia et Iure*, Disp. X, Sec. 1, n. 21, (Transl. as in Cronin, p. 59).
13. *Ibid.*, n. 32, 36.
14. *Ibid.*, n. 30, (Transl. as in Cronin, p. 64).
15. Cronin, *op. cit.*, p. 70.
16. V. Patuzzi, *Ethica Christiana sive Theologia Moralis*, (Bassani, 1770), Tom. III, Tract. V, Pars. V, Cap. X, Consect. sept.

17. Cronin, *op. cit.*, p. 77.

18. H. Noldin and A. Schmitt, *Summa Theologiae Moralis*, 3 Vols., (Oeniponte, Rauch, 1940-41), Vol. 2, p. 308.

19. E. Genicot and J. Salsmans, *Institutiones Theologiae Moralis*, 2 Vols., (Bruxelles, L'Edition Universelle, S.A., ed. 17, 1951), Vol. 1, n. 364.

20. H. Jone and U. Adelman, *Moral Theology* (Westminster: Newman Press, 1948), n. 210.

21. E. Healy, *Moral Guidance*, (Chicago: Loyola University Press, 1942), p. 162.

22. G. Kelly, "The Duty of Using Artificial Means of Preserving Life," *Theological Studies*, XI (1950), pp. 203-220.

23. G. Kelly, "The Duty to Preserve Life," *Theological Studies*, XII (1951), pp. 550-556.

24. Kelly, "Artificial," p. 204.

25. *ibid.*, p. 206.

26. *ibid.*, p. 207-08.

27. Kelly, "Preserve," p. 550.

28. Kelly, "Artificial," p. 219.

29. *ibid.*, p. 220.

30. *Homiletic and Pastoral Review*, XLIX, (1949), p. 904.

31. J. Sullivan, *Catholic Teaching on the Morality of Euthanasia*, (The Catholic University of America Studies in Sacred Theology, Second Series, No. 22, Washington, D.C.: The Catholic University of America Press, 1949) p. 72.

32. Kelly, "Artificial," p. 214.

33. Cronin, *op. cit.*, pp. 98-126.

34. *ibid.*, p. 105.

35. *ibid.*, pp. 127-28.

36. *ibid.*, p. 143.

37. *ibid.*, pp. 145-46.

38. *ibid.*, pp. 155-56.

39. *ibid.*, p. 157.

40. This chapter concludes with the work of Gerald Kelly and Daniel Cronin which preceded the allocution of Pope Pius XII mentioned above in note 1. A helpful summary of the theological commentary on that allocution, especially from European theologians, is found in: J. McCartney, "The Development of the Doctrine of Ordinary and Extraordinary Means of Preserving Life in Catholic Moral Theology Before the Karen Quinlan Case," *Linacre Quarterly*, 47 (1980), pp. 215-224.

Chapter 8

Principles for Moral Decisions About Prolonging Life

The Reverend Benedict M. Ashley, O. P., S. T. M.

When to Let Die?

Today the advances in medical technology make it possible to prolong a failing life after the body is no longer able to maintain its own life processes. Sometimes, it is even possible to prolong apparent life in a body which by traditional signs would have been considered a corpse. When are such medical procedures ethically justified? It seems to me that, in addition to the common principles relevant to any moral decision such as the Principle of Double Effect and the Principle of Cooperation, we can formulate four special principles which apply to this kind of problem.

Before developing these principles, it is well to say a word about the nature of "moral principles." Moral problems are practical problems. In practical matters, we should not expect to have the same clear-cut, certain knowledge that we sometimes have in theoretical matters, for example in mathematics or in chemistry. Practical matters involve the choice of an appropriate means to attain a goal already determined on. We usually find that there are several possible means of achieving a given goal, each of which has some advantages and some disadvantages, some benefits and some risks, some "spin-offs" and some undesirable side-effects. Moreover, our goals are not always perfectly clear, but are often clarified in the very process of trying to achieve them. Finally, the means to these goals are *actions* performed in a certain sequence, and each of these actions has to be taken in concrete circumstances which are never twice the same.

For the Christian, the goal of all human activity is union with God for ourselves and for all other human beings; yet this goal is mysterious, and the way to it shares in that mystery. The light of God's Word points to the goal and it sufficiently illumines the path to be taken, yet we have to walk by faith, in "fear and trembling." Consequently, when we speak of moral principles we are not talking about an exact recipe or prescription for living which can be mechanically applied to actual life-decisions, but about general practical truths which, along with the circumstances of a given action, need to be taken into consideration to determine whether that action is a morally appropriate means to the end. This does not mean, however, that these principles are merely "guidelines," because sometimes the honest application of a principle *absolutely* excludes certain possible means as morally wrong. For example, we can never directly kill an innocent human being, even to save the life of another human being dearer to us.

Life is a Divine Investment

The *first* special principle relevant to the prolongation of life is that because human life is not only a gift of God but an investment for which He demands a return (as we see in the Parable of the Talents, Matthew 25:14-30), *each of us must use his or her life to the last breath in such a way as to come ever closer to God* (that is the return of the capital) *and to help our neighbor to do the same* (that is God's interest on his loan). Suicide, therefore, is an act of injustice and ingratitude to God, a failure to appreciate His gift of life and to use it well in His service, a lack of trust that He will enable us to make good use of that gift to the end, even in trouble and anguish.

Such a principle must guide us if our goal is that promised by the

Christian Gospel. Even the secular humanist, however, needs an equivalent principle. If we are not certain of any other life than the one we have, and if that life is ours to dispose of as we will, without taking any Creator into account, all the more necessary is it for us to live that life to the end as best we can. Those humanists who have argued that they have a right to end their own life when they find it no longer worth living are acting inconsistently, since, by trying to control their own death, they are actually surrendering control of what life still remains possible for them. If human control over one's own life is our highest value, then self-destruction is a use of this self control to surrender self-control, to abandon what is most precious.

The Obligation to Live Well

The *second* principle is the *obligation to do whatever is required for the healthy functioning of one's own body,* since without this it is difficult to use the gift of life well. Each of us, individually, has this responsibility for our own health, a responsibility which we can ask others to help us to meet, as when we consult a physician, but which we can never simply turn over to someone else. We cannot say to a physician, "You care for me; you make the decisions about my health." We can use a physician as an instrument of our search for health, but we cannot lay on him the burden of the decisions we ourselves make about our health.

This principle takes on a special form when we come to the situation of patients who have learned that they have a terminal illness, that they have only a short time to live, and that medical science may be able to prolong this dying process for a while but probably cannot arrest it, or restore health. Obviously, in this situation, the problem for the patient becomes, "How can I make the best use of the remaining time and energy allotted to me?" Dying well is really living well with a dying body. Now we all know that we are all terminally ill, all living is dying; but there is certainly a great difference between living with a body which even when sick still retains the power of recovery and living with a body which has lost that capacity and is failing more and more.

Anyone faced with this situation still has a space of life which must be used well. The fear, the pain, the despair of this situation, like those of any part of our life, must be made occasions for creative living. When we have hope, we all find that we can take a lot, and, from that experience of struggle, we grow as persons. Looking back on such times, we would not like to live through them again, but we are proud that we did and usually we are convinced that we are more complete persons spiritually because of our survival. The difference for the terminal patient is that there is no hope.

For the Christian, of course, there is the hope of the resurrection, a hope that for many Christians is very nominal, but it is precisely at this time that this hope can become real. Only then does Christianity take on its full, experiential meaning. We can well think that it was only in His last hours that Jesus Himself in His humanness fully understood the whole truth of the Good News which He had preached. The secular humanist lacks that hope, but there remains for him or her at least this much hope (faint as it seems to the Christian), namely, to complete a well-lived life with courage and realism. In fact, the Christian, seeing a non-believer die this kind of courageous death, can well conclude that hidden in that apparently atheistic courage is actually an instinctive conviction that somehow life has had meaning, a conviction that is an implicit declaration of faith that there must be an unfailing God.

This determination to live out fully what remains of life presents to the patient the question of what kind of medical treatment is appropriate to his or her actual situation. Here it is, I believe, that much confusion has arisen in the medical profession. Physicians have been taught to fight to save a life, and to use whatever means they possess to do it. Consequently, they tend to think that these same means remain appropriate for the patient who is already dying. Actually, the kind of medical procedure appropriate when there remained hope of recovery may cease to have any real purpose when such recovery has become impossible. The patient now has to judge any treatment proposed by the physician by the test of whether, everything considered, this procedure will enable the patient to complete his or her living in the best way possible.

Obviously, patients will still need ordinary nursing treatment to keep them as comfortable as possible. Every other procedure, however, must be evaluated by weighing the benefits against disadvantages as regards the use of what life remains. The patient has got to ask whether it would be better to have eight weeks of life with additional suffering caused by surgery or other procedures intended to prolong life, or to have only four weeks with less pain. A patient has got to decide whether, in order to have greater clarity of mind, he or she is willing to take a certain degree of pain, or whether greater sedation will permit a peace of mind gained at some expense to full awareness, but more helpful in taking his or her last hours in calm resignation. No simple equation of the length of life with the best use of life can be made. Jesus used his life well, but quickly, and so have many other saints. On the other hand, for some a long life, prolonged beyond what seem to some "the years of usefulness," has been full of meaning because it has permitted the acquisition of reflective wisdom, of serene patience, of detachment from what is transient, and of firm trust in what is eternal.

We can sum up this principle by saying that for the terminal patient the question is not "How long can I live?" but "How can I best use the life that remains to me."

Informed Consent

I need not dwell long on the *third* relevant principle, the one which is fundamental in all medical-ethical decisions, namely, *the right and obligation of informed consent.* Because the patient has first responsibility for his or her own body, for the Gift of Life from God, no one else, not even the physician, has a right to do anything to that body without the patient's consent. Moreover, that consent cannot be simply a blank check to the physician, it must remain under the patient's control. The obligation of the physician, therefore, is to do nothing to the patient without first informing the patient of what he thinks should be done, with the significant alternatives (including doing nothing), and the probable risks and benefits of each.

I cannot insist too strongly that the physician has no right to decide for the patient whether or how life is to be prolonged by medical art. The doctor's right and responsibility extends only to informing the patient truthfully about his or her terminal condition and the possible ways in which this can be handled medically. The choice among these is the patient's, although this choice cannot be made prudently without honest and substantially complete medical information; yet it cannot be done on this information alone. Many factors, other than medical ones, are relevant to this decision, and the physician has no special expertise in regard to these.

Acting in Behalf of the Dying

The *fourth* and final principle is that, when the terminal patient is unable to make decisions about what medical procedures proposed by the physician are to be accepted or rejected, *the guardian of the patient (ordinarily the family) must make these decisions primarily in the patient's interest.* Thus, in the famous Karen Quinlan case, the primary consideration should always have been, "What will be of most benefit to Karen?". I say, however, "the primary consideration," because it would be inhuman and unreasonable to demand of the guardians that they totally ignore their own personal concerns in the matter. Obviously, those acting in behalf of a patient are also making sacrifices of time, emotional strain, and money. Such sacrifices have reasonable limits. Consequently, it is by no means wrong for the family of a dying patient faced with the prospects of a prolongation of life by an expensive medical procedure to take this also into consideration in deciding whether such expenditures are proportionate to the benefit the patient will receive. Indeed, this is not contrary to the reasonable interests of the patient who would hardly wish his or her family to be uselessly burdened. Every good family attempts to consider the interests of every member, but, in the effort to do this, fairness demands that the resources of the family be shared by all and not exhausted on a single member.

The importance of this principle becomes evident when we note how often the decision over whether to terminate special treatment of the terminally ill is not worked out in terms of benefit to the patient, but of benefit to the family or the physician. The real source of tension is often the family's effort to avoid the burden of decision, or their fear of guilt feelings, i.e., for the sake of their own emotional comfort. At other times, it is the physician's similar worries, along with his willingness to admit what appears to him to be a professional defeat. Rather, physicians should realize that the skillful medical care of the dying patient is a great part of their art, which in no way is measured by whether the patient dies or not, but by how well they die. A good physician is not one who always cures or saves life, but one who does what is appropriate, given the state of the art.

Application of the Principles

I now turn to describe the application of these principles in terms of the questions which a physician should put to himself in dealing with the terminally ill patient.

1). The first question, of course, is whether to inform the terminally ill patient, or, if the patient is no longer competent to understand, the family. Some physicians still hesitate to tell the patient, usually on the grounds that this will risk a shock which will further aggravate the patient's condition. Sometimes it is also argued that a patient does not really want to know. These "reasons" are more evasions of an unpleasant duty than a real concern for the patient.

The principle of informed consent requires that the patient be told, and be helped to face the reality of his or her situation. It is almost impossible to hide the truth from a dying patient whose fear and depression is greatly increased by the inability to discuss the matter openly. Those patients who "don't want to know" will probably continue to deny the facts even after they are told. The physician is not responsible for what the patient does with the information given him, but the physician is responsible to give that information honestly.

Naturally, it is very important *how* this information is given. In order to give it as compassionately and as understandably as possible, the physician may briefly postpone doing so until an opportune time, and he may even delegate this to a member of the family, a minister or even a nurse. Such delegation, however, should be an exception. Ordinarily, it is the physician who is in the best position to explain the whole truth of the matter in a way which the patient can receive with confidence.

2) The next question the physician must ask is how to inform the patient of the possible alternative ways of treating the patient during the dying process. If it is probable, as in cardiac cases, that the patient may have episodes of heart failure, the patient should be asked if he or she wishes to be resuscitated. If surgery or other painful or exhausting procedures are possible as a way of prolonging life, the relative risks and benefits of these should be explained. If it seems probable that the patient will become irreversibly comatose, then the patient should be asked for his or her consent to terminate the use of the respirator or intravenous injections when the physician no longer sees any benefit in such procedures. It should be explained that one possibility is simple "routine terminal care," i.e., keeping the patient as comfortable as possible without any attempt to prolong life.

3) The patient's worries about pain should be discussed and the physician should assure the patient that narcotics will be used at the patient's request without concern about addiction, short of direct killing. If a patient should request "mercy-killing", the doctor should firmly refuse, but assure the patient of constant care to make dying as easy a process as possible and should seek psychiatric and pastoral

assistance for the patient. In my opinion, the physician, by giving the patient an active part in determining the way in which the dying process will be managed medically, will greatly help the patient to use this time well and without unnecessary fears or a sense of utter helplessness.

4) In a very large part of all cases, however, the dying patient is *not fully competent*. The physician then must deal with the family. Here, it is extremely important that, in explaining the patient's condition and the decisions which have to be made, the physician puts the matter in the correct light. Too often, a family has been confronted with what appears to be the burden of deciding whether to "pull the plug" or not, i.e., to kill the one they love. As we have seen, this is not at all the decision that has to be made. What the physician needs to say is something like this: "We have been using the respirator with Karen in hopes that she would be able to respond, but we are convinced now that this is not helping, and it is only prolonging the inevitable. Since it is not helping, we are going to discontinue it and allow her to go peacefully, if you have no objections." Many families faced with this will be resigned. Those who say, "But isn't there anything more you can do?", should be told that there is nothing that will really be of benefit to Karen. Those who say, "I won't consent to stopping the respirator" should be told, "All right, we will continue it a little longer to see what happens, but then we will probably have to ask you again." Probably, when asked a second or third time, the family will have reconciled itself to the inevitable. In extreme cases, where the family insists on procedures which the physician believes are quite unreasonable, he retains the right to withdraw from the case.

To return to our first principle, we must all help one another in the process of living this earthly life, even living it to its very end. The really tragic dying is to die alone in the midst of a crowd of people who, because they themselves fear death, withdraw their personal presence when it is most needed. Even of Jesus dying it is written,

> Near the cross . . . there stood his mother, his mother's sister,
> Mary the wife of Clopas, and Mary Magdalene. (John 19:25)

Chapter 9

Prolonging Life: The Duty and its Limits

The Reverend John Connery, S.J., S.T.D.

The moral responsibility related to the question of prolonging life is frequently discussed today in terms of a so-called right-to-die. Since death is generally considered undesirable, those taking the rights approach find themselves in the curious position of defending a right to something people ordinarily try to avoid. They feel that they are justified because although death may be an evil, it is not the only evil, nor even the worst evil that can befall the human race, and hence can be desirable, at least as a lesser evil. It also comes to everyone, and so, seems to be something one can lay claim to as a right.

There is no inherent reason why rights language cannot be applied to morality or moral responsibility, since much of it is related to rights. But it seems more basic to speak in this area in terms of an obligation to life. At least this obligation should be explored first, since if it does exist, it would rule out, at least to the extent that it does, any right to die. Actually, it has been more in terms of an obligation to prolong life or preserve life that theologians have discussed this question since the fifteenth century.[1]

Treatises on moral theology discuss the duty to prolong life in the context of violations of human life, homicide and suicide, i.e., in the treatise *De homicidio*. They have generally held that respect for human life as a basic good demanded that no one deliberately destroy innocent human life, either his own or that of another.[2] On this score, they would condemn what is called mercy-killing or euthanasia. Even an otherwise good motive, such as mercy, could not justify taking innocent human life. But there was more to this duty. Respect for human life also imposed on everyone a duty to preserve his or her life. Theologians agreed that this duty extended to the ordinary or common means of preserving life, e.g., taking food or drink. Failure here would be tantamount to suicide, at least if it were deliberate or due to neglect. Thus, theologians would condemn even passive euthanasia if it were understood in this sense, i.e., omitting ordinary means to preserve life.[3] But they were also in agreement that, unlike the duty not to take human life, there was a limit to the obligation to preserve or prolong life.

Prolonging Life vs. Determining Death

Before going into this question further, it might be important to distinguish it from a different, though related, question; that of determining the time of death and the moral responsibility related to it. There has been a tendency to confuse these two issues in recent discussions. A number of cases have been discussed in the press in recent times where the issue was whether the person was dead or alive. This is not the issue we are dealing with here. The assumption in the present discussion is that the patient is still alive, and the issue is the obligation to keep him alive. The difference between the two issues can be illustrated by considering a decision whether to keep a patient on a respirator. The first question that might be raised in reference to this decision is whether the person is alive or dead. If he is dead, a decision to turn off the respirator would be proper. The criterion for determining the time of death would be key to this decision. But even if the patient were clearly alive, or even probably alive, the question of turning off the respirator might still be raised. But this time the issue would not be whether the patient is dead or alive, but whether there is a duty to prolong his or her life. The question we are dealing with in this chapter is not whether one may turn off a respirator because the person is dead, but whether one may turn it off even though he is still alive.

Historical Perspective

As already pointed out, theologians have always felt that human beings had some obligation to preserve life. At the same time, however, they maintained that this obligation was limited. It was limited, first, by the moral law itself; man would not be allowed to do anything morally wrong even if it was necessary to preserve his life. But there were further limitations on the obligation to preserve life. Even if the use of a particular means would be morally unobjectionable, while it might be used, it was not always of obligation. Antoninus, an early fifteenth century Dominican theologian, discussed the issue indirectly in terms of the obligation to obey a doctor.[4] Since the doctor, as such, has no authority over his patient, Antoninus argued that the patient has no strict obligation to obey him. He added, though, that it might still be imprudent not to obey a doctor, because of his or her expertise. Thus, if a sick person, either deliberately or out of neglect, were to eat or drink something that would cause his death, he would sin seriously. Although the sin might not be one of disobedience, it would be a violation of his obligation to preserve his life. Antoninus goes on to say, although not too clearly, that there is a limit to this obligation. He says explicitly that healthy people are not bound to live *medicinaliter,* since to the healthy all things are healthy.[5] The implication seems to be that healthy people do not have to be scrupulous about their health in their eating and drinking. But he adds that even a healthy person would sin if he deliberately took something harmful to his health. Briefly, what Antoninus seems to be saying is that while one has an obligation to his health, he should nevertheless be reasonable about it.

A successor of Antoninus, another Dominican theologian named Vitoria, also discussed the obligation to preserve life. Continuing what seems to have been the thought of Antoninus, he tells us that one is not obliged to obtain foods which are the best, the most expensive or the most exquisite to preserve life.[6] Neither is one obliged to live in the healthiest climate. By way of illustration, he advises that if a doctor advises a patient to eat chicken or partridge it is sufficient for him to eat eggs or other common dishes.[7] Apparently, chicken was a scarce item in those days and not easily available. At any rate, such advice would not be pertinent today since chicken would no longer be classified as a

126

delicacy or a rarity. Vitoria also discusses briefly the obligation to take medicine. He says that those who refuse to take medicine are not to be condemned since one can rarely be certain that it will work.[8] But if one is certain that a drug will save his life, he will sin mortally by not taking it. Even an effective drug, however, will not be obligatory if one has to continue to take it over a long period of time. Again, Vitoria clearly sets a limit to the duty to preserve life.

The first theologian to take up the question of surgery was Domingo Soto, a Dominican of the sixteenth century.[9] The problem he is discussing is the duty to undergo amputation of an arm or leg to preserve life. His answer is that no one could force a patient to undergo such torture. He is speaking, of course, at a time when anesthesia was not available. Again, one would not make the same judgment today, at least where anesthesia is available.

Ordinary/Extraordinary Means

Seventeenth century theologians formulated the principle dealing with the duty to preserve life in terms of a distinction between *ordinary* or *common* and *extraordinary* means.[10] According to this distinction, one would be obliged to use *ordinary* means to preserve life but, generally, would not be obliged to use *extraordinary* means. The distinction was based on the burden the use of some particular means would place on the patient (or others). If the burden was excessive, too heavy for the patient to carry, the means would be considered *extraordinary*, and therefore not obligatory. The general norm for gauging the burden would be the common reaction, although the sensitivities of the individual would also be taken into account. Thus, the embarrassment a particular woman might experience at the prospect of being examined by a male doctor might make such an examination an extraordinary means. In assessing a particular means, it made no difference whether the burden to the patient was experienced before, during or after the use of the means. Finally, the burden might take the form of great pain, physical or mental hardship, danger or even expense.

Some today are rather reluctant to accept great expense as a limitation on the duty to prolong life. To them, health is too important to be put in terms of financial investment. There is something to be said for this stand, but one must remember that what is sacrificed is not simply a certain amount of money but other things that money could buy, e.g., education, that may also be very important. Or one might be incurring crippling debts that could make life very difficult for a whole family.

We should point out at this juncture that the distinction between ordinary and extraordinary means which the theologian uses may not coincide with that used by the physician. To the physician, *ordinary* means may be *routine* means; whatever procedure is *customary* or *usual* in a particular case is considered ordinary. It is the *relation* of the means *to medical practice* that makes it ordinary; it has nothing to do with the *burden* placed on the patient . . . which is the interest of the theologian. It might well be that the two concepts would overlap in a particular case, so that a treatment that was routine from the viewpoint of the medical practice would be ordinary from the moral standpoint, at least in the sense that it was not difficult to get. But they are not co-extensive. A procedure that might be ordinary or routine, medically speaking, could be extraordinary by reason of the burden it places on the patient. An example of this might be the treatment for kidney failure called hemodialysis. The medical profession would consider this ordinary or standard treatment for kidney failure. And it might be ordinary treatment, even from the moral viewpoint, for temporary kidney failure. But if the kidneys are shut down permanently, hemodialysis can easily become too burdensome to a patient, particularly if he or she is elderly. In a counseling relationship, one might urge such a patient to put up with the burden for the benefit of prolonging life. But he or she could not impose a moral obligation on anyone to carry an excessively heavy burden. This case should make it clear that the theological distinction must not be confused with the medical distinction. Not all standard medical procedures are obligatory.

It might be appropriate at this time to point out that the reason underlying the moral distinction between ordinary and extraordinary means reinforces the position that the decision regarding the use of such means belongs to the patient rather than the doctor.[11] Only the patient can gauge the burden he experiences and judge whether it is too much for him. The doctor can acquaint him with the medical facts, but he can go no further.

Useful/Useless Means

Traditionally, the use of the distinction between ordinary and extraordinary means was not limited to terminal cases. Even if the use of a particular means, e.g., amputation, hemodialysis, etc., would

128

prolong life indefinitely, if it imposed too much of a burden on the patient, it would not be obligatory. So the decisive factor was not whether the treatment would benefit the patient or how long, but whether it imposed more of a burden than he could carry. Theologians, however, did use another distinction in dealing with the duty to preserve life and placed a limitation even on the obligation to use ordinary means. This distinction centered around the possible benefit to the patient. If there was little or no possibility that a treatment would benefit a patient, he or she would not be obliged to use it. The principle was a general one: *nemo tenetur ad inutile* (no one is bound to do something useless), but here it was being applied to the duty to preserve life. Judging from examples given, one can conclude also that theologians were speaking of terminal cases. If a person was dying and there was no real hope that the use of a particular means would prolong his or her life, except perhaps minimally, it would be considered useless, and hence not obligatory, even if it were otherwise ordinary. A seventeenth-century theologian exemplified· this point by the case of a person starving to death who had only one meal available. Since one meal would not make an appreciable difference in delaying death, it could not be considered obligatory. This limitation on the obligation to use ordinary means is especially important today in terminal cases, where death is imminent whether such means are used or not, e.g., in the use of such life-sustaining treatment as oxygen, intravenous feeding, blood transfusions, etc.

Many theologians today classify means that do not appreciably prolong life as extraordinary. Thus, they define as extraordinary means those that are excessively burdensome or offer no reasonable hope of benefit. My own preference is to keep benefit separate from burden. They are different issues, and usually apply to different kinds of cases. The question of benefit is raised largely in terminal cases; burden can be an issue even in non-terminal cases.[12]

Burden Variable

Whether medical procedures or treatments will be classified as ordinary or extraordinary, even from the theological viewpoint, will vary according to time and place. As was already pointed out, simple amputations were considered extraordinary means in the sixteenth century because of the pain involved. Where anesthesia is available, however, surgery would not be considered extraordinary, at least not because of the pain involved. Similarly, such procedures as giving oxygen, IV feeding, and blood transfusions, might have been considered extraordinary means fifty or a hundred years ago. Today they could hardly be considered such, except perhaps where they are not easily available. Finally, although procedures of this kind would generally not be classified as extraordinary means today if needed on a short term basis, e.g., to pull a patient through a crisis, long term use could make them such, e.g., long term use of an artificial respirator. As mentioned above, in terminal cases they might also be useless means.

Declaration on Euthanasia

The recent declaration on euthanasia by the Sacred Congregation for the Doctrine of the Faith confirmed the above tradition.[13] While recognizing the difficulties already mentioned with the use of the terms ordinary and extraordinary means, it reaffirmed the underlying principle. More specifically, it stated that it is always permissible to be contented with the common treatment which medicine has to offer. No one, therefore, can impose an obligation to use a remedy which, even though it may be in use, is either dangerous or too burdensome. Refusal of such treatments cannot be compared to suicide. It is rather the acceptance of the human condition, or a desire to avoid complicated medical treatment offering no proportionate benefit, or the intention of not imposing too great a burden on the family or community. Where death is imminent and inevitable, it is permissible to forego treatments that would only provide a precarious and painful prolongation of life, as long as the normal care due to the sick person in similar cases is not interrupted.

Right of the Patient to Decision

The obligation to preserve or prolong life belongs to the person himself. This is also true of the option to use extraordinary means; it is up to each person to decide whether to use or forego the use of such means. This offers no problem when the individual is acting independently, but if he or she is in a patient-doctor relationship, a conflict can arise. The doctor may want to use means that go beyond the obligation and the wishes of the patient. Even in this relationship, the decision belongs to and should remain with the patient. In a well-known talk given to a group of anesthesiologists in Rome (1957), Pius

XII stated that the doctor has only those rights over the patient which the latter gives him. If the patient, therefore, decides not to use extraordinary means, the doctor has no right to impose them on him, and if he does so, he is violating that patient's rights. (See Chapter 6 above.)

Once the principle is set down, it must be admitted that it is not always easy to determine the real wishes of the patient in this regard, especially in difficult situations. If a person is in great pain, a refusal of treatment may be more a reaction to this pain than a reflection of his wishes regarding life. It may be very difficult for a doctor in such cases to interpret properly the real wishes of the patient. It seems obvious that mistakes cannot be entirely eliminated in such interpretations; the most one can hope for is to keep them to a minimum. What is essential, however, is for doctors to keep in mind that the decision to use or forego extraordinary means is not their own; it must always be a justifiable interpretation of the real wishes of the patient.

Proxy Decisions

If the patient is comatose, or otherwise incompetent, it is up to a responsible relative to make the decision for him. A proxy decision of this kind is really the only way a patient who is not competent can exercise his right either to ask for extraordinary means or to forego them. The obligation of the proxy, then, is to make the decision the patient would make if he or she were able. What must be kept in mind is that the proxy does not have the freedom the patient himself has regarding the use of extraordinary means. His or her obligation is not determined by the distinction between ordinary and extraordinary means but by the wishes of the patient.[14] If the proxy were to decide against extraordinary means in a situation where the patient would want them, he would be doing wrong. Too often, in recent writing on this subject, authors have assumed that the proxy has the same freedom the patient has to forego extraordinary means.

But if the patient is incompetent, how does a proxy know what his wishes may be? A close relative should be in the best position to have this kind of knowledge. But if he does not, he may have to hazard a judgment based on the patient's *best interests*. Since one can legitimately presume that a competent patient would want what is in his best interests, a proxy will have good reason to believe that a decision made on that basis would accord with the wishes of his charge. To find out, in a particular case, what would be in the best interests of an incompetent patient, one may have to have recourse to decisions made by competent persons in parallel or comparable situations. If competent patients generally consent to certain means in spite of the hardships involved, a proxy has good reason to judge that the use of such means is also in the best interests of an incompetent patient, and that he would make a similar decision if he were able.

Quality of Life Considerations and Extraordinary Means

What if a patient is not only incompetent but also handicapped in some way, e.g., seriously defective or retarded? This is often referred to today as a *quality of life* consideration, and the question is whether it may be a legitimate factor in a proxy decision about the use of extraordinary means. I think a proxy could be justifiably influenced in his decision by a patient's handicap if it would make the use of the means considerably more difficult, or even more so, if it made their use ineffective. One can presume that the patient would have done this himself or herself, if competent.

The recent Spring case is a good example of how a handicap can add to the burden of treatment.[15] The inability of the patient, because of his senility, to understand what was going on made the hemodialysis treatment very trying, even resulting in violent reactions on his part. It is understandable that a proxy might not give consent to treatment in these circumstances even though the ordinary patient would generally consent to it. But there is no inherent reason why handicaps as such should make all treatment more difficult or ineffective. For instance, open heart surgery may not be any more difficult for a handicapped child than for a normal one. So one could not justify proxy decisions to forego extraordinary means based on the judgment that these means always impose a significantly greater burden on the handicapped person than on the normal person. And even in those cases where an additional burden is clearly present, the reason for the proxy decision to forego extraordinary means is not the burden as such but the interpreted wishes of the patient.

But what if the handicapped condition of the patient does not affect the use of the means? Could it still be taken into consideration in a proxy decision to refuse extraordinary means? Clearly, if a handicapped person were making the decision himself, he could legitimately forego extraordinary means, and the decisive factor might be his handicap. As to what actually happens, I am not sure that we have any decisive statistics. In other words, whether handicapped people forego extraordinary means more frequently than normal people may not be known. But I would be quite sure that handicapped people do not always turn down extraordinary means. So it would certainly not be legitimate for a proxy to turn down extraordinary means automatically because the person is handicapped.

Quality of Life and Ordinary Means

A more controversial question is raised today about the morality of *quality of life* considerations when the means in question are ordinary.[16] Some would ask further whether such considerations would justify even taking positive measures to end life.[17] The argument is that the duty to life should be related to the *quality of life* one is leading and that in some cases the *quality of life* can be so low as to remove any duty to preserve it. This question should not be confused with a different one that is not at all controversial. Theologians have traditionally allowed quality of life considerations in decisions about prolonging life if they were related to the means themselves. Thus, if a particular means, e.g., an amputation, would cause a drastic alteration of one's lifestyle, it might not be obligatory. Such a means would be classified as extraordinary because of the permanent handicap it would cause. In the controversial question we are dealing with, the handicap is not related to the means and the latter in themselves would have to be considered ordinary, e.g., the case of the mongoloid child in need of simple surgery. The question is whether the handicap in itself will affect the duty to preserve life.

The question could be relevant even to handicapped people who are competent. In practice, however, the controversy focuses largely on incompetent patients and proxy decisions. This may be due to the fact that some of the most difficult cases, e.g., persistent vegetative states, seriously defective infants, etc., necessarily involve proxy decisions. But the situation of the proxy differs in this case from the case we dealt with previously. Where the use of the means is optional, the wishes of the patient are the decisive factor, and the decision may go either way. But if the use of the means is obligatory, neither the patient nor his proxy have a choice. The proxy must either assume that his patient would not want to do anything immoral, or if he judges otherwise, he must dissociate himself from such a decision. But the moral question must be settled before he can make a decision.

Theologians, in the past, have not allowed quality of life considerations in themselves to interfere with the duty to life. The presence of a handicap would not justify either taking a life or neglecting ordinary means to preserve it. Either would be tantamount to suicide. This raises an immediate question: Why are quality of life considerations allowed if they are related to the use of the means and not apart from such a relationship? The basic difference would seem to be that in the one case the person is bringing the hardship on himself. When a person is afflicted with some handicap through no act or fault of his own, he certainly deserves sympathy, but he does not bring the handicap on himself. It is because a moral choice is involved in decisions regarding means to prolong life that related burdens become pertinent. There is a limit to the amount of burden you can reasonably expect a person to choose for himself. So there is a limit to the obligation you can put on a person in this regard. If one imposes an obligation that goes beyond that limit, he or she is obliging that person to more than he may be capable of.

So the difference between quality-of-life considerations related to means of prolonging life and those that are not is that, in the former, one who chooses the means in question brings the hardship on himself. While one should be free to do this, he should not be obliged to do so. Such choices are governed by the traditional distinction between ordinary/extraordinary means. But handicaps, in themselves, have never been considered reasons either for taking a life or neglecting ordinary means that would effectively preserve it. A proxy decision would have to be made within this framework.

Authority of Parents

Perhaps it should be mentioned, at this point, that parents do not have any special authority over their children in this regard by reason of their special relationship. They have no rights as parents to determine the life span of their children. As proxies, they are merely doing what any other proxy is obliged to do. They are exercising a right which belongs to the child himself. We are making this point precisely because the court in one of our states recently gave the impression that parents have the right to determine for the child whether or not he or she should get extraordinary means.[18] Certainly, the parents are the ones responsible for the child and have the right and duty to act as proxies. It would be wrong for the state to arrogate this right, except when necessary to prevent abuse. But the right and duty in question is the right to act as proxy, not a parental right to determine a child's lifespan.

Duty to Provide Means to Prolong Life

It is one thing to discuss the obligation of a patient to use means to prolong life (or the obligation of a proxy to make such a decision for the patient). It is quite another to discuss the obligation of others to *provide* such means to a patient. Again, recent writing on this subject has oversimplified this obligation by reducing it to the distinction between providing ordinary and extraordinary means. The impression is left that the obligation to provide means, like the obligation to use means, depends on the nature of the means: if the means are ordinary, there is an obligation to provide them; if they are extraordinary, there is no obligation. The obligation to provide means is much more nuanced than that. The nature of this obligation will differ according to the relation of the person providing the means to the patient. If that person is the patient's physician, he will have an obligation in justice to supply whatever means the patient reasonably requests. Because of their special relationship, parents will also have a special obligation to provide for the needs of their children. Others will have an obligation in charity to provide means to preserve life if the patient is in need of their help. Although these obligations are graded according to the relationship with the patient, none of them are absolute. In determining the limits of the obligation, another factor must be taken into consideration: the hardship to the donor or provider. No one, for instance, would be obliged to sacrifice his life to supply a patient's need. If someone were drowning and an attempt to save him would involve serious risk to my own life, while it might be a heroic thing to do, I would not be obliged to risk my life to save him. This would be true even of providing ordinary means.

I would not be obliged to give food necessary to preserve my own life to a starving man, although food is generally classified as ordinary means. On the other hand, if a patient wishes extraordinary means and cannot supply them otherwise, even a stranger might have an obligation to provide them if he could do so without serious hardship. And the obligation of the parent or doctor would be even more binding. So the obligation to provide means necessary to preserve life cannot be reduced

135

to the distinction between ordinary and extraordinary means. It is determined by the wishes of the patient, his relationship with the provider and the ability of the latter to relieve the patient's need without serious hardship.

A further question must be raised regarding the obligation to provide means to preserve the life of another. Does it cease apart from serious hardship to the provider? The assumption is that ordinary means are needed or that extraordinary means have been requested by the patient or his proxy. Could a person who might easily provide such means legitimately refuse to do so? It would certainly be wrong to refuse to give help if refusal involved discrimination. Thus, if a man was drowning and I could easily save him, it would be wrong to refuse to do so because he was black. But what if he is defective or handicapped? Again, it would be wrong to refuse help because I did not think him worth saving. This would also be discrimination. But what if I judged that it would not be in the best interests of society, or of his relatives, or even in his own best interests to prolong his life? Theoretically, at least, it would seem that the same degree of hardship that would excuse me from the obligation to provide help would continue to be an excuse even if it fell on someone else. I might refuse help out of concern for that party (relatives or community), claiming that providing help would not be in his or her best interests. But one would have to sort out his motives carefully in such a situation to make sure that a real concern for the others was operative rather than a discriminatory judgment. And the more committed the person might be to the patient (e.g., a physician or close relative), the less understandable would it be to be swayed by concern for others.

As far as the best interests of the patient are concerned, if the patient (or the proxy) wanted the help, one would have to presume that he or she considered it in his or her own best interests. A judgment on the part of the provider that help would not be in the best interests of the patient would then be contradictory. Theoretically, of course, it would be possible for the judgment of the provider to be correct and that of the patient or proxy wrong. But there are obvious hazards involved in making judgments about the best interests of others, especially when providing help is contingent on them. All of which seems to lead to the conclusion that when one can easily provide help to a patient in need, it is generally his or her duty to do so.

136

Other Duties to Dying

It should be noted, at this time, that the obligation to help another, whether of the doctor or the parent, or even of a stranger, goes beyond merely providing means to preserve life. A patient will have other needs, and these will continue to call for help even when the obligation to preserve life ceases. Paul Ramsey calls attention to this fact when he speaks of the obligation of "only caring" for the dying.[19] The only criticism I would have of his treatment is that one easily gets the impression from it that this latter obligation begins when the obligation to preserve life ceases. Actually, the obligation to help others in need is a general obligation that extends through life. A person may have many needs throughout his lifetime for which he himself cannot provide. The obligation of charity extends to any need the person himself cannot relieve. It continues even after the obligation to preserve life and the need for assistance in this regard has ceased.

One does not simply wheel a patient, at either end of life, into a corner and leave him there because it has been decided that the obligation to preserve his or her life has ceased. He is still a human being made in the image and likeness of God. He has a unique dignity, then, which must be respected. Those responsible for him must, out of respect for this dignity, keep him clean, comfortable and as free from symptoms that cause distress as is reasonable to expect. As long as he is alive (and even after), the obligation to charity will continue to call for relief of whatever other needs he or she may still have.

Conclusion

It would be impossible, in this chapter, to go into all the nuances of the obligation to provide help to people in dying situations. The purpose here has been chiefly to introduce the distinctions that should be made between the obligation of a person faced with a decision about prolonging life, the obligation of a proxy who has to make a decision for an incompetent, and that of a person whose help is needed to save another person's life. These are all related obligations, but they are also different. It is the judgment of the present writer that in recent writing they have been bunched together without adequate distinction. Each obligation has its own norms, and although they are related to the distinction between ordinary and extraordinary means, they cannot simply be reduced to it.

Notes

1. We are referring to the theologians in the Catholic tradition. It would be impossible and pointless to try to name all of them, however, Chapter 7 above outlined much of their work.

2. Taking life as punishment for certain crimes, although it is now being questioned, has been allowed in the past. Similarly, taking life in self-defense against unjust aggression is permissible. But if one had committed no serious crime and was not engaged in unjust aggression, that is, if he was "innocent", it was never permissible to take his life.

3. Passive euthanasia might include omission of extraordinary means. As will be seen, understood in this sense, it would not be objectionable. But the ambiguity of the term makes it morally unsuitable.

4. Antoninus, *Summa Theologica*, Tom. 3, t. 7, c.2 (Graz: 1959).

5. It would be impossible to translate the meaning of this word simply. It would seem to mean that one does not have to take food as he does medicine or treat it as such.

6. Francisco de la Vitoria, *Reflectiones Theologicae,* IX, De temperantia, n. 12 (Lyons: 1557).

7. Francisco de la Vitoria, *Comentarios a la Secunda Secundae de S. Thoma,* q. 147, a. 1 (Salamanca: 1952).

8. Vitoria, *Reflectiones,* op. cit., De temperantia, n. 1.

9. Domingo Soto, *De Iustitia et Iure,* Lib. 5, q. 2, a. 1 (Venice: 1568).

10. Ioannes De Lugo, *Disputationes Scholasticae,* VI: *De Iustitia et Iure,* Disp. 10, nn. 29-30 (Paris: 1869). In an address given to an International Congress of Anesthesiologists in Rome, Pius XI applied these norms to the question of resuscitation. *See The Pope Speaks,* 4, (1958), pp. 393-98.

11. It will be seen that the basic reason why this decision belongs to the patient is that it is *his* body, and therefore *his* duty or option.

12. Although I think there is good reason for keeping the two notions separate, I do not consider it morally objectionable to combine them.

13. May 5, 1980. See Appendix I.

14. We are speaking here of the legitimate wishes of the patient. A proxy would not, of course, be allowed to cooperate with a patient's desire to forego ordinary means, much less to end his life.

15. In re Earle N. Spring, Commonwealth of Massachusetts (1979-80).

16. Richard A. McCormick, S.J. has suggested that the quality of life can be so low in some cases that the obligation to use ordinary means to sustain it ceases (America, July 13, 1974, pp. 6-10).

17. Daniel Maguire holds that in some cases, it is permissible to choose death, i.e., put an end to life (*Death by Choice,* Garden City, Doubleday, 1974, p. 112).

18. In re Phillip Becker, Cal. Rptr. 48, 1st App. Dist., Div. 4, 1979.

19. *Patient as Person* (Yale University Press, New Haven, 1970).

Chapter 10

Prolonging Life
Conscience Formation

The Reverend Lawrence T. Reilly, S. T. D.

Dying is a time of anxiety. The dying person experiences fear of the unknown, fear of leaving loved ones, fear of pain and fear of isolation. People who were accustomed to being at least in partial control of their own lives suddenly feel helpless and totally dependent on others.

Families, especially parents, children, and spouses, must face the terrible reality that they will have to live without their loved one. They can't imagine what life will be like without the person who has been so central to their lives, so important to them. They, too, experience fear and anxiety. They try to hide their true feelings in an attempt to be loving, supportive, and encouraging. They fear their fear. They cannot share their deep emotions with their dying loved ones.

Nurses, doctors, and other health care workers also fear death. Their professional lives are directed toward cure and restoration of health. Although they discipline themselves to stay calm in the face of death, many experience a sense of helplessness and failure.

This anxiety, fear, and helplessness frustrate efforts to make good decisions about care of dying persons. Although anxiety and fear can seldom be completely overcome, careful formation of conscience can considerably reduce the tension and anxiety that accompany dying. We must prepare for death. We must think about how we intend to live our own dying and how we intend to live through the dying experience of those we love. We must also pray, asking God to guide and help us.

All those who make decisions about care of the dying have a responsibility to form their consciences well in the light of objective moral norms and through reflection on practical situations they will have to meet. Those whose consciences will guide decision-making during the dying process include patients, families, nurses, physicians, chaplains, and administrators. In an analogous sense, the hospital itself also has a conscience which is expressed in its policies and procedures that govern care of the dying and critically ill.

Every human action is influenced by conscience. We have a sense within us that this particular action is best and we do it. Sometimes our consciences are troubled. We're not sure what to do, but we must act now and we act. But our action troubles us because we were not sure; our troubled conscience continues to trouble us. When we do something that is clearly wrong, our consciences reproach us. We're not at peace because our consciences will not leave us rest.

Not all consciences are well-formed. A poorly formed conscience can lead a person to seriously injure himself or others. During a recent television discussion, a Jewish rabbi expressed his dismay at the emphasis placed on the importance of following one's conscience by the priests and ministers who were with him. He said that the Holocaust was a result of "following conscience." The Nazis' consciences permitted them to do anything that they thought necessary for the furtherance of the Aryan race. The rabbi insisted that emphasis on "following one's conscience" should be balanced by equal emphasis on "forming one's conscience properly." The Church insists that we have a serious moral obligation to form our consciences well and to follow our consciences.

The word "conscience" is familiar. It usually refers to the conscience of an individual person. But the word is used in broader senses, too; for example, the conscience of a nation, of a people, of a country, of a Church, etc. The conscience of a hospital refers to the support that a hospital gives to good decision-making. When a hospital is ordered in

140

such a way that it frustrates good decision-making, it does not have a good conscience. When everyone in the hospital is imbued with respect for the personal dignity of each patient, fellow employee, and visitor, and when the hospital's daily life, programs, and policies encourage and support this respect, the hospital has a good conscience.

But conscience remains an ambivalent term. It has been defined and described in many ways. One theologian, Rudolf Hofmann, states:

> In conscience, man has a direct experience in the depths of his personality of the moral quality of a concrete personal decision or act as a call of duty on him, through his awareness of its significance for the ultimate fulfillment of his personal being.[1]

He also says that:

> Conscience brings to mind the objective moral norm in its relation to the concrete decision to be made in the present situation.[2]

The formation of a good conscience depends on instruction, prayer, personal experience, and informed reflection. Three important elements of reflection should be: objective moral norms, concrete situations, and the ultimate fulfillment of personal being.

What are the objective moral norms that must always be considered in care of the critically ill and dying?

1. We must respect life as a gift of God and take reasonable means to protect and preserve it.

2. We must accept death and view it as a transition to the fullness of life in God.

3. We must help one another to live well and to die well.

These three norms are fundamental. They must always be kept in mind by those called upon to make life-prolonging decisions. These norms don't lead to inevitable concrete decisions, but they help decision-makers keep seemingly contradictory values before their minds. The concrete decision must contain a reasonable balance of all the values found in the norms.

The primary decision-maker in life-prolonging decisions is the person whose life is in question. It is not acceptable to say, "I'll do whatever the doctor says. The doctor knows best." The doctor does not know what is best. The doctor's field of competence is limited. A physician must provide as accurate and careful a diagnosis as possible.

He must try to describe the illness or injury in comprehensible language. Then, insofar as his knowledge and experience allow, he must try to describe the progression of the illness and effects of the injury. He then discusses the various forms of treatment that are available. It is the patient who has the moral obligation to choose treatment. The patient should not impose this obligation on the physician.

Unfortunately, many dying patients cannot make decisions or communicate them. Some have lost consciousness; others, though conscious, cannot communicate their desires. Some are so confused that they are incoherent or irrational. Others are so afraid and so ill-prepared for death that they refuse to face reality and refuse the help of those who could assist them in making good decisions.

In these painful situations, the moral obligation and responsibility for decision-making fall on the person or persons who can be presumed to know what the patient would want. This means persons united to the dying person by love or blood, that is, spouse, parent, or child — in that order. When no such person is available, or when such persons seem to be acting in their own interest rather than the patient's best interest, the community assumes responsibility for good decision-making and for acting in the patient's best interest. The community may be represented by the hospital or a judge, depending on the circumstances.

All these persons, patient, family members, health care workers, community representatives, will be able to make good decisions only if they have worked ahead of time at the proper formation of their consciences.

What are some important elements to keep in mind? First and foremost, the sick person is a child of God. He comes from God, is created in God's image, and is called to the fullness of life in God. His life here on earth is a preparation for his risen life in heaven. This life is enriched by relationships of love, relationships with God, with others, with himself and, in a certain sense, with the material world. Human life on earth is meant to support and facilitate relationships of love.

In contemporary health care facilities, highly skilled nurses in intensive care units, cardiac care units, thermal and burn units, oncology units and neonatal units give round-the-clock care to persons whose lives are threatened by disease or injury. The basis for this care is the conviction that life is worth saving, that continued life is a good. In surgeries and emergency rooms, the same conviction supports the use of other specialized skills.

Health care providers are challenged to give as much care, concern, and skill to helping people die well when their lives are ending, as they give to people whose lives can be preserved and restored. This means providing an atmosphere in which a dying person will be physically as comfortable as possible, an atmosphere in which a person can also be comforted mentally, emotionally, and spiritually. Ideally, this comfort will be provided by family and health care professionals (including pastoral care personnel). The purpose of efforts to provide this atmosphere of comfort is to assist the dying person to prepare well to leave this life and to meet God face to face.

Everyone who works in health care knows that there are many situations in which it isn't easy to decide when a person is dying, when death is imminent. Skilled medical and nursing care in America allows people to return to happy, fulfilling lives: people who, in another age or in other places, would certainly have died. Yet death still occurs eventually.

Roman Catholic moral theology insists that all persons have a serious responsibility to take ordinary means to preserve their health and their lives. No one is morally obliged to take extraordinary means. Ordinary means are those which do not place excessive physical, mental, financial, or spiritual burdens on the patient or the patient's family. Extraordinary means are those which do create grave burdens. What is an excessive burden? The answer to that question differs from situation to situation. Although it is difficult, the question can be answered in a satisfactory manner if all persons concerned weigh the facts in a calm and responsible way.

Because the expressions "ordinary means" and "extraordinary means" can be confusing, some theologians and the Sacred Congregation for the Doctrine of Faith also use the expressions, "proportionate means," and "disproportionate means." Father John Connery has frequently spoken of "burden" and "benefit." Does the benefit to the patient justify the burden? Is there a due proportion between the benefit we hope to gain and the burden we have to bear?

It is important to avoid two extreme approaches:

1. Automatically doing everything medical science can do and at any cost.
2. Judging that an individual's life is no longer "worth living" and abandoning the person or directly ending his life.

Neither of these extremes is morally acceptable.

What are some of the situations surrounding death that cause problems of conscience? The most common conflicts of conscience in American health care are centered on the use of drugs, the definition and determination of terminal illness, code-no-code policies, the supportive care concept, the withdrawal of life-sustaining mechanisms, truth-telling, and lack of unanimity among decision-makers and their advisors in crisis situations.

Sometimes a patient's suffering is so great that it can only be alleviated by medication that is addictive or even shortens life. Although we cannot give drugs whose purpose is to end life, we can administer drugs whose secondary effect is addiction or a shorter life, provided the primary purpose is to make a patient more comfortable and better able to prepare for death.

The use of drugs is complicated by the fact that their effects often differ from person to person. Dr. Cecily Saunders and the hospice movement have encouraged the use of drugs to alleviate pain, even when their side effects are disquieting. Dr. Saunder's position is that when a pain-relieving drug helps a person to focus attention on something other than pain, the drug is a benefit to the patient. Her own experience at St. Christopher's and elsewhere has strengthened her conviction that pain-relieving drugs can help dying people remain in richer contact with God and those around them. Addiction of someone who is dying is a completely different phenomenon from drug addiction of a person who can be expected to recover and return to a relatively normal life. In the first situation, the drug can be a blessing; in the second, a curse.

What is a terminal illness? One that leads to death. But how can we determine that a person is terminally ill when some people recover from illnesses that take the lives of others? Even serious illnesses that usually lead to death are sometimes cured or temporarily remitted.

Every hospital needs a working definition of terminal illness and guidelines to help determine when terminal illness may be present. Medical-moral committees can provide these definitions and guidelines and seek approval of them from medical and nursing staffs. This does not remove responsibility from the physician, but it helps him to determine when he should talk to patients and families, so that they can begin to prepare for death. Physicians who find this an intolerable burden should be offered help by the hospital. Nurses, social workers and chaplains have frequently received special training in talking to patients about terminal illness. Hospital policy should ensure that the terminally ill are neither left in ignorance, nor deprived of the help they need to face their illness and possible death.

For many years, large numbers of physicians believed that sometimes the truth was bad for people's health. The truth created fear and caused patients to abandon hope. Today, when so many health care professionals are well-equipped to assist patients in dealing with fear and to help them place their hope in God's promise of eternal life, there is no excuse for withholding the truth from patients.

Automatic coding of patients for emergency resuscitation is another practice that needs to be reviewed. Once again, the hospital's medical-moral committee should take the initiative in formulating a code-no-code policy. When approved by administration, medical, and nursing staffs, this policy can be the subject of in-service education at all levels of hospital life. Is it right and good to code patients against their will or to code patients who are not expected to live much longer? The wave of protests against widespread coding practices from many nurses, social workers, and chaplains clearly indicates a conflict of conscience that needs resolution. Coding policies must reflect true respect for the spiritual and physical dignity of patients.

Some have expressed the fear that a "no-code" indication will lead to poor care or no care at all. This fear can be alleviated by a supportive care policy, such as one being formulated at St. Alphonsus Hospital in Boise. Rather than write "no code," the physician can write "supportive care only." The hospital's policy will provide clear procedures for sensitive, supportive care of the dying. Needless to say, a decision not to code or to code should, when possible, be made by the patient, family, and physician together.

The courts have been active in decisions regarding the withdrawal and continuation of life-sustaining mechanisms. Legal and medical literature on the subject is abundant. What is the role of the courts? When is a person dead? What is true brain death and what are the best criteria for determining brain death? These questions continue to be debated. The courts are called upon for help when patients, families, nurses and physicians cannot agree, when their consciences lead them to conflicting conclusions about what is best for a patient. Must a patient be dead before life-sustaining mechanisms are withdrawn? A patient has no moral obligation to remain attached to life-sustaining mechanisms when they become an extraordinary burden. If hospital policies have

145

been carefully written, they will considerably reduce the anguish of those who care for patients who rely on machines for continued life.

Lastly, a word about family members who abuse their dying loved ones. When a dying patient has clearly indicated that he does not wish further treatment but only supportive care, and a family member insists that "everything possible" be done, what should the hospital do? When doctors and nurses have serious reason to suspect that family members are not making decisions on the basis of what is best for the patient, but on the basis of what is best for themselves, what should the hospital do? Someone must speak on behalf of the patient. If it is clear that the family is not doing so, the hospital should have mechanisms in place to protect the patient from his family. Respect for the patient's dignity should move the hospital to become the patient's advocate.

Conscience formation is a life-long task. We help one another by sharing our experience, our knowledge, and our convictions about care of the dying. Small group discussions can be an effective method of conscience formation in the hospital. They offer an opportunity to health care professionals to reflect on their common experience in caring for critically ill and dying persons. This common experience should be broadened by reflection on moral norms and on the ultimate purpose of life: full union with God. The norms come from the Church's reflection on its experience of life in faith. This reflection should be made available through educational programs in the hospital and be integrated with the day-to-day experience of the hospital's staff. Conscience formation takes time and effort, but it results in better care for patients and more peace of mind for those who give the care.

Notes

1. Rudolph Hofmann, "Conscience," *Sacramentum Mundi*, Vol. I (New York: Herder and Herder Publishing, 1968), p. 411.
2. *Ibid.*, p. 413.

Chapter 11

Euthanasia, The Right to Life and Termination of Medical Treatment: Legal Issues

Dennis J. Horan, J. D.

The law ordinarily works by reason and analogy to apply existing legal principles to newly-perceived legal problems.[1] In doing so, it neither slights the present, nor unduly sacralizes the past. Termination of medical treatment is one of these problems. In a few short years, courts and legislatures have grappled with the legal principles involved in an attempt to create a societal consensus or, as some may phrase it, a secular solution to this newly perceived problem.

The interests to be considered in the termination of treatment problem are those of the patient, the family, the state, the physician and the involved medical institution. Proposed solutions to the problem sometimes focus on one of these interests while ignoring others. For example, some commentators emphasize the interests of the family and argue that the broadest powers possible to terminate medical treatment, consistent with the law, should repose with the family in order to solve the problem on a familial basis.[2] Other commentators note that in the reported cases, parents have often been adverse to their children's interests in cases where the law has otherwise recognized the child's right to necessary medical treatment, in spite of mental retardation or other physical deficiencies.[3] Therefore, a significant difficulty the law faces in resolving the termination of treatment problem is the balancing of the competing societal and personal interests which converge in this issue. This is particularly true when determining the rights, duties and obligations surrounding the incompetent and children.

My perception of the cases and statutes leads to a very modest conclusion: That no matter how inartfully drafted in a statute, or clumsily stated in an opinion, there is developing an underlying basic consensus in approach to the termination of treatment problem. That consistency is best displayed by the struggle engaged in by the courts which, in considering this issue, have cautiously enunciated legal principles applicable to termination of treatment cases with certain narrow exceptions. These courts have uniformly recognized the competent adult's right to refuse medical treatment.[4] When children or incompetent patients are involved, the problem of terminating medical care is much more complex since it is not a decision made by the patient, but rather by those who are concerned with the patient's care. In this sense, the courts have uniformly discussed termination of medical treatment only in the context of patients not capable of deciding for themselves; that is, children and the incompetent.

In addition, such discussion has occurred only in cases in which the courts have found to involve terminal patients. This remains true even though one may factually dispute that, as to a given case, the patient was truly terminal in the sense that death was imminent and certain, rather than, as some cases seem to consider, "merely" hopeless and certain, but would occur some time in the distant future. The courts have implicitly indicated, therefore, that they realize that allowing termination of medical treatment in non-terminal cases, where treatment is otherwise necessary and beneficial, would be to legalize euthanasia.

Under the American law, euthanasia is a homicide.[5] Even though one who commits euthanasia bears no ill will towards his victim (the patient) and believes his act to be morally justified, he nonetheless acts with the necessary malice under our homicide laws, if he is able to comprehend that his conduct is prohibited by society, regardless of his

148

personal belief. The motive of the perpetrator is rejected as an ameliorative fact in American law. If the facts establish that the killing was done wilfully, that is, with intent and as a result of premeditation and deliberation, our law calls it murder regardless of what the defendant's motive may have been.[6]

The homicide laws, therefore, constitute one aspect of the legal issues surrounding termination of medical treatment which bear strongly on the legal resolution of the problem. The legal resolution of the problem will not necessarily conform to the moral resolution of the problem, since the courts and legislators operate in a different context than the moralist. The courts and legislatures operate under all strictures of the civil and criminal law. They cannot fashion a solution which would violate the constitution or disrupt the overall efficacy of other areas of law which converge on this problem. For example, they cannot fashion a solution to the treatment problem which violates the patient's fundamental right to life or the criminal law's absolute prohibition against unjustified killing. Nor can they overlook certain tort principles of law which seek to protect patient autonomy in medical decisions.

The problem, therefore, that courts and legislators have faced is the creation of a solution to this question: When, if at all, may medical treatment be terminated by one person for another? In attempting an answer, they have steered carefully to avoid violating basic rights of persons or transgressing other well defined areas of the law such as the homicide laws.[7]

Legislative Approaches to Termination of Medical Treatment

A) The California Scheme

Legislative attempts to solve the termination of treatment problem began in 1976 with the passage of the California Natural Death Act.[8] By 1977, seven other states had passed similar "Living Will" or "Natural Death" legislation.[9] Since then, only three other states have done so: Alabama, Kansas and Washington.[10] Texas and North Carolina have recently amended their statutes.[11] Generally speaking, such legislation allows a person to execute a directive to his physician for the purpose of withholding medical treatment at some later date, usually when the patient has reached a terminal state and is unable to exercise his right to refuse medical treatment.

These statutes have been analyzed elsewhere as to many of their deficiencies.[12] Two problems are, however, especially worthy of comment. *First,* to the extent that such statutes mandatorily attempt to direct the conduct of the physician at some future date, they fail to consider the physician's own medical judgment concerning the appropriateness of treatment. Such legislation should, at least, provide that the desires of the patient be expressed in a manner which will assist the physician in handling the terminal case. The *second* related problem is that such legislation is likely to inhibit the physician's effort to treat the dying patient with dignity, grace and a measure of humanity in a fundamental way. Whenever a statute is enacted regulating conduct, especially where punitive sanctions are available for non-compliance, the effect is to chill and inhibit similar conduct, otherwise legal, but not now in conformity with the requirements of the act. Thus, physicians may be reluctant to withdraw or withhold life-sustaining treatment unless a directive has been executed by the patient, even though there is no legal obligation to extend heroic or useless care. If even twenty percent of the population executed a living will within the requirements of the given statute — an optimistic figure in view of the small percentage who execute documents for disposition of property — the remaining eighty percent must suffer the consequences. California attempted to mitigate this problem through the enactment of Section 7193, which indicates that its "Natural Death Act" does not impair or supersede any prior right or responsibility the person possesses to effect the lawful withdrawal of life-sustaining procedures.

Whether such statutes are even necessary is open to serious question. They create more legal problems than they solve, do not aid the family or physician in solving with dignity the dying problem, and are sometimes sloppily drafted. Moreover, they do not show an understanding of the nature of the legal-medical principles which are applicable.

The California Act requires that the adult must be in a "terminal condition" before the directive to the physician is effective. Terminal condition is defined as an incurable condition caused by injury, disease or illness which, regardless of the application of life-sustaining procedures, would, within reasonable medical judgment, produce death, and where the application of life-sustaining procedures serves only to postpone the moment of death of the patient. A life-sustaining procedure is defined as a procedure or intervention which utilizes mechanical or other artificial means to sustain, restore, or supplant a vital function

150

and which, when applied to a qualified patient, would serve only to artificially prolong the moment of death, and where, in the judgment of the attending physician, death is imminent whether or not such procedures are utilized. If such legislation is to be passed at all, these safeguards are essential since they keep the act within the proper standards of medical care and treatment in our society. When truly limited to a "terminal condition" under the standards stated in the California Act, such legislation, although unnecessary, does not violate any of the legal values we seek to preserve. It does not legalize mercy killing or assisted suicide. It does not leave the aged defenseless, or the handicapped newborn at risk. It does not destroy the ethical basis of medicine: "to do no harm." Under these circumstances, our concern must be to see that these safeguards are not changed by amendment. However, other acts which have not been so carefully drafted do not contain even these most basic of safeguards.

B) The Arkansas Scheme

The tight drafting of the California Act should be contrasted with the loose drafting of the Arkansas Act.[13] Section one of the Arkansas Act creates a right to die with dignity and to refuse medical treatment. The common law already gives the right to refuse medical treatment which is probably not as absolute as is usually thought, but the exception need not deter us here. The decision to reject medical treatment, even in terminal cases when done by a competent adult, cannot properly be construed as suicide or euthanasia,[14] and it is not a right that needs statutory authority.[15]

Section two allows the creation of a directive to reject any "artificial, extraordinary, extreme or radical medical or surgical means or procedures calculated to prolong his life." The act does not state that the illness must be terminal, and does not define the critical terms, "artificial," "extraordinary," "extreme," or "radical." Since it is not limited, the act applies at any time and under any circumstances. One assumes that the Arkansas legislature would be shocked if they understood the radical departure from existing law that results from a literal reading of the statute. Presumably, the Arkansas Supreme Court, if called upon to interpret the statute, would interpret it to apply only to a terminal illness. This construction can legitimately be read into the Act because of the phrase "calculated to prolong his life." Prolongation is a word usually used only in discussions concerning terminal illness.

151

Section three of the Arkansas statute allows a parent or guardian to execute a directive for anyone, even a minor, who is mentally unable to execute one "or who is *otherwise* incapacitated." Needless to say, "otherwise incapacitated" is undefined. The abuses capable under such an act are beyond imagination. In addition, the act gives preferences as to who may execute the directive on behalf of another, even to the extent of allowing a majority of the children to do so, if a spouse is unwilling or unable to act.

The Arkansas statute is ill-conceived, ill-defined, and sloppily drafted. It is an unconstitutional withdrawal of the protection of life without due process or equal protection and is subject to repeal on those grounds. It is tantamount to the legalization of euthanasia which, under American law, is homicide. It is this type of statute that illustrates the dangers in death legislation, which must be carefully monitored at every legislative level. If there must be such legislation, then effort must be made to ensure the necessary safeguards. Such legislation must be effective only in truly terminal cases; must not allow withdrawal of sustenance; must not allow withdrawal of ordinary medical means which are beneficial; must apply only to adults; must not seek mandatory control over the physician's judgment in some future undetermined circumstances; must not require complex procedures, as are usually found in the probate court; must ensure that consent was given voluntarily where consent is involved; must prohibit mercy killing; must prohibit assisted suicide and must not confuse the difference between "brain death" and irreversible coma.

Withdrawal of medical treatment for the terminally ill does not need legislative support. Indeed, several of the acts under consideration here contain specific sections indicating that the execution or nonexecution of a directive does not supersede any existing legal right or legal responsibility which any person may have to effect the withholding or non-use of any medical treatment in any otherwise existing lawful manner. Such statutory provisions indicate rather clearly that, in the minds of those legislatures, withholding treatment is legal under certain circumstances when done in conformity with existing medical-legal standards. What, then, are the current legal-medical standards for the termination of treatment? Several recent cases have dealt with the withholding or withdrawal of medical treatment and have enunciated the applicable legal standards. A review of these decisions is necessary at this juncture in order to assist us to understand the emerging consensus in the termination of medical treatment problem.[16]

Judicial Approaches to Termination of Medical Treatment *In Re Quinlan*

Karen Ann Quinlan was a 21-year-old woman who was brought unconscious to the hospital. She was placed on a respirator but remained in a comatose condition. Ultimately, her father sought court approval for her withdrawal from the respirator over the objections of the attending physician and hospital. In *In Re Quinlan,* the Supreme Court of New Jersey held that the father was a proper guardian and that he was authorized to terminate the respirator treatment if: (1) he obtained the concurrence of the responsible attending physicians, who must conclude that there is no reasonable possibility of Karen's ever emerging from her present comatose condition to a cognitive, sapient state, and, (2) if he obtained the same type of agreement from a hospital ethics committee.[17]

The *Quinlan* case was litigated on the basis that Karen was in a terminal state.[18] That this proved to be a factual error is significant only to show how mortal judges and litigants are. It is important, however, to note the stress which the court placed on its conclusion that Karen was in a terminal state.

The *Quinlan* court recognized the right to refuse medical treatment based upon a constitutional right of privacy which the court found to be implicit in both the federal and New Jersey constitutions. The court held that Karen's right of privacy — her right to refuse medical treatment — could be asserted by her guardian and family on her behalf only under the particular circumstances of this case. The court also concluded that, in the future, these matters could prospectively be handled by the family, the physician and the hospital ethics committee without application to a court.

It must be clearly understood, however, what the New Jersey Supreme Court allowed and did not allow. It did *not* allow the father, the guardian, or the parents to *direct* the type of treatment or lack thereof which the physician must then carry out. It did not allow the father, guardian, or parents to *direct* that the respirator be discontinued. What it did allow was very narrow. It allowed the father to be appointed as the guardian but then gave him only one limited right:

> To appoint Joseph Quinlan as guardian of the person of Karen
> Quinlan with full power to make decisions with regard to the
> identity of her treating physicians.[19]

Contrary to much popular belief, the *Quinlan* case does *not* stand
for the proposition that the parent, guardian or family can *direct* the
physician in the exercise of his medical judgment. The Quinlan court
gave the parent/guardian the right only to hire and fire the physicians
on the case. As to the treatment, however, it limited the guardian to
concurring with the physician's judgment to terminate treatment, if such'
was the physician's judgment and such judgment was concurred in by
the hospital ethics committee under *Quinlan*. Should the physician
disagree, the only power to be exercised by the family would be to fire
the physician. The family may not force the physician to treat nor not
treat without considering his medical judgment. Those are matters that
remain within the sound use of his medical judgment. The family
cannot direct him how to exercise that judgment. Nor can the courts.

There is no question that the body of the opinion, as distinct from
the holding, allows the guardian to reject medical treatment on behalf
of the ward. The opinion clearly, however, limits the exercise of the
power to a terminal situation where the physician's medical judgment
concurs that such termination is good medical practice. It further
requires concurrence by a medical ethics committee.

Nor does *Quinlan* stand for the proposition that the physician may
not continue to treat an incompetent unless he has obtained the continuing informed consent of the parent or guardian. Consent to treat is
necessary, but the role of consent and informed consent in termination
of treatment cases has been misunderstood. It does not mean that the
physician's power or right to handle the incompetent's case must cease
if not supported by an informed consent of the parent or guardian. No
court has gone that far.

The courts have not specifically adopted the competent's right to
reject medical treatment to the incompetent. First, the courts have
limited the exercise of the incompetent's right to reject medical treatment by another person through substituted judgment or a "best
interests" standard to terminal cases. The competent patient can exercise that right at any time. Second, the courts have limited the exercise
of the right on behalf of the incompetent to those terminal cases where
no curative medical intervention exists, or where treatment would only
prolong an inevitable and imminent dying state. Such cases are aptly

154

described as terminal and hopeless. The competent adult patient is not so limited. With narrow exceptions, he or she may reject medical treatment at will.

The origin of the physician's power to treat arises from the initial consent. Once treatment commences, however, the physician has a duty not to abandon his patient, although he may resign from the case after having arranged for appropriate follow-up treatment. That duty, as expressed in community medical standards by applicable tort laws, plus the physician's ethical duty to do no harm, and the proscription of the homicide laws, constitute the parameters within which the physician handles the terminal case. If he violates these parameters, he becomes subject to civil suit or criminal liability. Within these parameters, he is guided by his medical judgment and the ethical constraint to do no harm to the patient.

However, the role of consent in medical treatment cases should be understood. The legal relationship between a physician and patient is contractual. The physician cannot commence treatment without the creation of that contractual relationship by a consent from the patient, either express or implied. In emergency situations, the law presumes such a consent since the treatment is for the benefit of the patient. Once the initial consent occurs, however, it is presumed thereafter that the patient consents on a continuing basis until the necessity for some more radical form of medical interventions, such as surgery, becomes necessary. Then a more particularized consent is necessary and is obtained.

It is from this particularized consent that the doctrine of informed consent has emerged in tort law. Generally speaking, for a consent to be "informed" the patient must be told the nature of the treatment, the risks involved, and the alternative forms of treatment, if any. A failure to do so may create a cause of action in tort against the physician when a risk materializes causing injury which the patient might have otherwise avoided by rejecting the treatment had he known of the risk. This cause of action is known as a lack of informed consent case.[20] Ordinarily, it has little significance in medical malpractice cases.[21] There is much confusion about the nature of the action. In addition, most states have adopted a negligence standard for informed consent cases which requires the plaintiff to prove by expert testimony that community medical standards mandate that the risks be revealed. If community medical standards do not require revelation of the risk, then a failure to do so does not create liability on the part of the physician. Thus, the necessity for informed consent is not a legal absolute as some moralists seem to think. It may be a moral absolute but it is not a legal absolute.

The law presumes that incompetents and children do not have the mental capability to give consent and requires, therefore, that parents and guardians consent on behalf of children and wards. However, the legal significance of the consent by the parent or guardian is important to an understanding of the role of consent in termination of treatment cases. The law presumes that the parent or guardian can only consent to treatment which is *beneficial* to the patient. The same is true for the refusal to consent. A parent or guardian may not withhold or refuse consent to necessary or lifesaving medical treatment. Should a parent so refuse, the physician's obligation to treat is not vitiated. This is so because the civil cause of action in tort belongs to the child, not the parents. This will become clearer when the case of John Storar is considered later in this chapter.

Superintendent v. Saikewicz

The second most important case in this area of the law, while agreeing with most of what the *Quinlan* court said, severely criticized it for not requiring that all such decisions to withhold or withdraw treatment be made by a court of competent jurisdiction.

The *Saikewicz*[22] case involved a 67-year-old man with an I.Q. of 10 who had been institutionalized all his life and had contracted acute myeloblastic monocytic leukemia for which the usual treatment is chemotherapy. The involved medical institution petitioned the court for a guardian to make the necessary decision regarding the use of chemotherapy in treatment of the disease. The guardian and the attending physicians recommended against the chemotherapy and the Supreme Court of Massachusetts ultimately affirmed this decision.

Like the *Quinlan* court, the *Saikewicz* court treated this as a case involving a terminal patient. Indeed, during the 18 months between the entry of its first order of affirmance and the publication of its opinion, Mr. Saikewicz "died without pain or discomfort."[23]

The court agreed with the *Quinlan* holding that constitutional right of privacy was applicable. In addition, the *Saikewicz* court felt that the best interests of the incompetent were to be considered and that this substituted judgment could be applied to the facts of the case. In affirming the decision of the guardian and the physician not to treat, the court seemed to lean heavily on the inability of an individual of diminished intellectual capacity to comprehend and cooperate with the onerous and difficult treatment of chemotherapy. The court criticized *Quinlan*, however, for allowing family and physicians to make such decisions without court authority, and explicitly stated that court approval of such decisions must be sought. This aspect of the decision has been severely criticized, and its importance qualified, by the later *Dinnerstein*[24] and *Earle Spring*[25] decisions.

In *Saikewicz*, the trial judge had agreed with the guardian's decision not to treat on the basis of the patient's (1) age, (2) inability to cooperate, (3) adverse side effects, (4) low chance of remission, (5) suffering caused by chemotherapy, and (6) quality of life remaining. The Supreme Court of Massachusetts agreed with the first five reasons but rejected any quality of life consideration in these cases.

The *Saikewicz* court stated that the state's interest in such a patient is limited to (1) the preservation of life, (2) protecting the interests of innocent third parties, (3) the prevention of suicide, and (4) the maintenance of ethical integrity of the medical profession. It found none of these interests violated in this case and, therefore, ruled that the state had no intervening interest.

The court limited the application of the *Saikewicz* rule allowing treatment to be withheld to those cases where the patient has (1) an incurable and terminal illness, and (2) where there exists no life-saving or life-prolonging treatment or (3) where the treatment, if available, would only effect a brief and uncertain delay in the natural death process.

It posits these as the applicable legal standards to be applied by the courts: (1) There exists in all persons a right to reject medical treatment under appropriate circumstances, (2) this right extends to an incompetent under conditions previously stated above, and (3) may be exercised on his behalf when it is in his best interests, (4) but those best interests may not include quality of life considerations.

The court was quick to reject quality of life considerations stating that:

> . . . the chance of a longer life carries the same weight for Saikewicz as for any other person, the value of life under law having no relation to intelligence or social positions.[26]

157

Matter of Dinnerstein

The furor created by the requirment in *Saikewicz* that court approval be sought for any decision to withhold treatment quickly caused a Massachusetts appellate court to temper such a harsh rule by the application of common sense. In *Matter of Dinnerstein*,[27] it was held that court approval for termination of treatment need not be sought unless life-saving or life-prolonging treatment alternatives are available and the decision was against use of those treatments. The *Dinnerstein* case involved a physician's request to a court concerning the legality of a no resuscitation order. The patient was a 67-year-old woman suffering from Alzheimer's disease. In addition, she suffered a stroke and was in an essentially vegetative state, immobile, speechless, unable to swallow without choking, and barely able to cough. She had a serious life-threatening coronary disease, and her condition was hopeless. Her physician recommended that if cardiac or respiratory arrest occurs, resuscitation efforts should not be undertaken. Her family agreed. The guardian appointed by the court opposed the order.

The *Dinnerstein* court found the do-not-resuscitate order to be appropriate. It explained that *Saikewicz* did not mean that treatment may only be withheld by court order since that would be to ignore the sound exercise of medical judgment. It explained *Saikewicz* thus:

> . . . that when the [Saikewicz] court spoke of lifesaving or life-prolonging treatments, it referred to treatments administered for the purpose and with some reasonable expectation of effecting a permanent or temporary cure of or relief from the illness or conditions being treated. Prolongation of life as used in the *Saikewicz* case, does not mean a mere suspension of the act of dying, but contemplates, at the very least, a remission of symptoms enabling a return towards a normal, functioning, integrated existence.[28]

The *Dinnerstein* court emphasized that the facts of this case indicated that it was hopeless and that death must come soon. It described the medical condition as one where the patient is in the terminal stages of an unremitting, incurable mortal illness.

The *Dinnerstein* case, said the court, did not present the type of significant treatment choice which is made by the patient, if competent to do so, in the light of sound medical advice and where life-saving forms of medical intervention exist. In those circumstances, the court indicated that a decision *against treatment* would require judicial approval.

158

Where the case presents a question within the competence of the medical profession as to what measures are appropriate to ease the imminent passing of an irreversibly, terminally ill patient in light of her history and family wishes, that question, the court said, is one not for judicial decision, but one for the attending physician. The *Dinnerstein* court, finally, pointed out that the court should only become involved if there is a contention that the physician failed to exercise the necessary degree of skill and competence.

Several other cases of significance have been decided recently. The *Earle Spring*[29] case has been decided by the Supreme Court of Massachusetts, which is the same court that decided *Saikewicz, Dinnerstein* having been decided by a Massachusetts appellate court. In addition, the New York Court of Appeals, the highest judicial authority in that state, has decided the *Brother Fox* and the *John Storar* cases.

Matter of Spring

The *Earle Spring* case was decided by an order entered January 14, 1980 by the Supreme Court of Massachusetts. However, the opinion was not issued until May 13, 1980, and by that time Mr. Spring was deceased. Earle Spring, an incompetent person, was receiving life-prolonging hemodialysis treatment. On the petition of his wife and son, who was his temporary guardian, a judge of the probate court found that the ward "would, if competent, choose not to receive the life-prolonging treatment" of hemodialysis. That court entered an order allowing the attending physician, together with the ward's wife and son, to make a decision with reference to the continuation or termination of dialysis. The Court of Appeals affirmed. However, the Supreme Court of Massachusetts concluded that it was an error to delegate the decision to the attending physician and the ward's wife and son. It issued an order reversing the judgment of the probate court and remanded the case for entry of a new judgment ordering the temporary guardian to *refrain* from authorizing any further life-prolonging treatment except by further order of the probate court. If there was evidence of significant change in the condition of the ward or in the treatment available for him, then the probate court was authorized to revise its findings and judgment. The important point, however, is that, according to the Massachusetts Supreme Court, authority to terminate treatment must be sought from the court and cannot be delegated to the family or to anyone else. This the court emphasized in the opinion.

Mr. Spring was born in 1901 and had been married for 55 years before these events. He was suffering from end-stage kidney disease which required him to undergo hemodialysis three days a week for five hours a day. He also suffered from chronic organic brain syndrome or senility, and was completely confused and disoriented. The court described the illnesses as follows:

> . . . both the kidney disease and the senility were permanent and irreversible; there was no prospect of a medical breakthrough that would provide a cure for either disease.[30]

The court further described the treatment as being unable to cause a remission or to restore him even temporarily to a normal cognitive integrated functioning existence. The court reviewed many of the decisions in this area and concluded that a consensus was growing. It stated that a person has a strong interest in being free from nonconsensual invasion of his bodily integrity and a constitutional right of privacy that may be asserted to prevent unwanted infringements of his bodily integrity. The same right is extended to an incompetent person to be exercised through a substituted judgment on his behalf by the court. The decision should take into account the actual interests and preferences of the ward, and should try as much as possible to be the decision that the ward would have made.

The court was very concerned with discussing the procedure for making these decisions in light of the heavy criticism leveled against the *Saikewicz* opinion by medical and legal commentators. In describing its *Saikewicz* decision, the court indicated that it disapproved the delegation of the ultimate decision-making responsibility to any committee, panel or group, *ad hoc* or permanent. It reaffirmed its reasoning and decision in *Saikewicz*. It describes *Saikewicz* as follows:

> We also indicated that, if the judge in such a case was not persuaded that the incompetent individual's choice, as determined by the substituted judgment standard, would have been to forego potentially life-prolonging treatment, or if the interest of the state required it, the treatment was to be ordered.[31]

The court distinguished *Saikewicz* from the *Spring* case on the theory that the *Spring* case did not involve state action since the patient was not in state custody. Lest one misunderstand the thrust of its opinion, the court again reaffirmed its position that only courts could make such ultimate decisions:

160

Again we disapprove shifting of the ultimate decision-making responsibility away from the duly established courts of proper jurisdiction.[32]

It repeated several times that *Earle Spring* was suffering from what it described as an incurably fatal disease. It described the treatments as intrusive and life-prolonging rather than life-saving; "there was no prospect of cure or even a recovery of competence."

However, showing its sensitivity to the barrage of criticism leveled at its *Saikewicz* opinion, the court tried to mitigate its absolute position by implying that judicial approval need not be sought in every case:

> Neither the present case nor the *Saikewicz* case involved the legality of action taken without judicial authority, and our opinions should not be taken to establish any requirement of prior judicial approval that would not otherwise exist.[33]

In further discussing the necessity for judicial approval, the court tried to show that acting to withhold treatment in terminal, hopeless cases held no practical or real risk of prosecutorial action:

> It is reported that apparently no prosecutor has proceeded to trial in a case where a physician chose to terminate life-preserving treatment or omit emergency treatment in a hopeless case.[34]

Continuing in this back-tracking from *Saikewicz*, the court pointed out that not even court approval is a guarantee of absolute immunity:

> Whenever a physician in good faith decides that a particular treatment is not called for, there is a risk that in some subsequent litigation the omission will be found to have been negligent. But the standard for determining whether the treatment was called for is the same after the event as before; negligence can not be based solely on failure to obtain prior court approval, if the approval would have been given. Consent of the patient may not always immunize the physician from a charge of negligence. . . . Immunity afforded by court authorization would seem to be subject to similar limitation, for example, if the physician is negligent in implementing the court order. Thus absence of court approval does not result in automatic civil liability for withholding treatment; court approval may serve the useful purpose of resolving a doubtful or disputed question of law or fact, but it does not eliminate all risk of liability.[35]

The *Spring* opinion both reaffirmed *Saikewicz* and yet went out of its way to imply that Saikewicz was in some unexplained way limited in its breadth and impact. Perhaps sensing the confusion that the *Spring* opinion would cause, the court asked itself this question: "What, then, is the significance of our disapproval of a shift of ultimate responsibility away from the court?"[36]

The answer it gives is a legal one, of doubtful assistance to anyone trying to work their way through the difficult questions involving termination of medical treatment and the concomitant potential exposure to criminal or civil liability. The court says this:

> When a court is properly presented with the legal question, whether treatment may be withheld, it must decide that question and not delegate it to some private person or group. Subsidiary questions as to how to carry out the decision, particularly a purely medical question, must almost inevitably be left to private decision, but with no immunity for action taken in bad faith or action that is grievously unreasonable.[37]

Such language invites every physician involved in a terminal case to file suit. How else can the physician or medical institution otherwise prudently avoid civil and criminal liability? Is this what the Massachusetts Supreme Court really wants?

The last few pages of the opinion are a plea by the court to the Massachusetts Probate Courts to accelerate all decisions in these cases. In view of the length of time it took to litigate the *Spring* case, the plea lacks credibility, and supports the criticism of the *Saikewicz* case that the courts are incapable of handling the decision-making process in terminal cases. If anything, the *Earle Spring* case proves the truth of that criticism.

The Brother Fox and John Storar Decisions

On March 27, 1980, an intermediate Appellate Court in New York decided the *Brother Fox* case.[38] Brother Fox was an 82-year-old member of the Roman Catholic Order of the Society of Mary, who had been in a permanent vegetative coma since October 2, 1979, when he suffered a cardiac arrest during surgery, which resulted in severe and irreversible brain damage. The head of the order, Rev. Philip K. Eichner, instituted a proceeding under New York law to have Brother Fox declared incompetent and to obtain judicial approval for the withdrawal of his respirator. Such an order was issued by the trial court, but its effect was stayed, pending the outcome of the appeal. Shortly after oral argument of the appeal, Brother Fox died. The Appellate Court decided the controversy anyway, holding that Father Eichner, as a committee of the incompetent under New York law, was entitled to the relief sought.

The New York Appellate Court rejected the trial court's position that the constitutional right of privacy was not involved. The trial court had decided the case based on applicable medical/legal principles based on the common law and had granted the relief sought. The appellate court also granted the relief, but only after indicating that the right to refuse medical treatment was a part of the constitutional right of privacy, which might be exercised on behalf of the incompetent by someone else. The Court also indicated that that decision could only be made under court auspices and by means of an elaborate procedure wherein all interested parties, including the State's Attorney, had a right to present evidence. The Appellate Court had set up certain standards before treatment could be terminated. These standards were:

1. The patient must be terminally ill;
2. He must be in a vegetative coma, characterized by the physician as permanent and irreversible;
3. He must lack cognitive brain function;
4. The probability of his ever regaining cognitive brain function must be extremely remote.[39]

It then required that the standard to be met by the evidence is that of clear and convincing evidence, which is the highest standard under civil law.

The Brother Fox case was appealed further, and in March of 1981, the highest court in the State of New York rendered its decision not only in the Brother Fox case, but also in the matter of John Storar.[40]

John Storar was a profoundly retarded 52-year-old with the mental age of about 18 months. At the time of the proceeding, he was a resident of the Newark Developmental Center, which had been his home since the age of 5. Blood was detected in his urine and, as a result of diagnostic tests, he was found to have cancer of the bladder. It was recommended that he receive radiation therapy, which the hospital refused to render without the consent of a legal guardian, in this case, his mother. Initially, she gave her consent and radiation therapy was commenced and the disease went into remission.

In March of 1980, there was a new flare-up, and the physician diagnosed the cancer as being terminal, concluding that, after using all medical and surgical means available, the patient would nevertheless die from the disease. The mother was asked permission to administer blood transfusions. Initially, she refused but then changed her mind. For several weeks John Storar received blood transfusions, but then the mother requested that they be discontinued. The Director of the Center filed suit to seek authorization to continue the blood transfusions.

The Court of Appeals (New York's highest court) decided the *Storar* and *Brother Fox* cases in a single opinion. In the case of Brother Fox, it held that termination of the treatment was warranted. In the case of John Storar, it held that termination of the treatment (blood transfusions) was unwarranted. In both cases, the Court rejected the doctrine created by *Quinlan* and followed by *Saikewicz* that the right to refuse medical treatment was a part of the constitutional right of privacy. Instead, the Court noted that, although several Courts have so held, "this is a disputed question which the Supreme Court has repeatedly declined to consider. . . . Neither do we reach that question in this case because the relief granted to the petitioner, Eichner, is adequately supported by common law principles."[41] The Court found that the sensitive question of whether or not discontinuing life-sustaining medical treatment may be made by someone other than the patient ". . . is not presented in this case because Brother Fox made the decision for himself before he became incompetent."[42] Even by the highest standard applicable to civil cases — clear and convincing evidence — the Court found the result compelled by the fact that Brother Fox had clearly and unequivocally announced his decision against medical treatment under these circumstances, while he was still competent to do so. The Court indicated that his desire, as clearly announced, could be followed and treatment terminated.

However, in the case of John Storar the Court reached a different conclusion. John Storar was never competent at anytime in his life and, therefore, there was no clear and convincing evidence, nor any evidence whatsoever of his desires with regard to the termination of the life-prolonging treatment in his case. Since, mentally, John Storar was an infant, the Court decided that the only realistic way to assess his rights in the case was by looking at legal principles applicable to cases involving infants. Thus, the Court followed these longstanding legal principles:

A parent or guardian has a right to consent to medical treatment on behalf of an infant. . . . The parent, however, may not deprive a child of lifesaving treatment, however well intentioned . . . Even when the parents' decision to decline necessary treatment is based on constitutional grounds, such as religious beliefs, it must yield to the State's interest, as *parens patriae*, in protecting the health and welfare of the child. . . . Of course it is not for the courts to determine the most effective treatment when the parents have chosen among reasonable alternatives. . . . But the courts may not permit a parent to deny a child all treatment for a condition which threatens his life. . . . The case of a child who may bleed to death because of the parents' refusal to authorize a blood transfusion presents the classic example. . . . (citations omitted)[43]

In the *Storar* case, there were two complications which threatened John Storar's life. There was the cancer of the bladder, which was incurable, and would probably claim his life eventually. There was also the related loss of blood, which posed the risk of an earlier death. One of the experts had compared transfusions to food; they would not cure the cancer, but they could eliminate the risk of death from another treatable cause. The Court concluded that no court could allow an incompetent patient to bleed to death because someone, "even someone as close as a parent or sibling, feels that this is best for one with an incurable disease."[44] Consequently, the Court determined that it would be inappropriate to allow anyone to refuse to continue the blood transfusions to Mr. Storar.

On the issue of whether or not court intervention was always necessary, the Court of Appeals of New York concluded that interested persons may apply to the Court for permission to terminate treatment since they need not act at their peril. The court emphasized, however, that any such procedure is optional.

Neither the common law nor existing statutes require persons generally to seek prior court assessment of conduct which may subject them to civil and criminal liability. If it is desirable to enlarge the role of the courts in cases involving discontinuance of life-sustaining treatment for incompetents by establishing, as the Appellate Division suggested in the Eichner case, a mandatory procedure of successive approvals by physicians, hospital personnel, relatives, and the courts, the change should come from the legislature.[45]

While some commentators have criticized the *Storar* case,[46] others, such as Prof. William Curran of Harvard, have found its conclusions:

> refreshingly clear and wholly convincing. It is directly contrary to the contrived argumentation of the *Saikewicz* case . . .[47]

Prof. Curran also makes a most interesting comment about the *Storar* case vis-a-vis the other cases we have been discussing in this article:

> The unusual nature of this matter is also found in the fact that of all the right-to-die cases that have been brought to court around the country up to this writing, *Storar* is the only major decision of a highest court that has refused to allow the patient's death to occur as result of judicial inquiry. Despite· their often impassioned rhetoric about protecting life and requiring courts to intervene, the *Quinlan, Saikewicz, Perlmutter, Spring, Severns* and *Eichner* cases — the series of decisions that provoked the broadside of medical, ethical, and legal commentary — have all approved actions to remove treatment that was presumed to result in death. The *Storar* matter may well be a turning point in judicial intervention in this field.[48]

What Curran found contrived in *Saikewicz* was the application of the substituted judgment doctrine where a court attempts to determine what a person with lifelong profound retardation would have wanted if he could have made a rational decision. This issue will be discussed at some length later in this chapter.

Other Recent Cases

Recently, the Supreme Court of Delaware decided a case involving these issues. In *Severns* v. *Wilmington Medical Center*[49] the court followed the lead of *Quinlan* and *Saikewicz* by holding that a Court of Chancery has jurisdiction without specific legislative support to grant a guardian the power to withdraw medical treatment in an appropriate case after an evidentiary hearing. The court, however, asked the legislature "to enact a comprehensive state policy governing these matters which are, in the words of *Quinlan*, of transcendent importance."[50]

The Delaware court returned the *Severns* case to the trial court for an evidentiary hearing and a determination as to whether the relief should be granted in the circumstances of this particular case.

The Delaware Supreme Court did not see the issues involved as an application of currently existing legal-medical precedents or current ethical standards. Instead, it found the requested relief (termination of life-saving medical treatment) "novel to Delaware and, relatively speaking, it is new in our civilization."[51] What does the court mean? Does the court mean by that expression that it supposes that its order allows the purposeful termination of human life? Does not the court understand the important ethical and legal distinction between letting a terminal patient die when continued "treatment" is not beneficial and the outcome is hopeless, and the otherwise purposeful taking of a human life?

The Delaware Court raises other serious questions: "what is a life-sustaining system for a person who has been comatose for many months?"[52] The court then wonders whether medicines or food are included.

The *Severns* case, while not deciding any of the factual issues involved, leaves one with the uneasy feeling that the comatose patient now finds himself on a slippery slope with the courts gently pushing towards the legalization of euthanasia. Such is the ultimate consequence of an inability to distinguish between the truly terminal case in the application of the legal principles allowing the termination of medical care. Once termination of treatment is allowed by the courts in non-terminal cases and for other than medical reasons, the door is open to legalized euthanasia.

The misunderstanding possible is best illustrated by an unreported New Jersey case recently brought to our attention. A retarded child several months old was suffering from a medical condition which caused brain seizures which were controlled by Phenobarbital. The parents did not want the medication continued. The attending physician agreed as did the hospital ethics committee. The physician withheld the Phenobarbital, the assumption being that the child would die of the seizures in a matter of weeks. The rationale for withholding the medication was said to be the Quinlan case. We have been advised that this is not an isolated case in New Jersey.

In fact, this child was not dying and was not a terminal case. There existed a well-known form of medication which controlled the underlying condition and was beneficial to the child. Withholding of treatment under those circumstances is *not* supported by the Quinlan case. Such conduct is a homicide as well as an intentional tort. Withholding treatment in this case caused the child's death, as surely as would the injection of a poison in its veins. This was not a terminal case; it was the decision to withhold the Phenobarbital which made the case terminal. The case illustrates the danger of legalizing euthanasia if the principles for withholding medical treatment to the incompetent are not limited to the truly terminal situation.

These decisions should be contrasted with the decision of the Supreme Court of Massachusetts in the famous *Chad Green*[53] case. Chad, at age 20 months, contracted leukemia. His parents refused to give him the appropriate treatment which was chemotherapy. The Supreme Court of Massachusetts affirmed a lower court decision taking custody from Chad's parents for the purpose of giving him chemotherapy. The court distinguished *Saikewicz* because here the treatment being withheld was both life-prolonging and life-saving. Under these circumstances, the state's interest in protecting life overrides the parents' rights to direct the medical treatment of their child. The child's best interests also militate against nontreatment. For these reasons, the court took custody from the parents for the purpose of requiring treatment.

So too, in the baby *Houle*[54] case, the court appointed a guardian to give consent for surgical correction of a tracheal esophageal fistula of a five-day-old infant whose parents refused consent. More recently, a New York court has ordered treatment even against the parents' wishes in a spina bifida case.[55] The results in these cases where treatment is ordered by the court should be contrasted with the previously discussed cases where treatment was terminated. A significant difference between these cases where treatment was ordered by the courts, and previously discussed cases where it was not, is that the physicians took the position that treatment was necessary and warranted, and that the treatment held out reasonable hope of benefit. These cases help us to understand the growing consensus under discussion in spite of the procedural difference between *Quinlan* and *Saikewicz*.

The Right to Refuse Medical Treatment and The Right to Privacy

The competent adult patient may ordinarily reject medical treatment even if the rejection means ultimate death. Such conduct has never been considered to be suicide, nor is the physician guilty of homicide or abandonment of his patient. That right is tempered only by state interests in the preservation of life, the need to prevent suicide, and the requirement that the law help maintain the ethical integrity of medical practice. Those state interests are ordinarily not found present in truly terminal cases involving adults. An example of such a situation is *Satz v. Perlmutter*[56] where the Florida Supreme Court held that a 73-year-old patient, mortally ill from amyotrophic lateral sclerosis, could knowingly direct his removal from the respirator, even though death would follow in an hour. The Florida Supreme Court defined the issue as the right to refuse extraordinary medical treatment where the family also consents.

The right to refuse medical treatment need not be considered a constitutional right of privacy, nor does it need legislative support. Such a right exists in view of the common law of torts which prohibits any unconsented touching of one's body by another, except in emergency situations, but, even then, only for the benefit of the one touched. Prior to *Quinlan* and *Saikewicz*, it was not felt necessary to discuss the right to refuse medical treatment as a constitutional right. Nor need it be.

However, since *Quinlan*, and when discussing the rights of the terminally ill incompetent patient, almost all courts except the New York Court of Appeals in *Brother Fox* and *John Storar* have found the right to refuse medical treatment as a part of the constitutional right to privacy. This is unfortunate, since it was not necessary to go this far, and finding the right to be of constitutional dimensions lays a heavy burden on state legislative experimentation in this area, if not entirely voiding it.

It is also important to note the weakness of the basis for asserting a constitutional right to refuse treatment even for the competent. There has never been a United States Supreme Court decision asserting the existence of such a right. Nor has it been demonstrated on what basis such a right might be constructed, either through logic or through the marshalling of historical evidence demonstrating that the Framers intended it to be protected either by the Bill of Rights or by the Fourteenth Amendment.

Surely those advocating the "recognition" of an entirely new and, until recently, unknown constitutional right bear a heavy burden of showing why it should be created. Neither the courts of New Jersey or Massachusetts have supported its creation by much more than an *ipse dixit*.

In the *Fox* case, for example, the Appellate Division held that, under the Constitution, Brother Fox's respirator can and should be terminated in accordance with his right of privacy as exercised by his committee. Even if, *arguendo*, a constitutional right exists with regard to a decision by the patient alone to terminate medical treatment, the conclusion that this right may be exercised by a third party is bad public policy and is based on a misunderstanding of the nature of the right to privacy.

The right to privacy is, by its very nature, personal because it relates to an individual choice based on the individual's own perceptions of his or her own interests. In *Whalen* v. *Roe*,[57] the Supreme Court characterized the constitutional right of privacy as involving "two different kinds of interests. One is the individual interest in avoiding disclosure of personal matters, and another is the interest in independence in making certain kinds of important decisions."[58]

The application of the privacy right to which the courts have closely analogized the treatment-refusal right was the abortion-related right recognized in *Roe* v. *Wade*.[59] In its most recent relevant pronouncement, the Supreme Court characterized this right as "freedom of personal choice in certain matters of marriage and family choice."[60]

Similarly, the "right to refuse treatment," assuming, *arguendo*, its existence as an element of the constitutional right of privacy, should more properly be seen as a freedom of personal choice concerning what available treatment to accept. What is truly involved here is the *choice* to: (1) accept medical treatment, (2) refuse medical treatment, (3) terminate already existing medical treatment, and (4) choose among alternative medical treatments.

When the privacy right arguably involved is thus understood, it emerges not as an affirmative, substantive protection against particular treatment, but rather as an autonomy-respecting protection against unwanted treatment, and equally, against unwanted termination of treatment. Viewed in this light, the crucial essence of the right is the individual's freedom of choice.

Because the essence of such a right is in the autonomous choice of the individual, to allow substitution of judgment by others purporting to exercise the right on behalf of that individual is not to vindicate that right, but to obviate it. What would be said of a claim that when someone was, by reason of incompetence, unable to vote, a committee must be empowered to cast that vote for him or her, or else the incompetent would unconstitutionally be deprived of the right to vote? A freedom of choice is precisely that: a protection from state interference with a choice one has made. Where no choice is or can be made, there is no constitutional right at issue. If one is unable to make the choice by virtue of incapacity or incompetence, there can be no interference with any right of choice by the state, for the state is not responsible for that incapacity.

The Constitution accords a variety of substantive rights, for example, the right to a jury trial or to the assistance of counsel in one's defense against criminal prosecution. Such rights may often be waived by the person protected by them, but the waiver must be knowing and intelligent. In the absence of such a waiver, a choice to exercise them is presumed. Thus, a defendant who stands mute when asked to plead, or to elect between a jury and a bench trial, is presumed to plead "not guilty" and is given a jury trial if mentally able to stand trial. The Constitution does not permit, let alone compel, the substitution of judgment by which an incompetent defendant could waive such rights "in his best interests." Such a waiver is personal, and must be freely and intelligently made by the individual.

In termination of treatment circumstances, the right to choose concerning one's treatment, arguably an aspect of the right to privacy, is not the only constitutionally protected right at stake. Also involved is the right to life, and the right to equal protection of the law in protection of that right. While the privacy right to "independence in making certain kinds of important decisions,"[61] is value neutral (it simply protects the *choice* of the patient, whatever the choice may be), the right to life is not. The right to life is an affirmative right, just as is the right to a jury trial or the right to the assistance of counsel, and a waiver of life can no more be a proper subject of substituted judgment than can the waiver of a jury or of the assistance of counsel. The legal fiction under which a court or some third party purports to exercise a right of treatment choice, by substituting its judgment of what the individual "would have chosen, if competent" in order to demand termination of treatment, is an intellectually incoherent approach that both vitiates the asserted privacy right and violates the right to life and equal protection of the law.

Thus courts have held that a patient's presumptive right to refuse treatment — a right which, as shown above, cannot exist when the patient is incompetent — may be employed by a third party to deprive the patient of his or her right to life; a right whose existence is not altered or diminished by the patient's incompetence. This illogical

171

conclusion seems based solely on an impulse to obtain, at all costs, the termination of treatment in incompetents.

Moreover, the conclusion that the freedom of an individual to choose or to refuse treatment can be transferred to a third party is not even self-consistent. The common law right to refuse treatment includes the right to refuse *any* form of treatment for oneself, regardless of whether or not one is terminally ill. If this is understood as the nature of the postulated constitutional right as well, and if this right can and must be transferred to another whenever one is incompetent, then there is no logical barrier to concluding that third parties must be able to refuse any and all treatment for the incompetent and incapacitated, regardless of whether or not the treatment could effect a cure or alleviate pain, and regardless of whether or not the incompetent patient is terminal. This would amount to involuntary euthanasia for the incompetent. The courts of New Jersey and Massachusetts which have confronted this issue have, thankfully, not been willing to carry their constitutional doctrine of a right to privacy — exercised by substituted judgment — to this logical, if clearly unacceptable, conclusion. They have wisely limited the exercise of this poorly conceived constitutional right to those terminal cases where curative medical intervention does not exist.

But the danger — and inherent logic — of its future assertion should counsel all courts against adopting the conclusion that a constitutional right of the incompetent mandates granting third parties authority to terminate treatment for them.

Apart from the theoretical incoherence of constitutionally mandating the delegation of a choice right which is inherently personal in nature, such a delegation carries a great potential for abuse. The decisions of those who are delegated this authority may well be influenced by their own values and interests rather than those of the incompetent. The value judgments potentially involved in balancing between the expense, pain, and extreme forms of bodily intrusion associated with some medical treatment, on the one hand, and the prolongation of life, on the other, are intensely personal and subject to a multitude of varying and conflicting resolutions.

Not only is there no guarantee that the value system of a third party will not substantially differ from that of the incompetent individual whose life is in his or her hands, but there may also be a direct conflict of interests. If the third party is a relative, or group of relatives, there may well be a financial advantage to terminating treatment. Less crassly, but with equally grave consequence, there may be a psychological or aesthetic burden to the relative or relatives associated with the incompetent remaining long and indefinitely in that state. If the state is directly involved, or if there is some hospital committee given authority, the decisions will almost certainly be influenced by cost-benefit considerations that have nothing whatever to do with what choice the patient would have made.

To say that such a situation is not merely constitutionally permissible, but constitutionally compelled, in order to vindicate the rights of the incompetent, is to violate fundamental rights and interests under the guise of protecting them. What then becomes of our consensus, or modest conclusion?

The Emerging Consensus

For the incompetent patient, the consensus seems to be that medical treatment may be terminated by a physician when, in his medical judgment, treatment is useless, which is to say that it offers no medically reasonable hope of benefit. Treatment may then be terminated, and the patient allowed to die as the natural consequence of the underlying disease process. The physician is not mandated by the law to render useless treatment. This standard is the same for the competent and the incompetent patient, but is not dramatically at issue in cases involving competents and so is seldom discussed in those terms.

By "useless" it is meant that the continued use of the therapy cannot and does not improve the prognosis for recovery. Even if the therapy is necessary to maintain stability, such therapy should not be mandatory where the ultimate prognosis is hopeless. This does not mean that ordinary means of life-support, such as food and drink, can be discontinued merely because the ultimate prognosis is hopeless. It does mean, however, that physicians can use good practical common medical sense in determining whether or not treatment is efficacious and, if it is not, then to cease the treatment. When the patient is terminal and the end is near, society, through the physician, should be concerned with easing the difficult burden of death with loving care and concern, and not with unduly prolonging the inevitable by officious death bed burdens through over-treatment, over-legislating and requiring court approval for conduct which is better guided by common sense.

173

By "hopeless," it is meant that the prognosis for life (not meaningful life) is very poor. The fact that someone may not return to "sapient or cognitive life" may or may not fulfill the requirement, depending on other medical factors, but in and of itself it does not. Merely being in a coma is not the equivalent of being in a terminal state. The courts have trouble understanding this. However, at this time, we are trying to determine principles by which future medical decisions can be made, and are not interested in mistaken or disputed facts. As was said by the Supreme Court of West Germany:

> Where human life exists, human dignity is present to it; it is not decisive that the bearer of this dignity himself be conscious of it and knows personally how to preserve it.[62]

Withdrawal of treatment and the subsequent death of the patient under these circumstances is not violative of any law, civil or criminal.

The physician who withdraws treatment from the terminally ill patient for whom death is imminent should not be held criminally or civilly liable for such conduct, when the "treatment" merely unduly prolongs the life of the dying patient without holding out any reasonable hope of benefit. Whether treatment is beneficial to the dying patient is, first of all, a matter of medical judgment to be made by a physician. When the physician decides that such treatment is useless, it may be discontinued without fear of liability either criminal or civil.

There are no public policy considerations that warrant imposition of a duty to employ useless treatment; the medical profession does not regard the use of useless or non-beneficial treatment to be medically indicated, or to be "usual or customary" (indeed, the use of such treatment would be contrary to good medical practice); and there is no case law, civil or criminal, that warrants imposition of such a duty.

The physician who withdraws or fails to employ treatment that only briefly forestalls imminent and inevitable death does not legally cause the death of his patient. Such conduct merely allows the underlying disease or illness to run its natural and inevitable course. When treatment that would merely prolong the dying process of a terminally ill patient is appropriately withdrawn or is not employed, this does not legally cause the death of the patient since the patient's death is imminent and would occur in any event. However, the physician's duty to give palliative care, such as food or painkillers, continues even for the terminal patient.

By merely holding that the physician, under such circumstances, is not criminally or civilly liable because he has no duty to employ such treatment, and because he may not legally be deemed to have caused death, courts would avoid the illogical, erroneous, and dangerous rationale which they have pursued under the aegis of an asserted "right of privacy" exercised by way of substituted judgment.

With his obligations under the civil and criminal law thus carefully and clearly defined, the physician would not be obliged to resort to the costly and time-consuming judicial procedure suggested by the *Saikewicz* and *Fox* cases each time he or she withdraws or fails to employ treatment that would only momentarily forestall the time of inevitable death. This solution does not diminish the rights of the patient.

Court intervention is only necessary where the decision is against treatment, and where there does exist life-prolonging or life-saving treatment. Those courts which require court authority before a physician can terminate medical treatment misapprehend the physician's role in these cases. The physician cannot be mandated in the exercise of his medical judgment by the family or the guardian or the court. When, in the exercise of his medical judgment, the physician determines that treatment is useless and the case is hopeless, he may discontinue it. Indeed, he would be violating his own standards of medical practice were he to do otherwise. The fact that the case is a terminal one does not alter the situation. He may terminate the treatment (having decided that it is useless), even if the underlying illness then causes the death of the patient. The family and guardian may concur in that decision, but cannot direct it against the physician's medical judgment. The Massachusetts Supreme Court would go even further and say that, where incompetents are involved, cessation of treatment can only be directed by a court when, after a court proceeding, the court determines that it is in the best interest of the incompetent to do so. Although it has not faced the issue yet, it would presumably say so even against the judgment of the physician, if it were convinced that this is in the best interest of the incompetent.

For the great majority of cases where termination of treatment is warranted, the opinion of the *Dinnerstein* court is the correct one: in the ordinary and usual case where a patient is dying, the choice of treatment is the physician's, and he does not need court authority to do what he, as a responsible physician, has been trained to do: make medical judgments. If that judgment is so ill-used as to violate the homicide or tort laws by abandoning his patient or committing mercy killing, then the law is prepared to deal with those situations as it should. But those situations are not our case. The law should not seek to control an area as sensitive as the death bed by requiring officious and intermeddling standards of legal conduct before medical judgment can be exercised.

Conclusion

The courts and legislatures exercise their proper functions when they set the societal standards for the withdrawal of treatment. This the courts have adequately done in the cases discussed in this paper, in spite of some mistaken facts or procedural confusion. They have properly required that, before treatment may be withdrawn, the patient must be in a terminal state where death is imminent and there exists no form of life-saving medical intervention or where the treatment would only uselessly prolong the dying state without hope of benefit or recovery. These judgments are to be made by the attending physician, and may be concurred in by the family. In those rare cases where there arises a dispute between the physician and family such that it cannot be otherwise resolved, then court proceedings may be necessary.

Requiring court approval in every case, as the *Brother Fox* appellate court opinion did, or when immunity (perhaps illusory) is desired, as do *Saikewicz* and *Spring*, is an inappropriate solution to the problem. Neither the physician nor the dying patient can wait for the slow wheels of justice to grind out a solution. The courts have created a standard, and they must now be satisfied with letting the medical profession exercise its judgment within the parameters of that standard. If physicians violate those standards, then the homicide and tort laws will be called upon to correct the situation. The courts err if they think they can possibly impose upon society an unrealistic and unworkable burden which would require court approval before treatment can be terminated.

Notes

The author wishes to express his indebtedness to, and recognize the assistance of John D. Gorby, Thomas Marzen and Stephen D. Hurst in the preparation of this chapter.

1. Levi, Edward, *The Sovereignity of the Courts,* Occasional papers from the Law School, University of Chicago, No. 17, at p. 16 (1981).

2. McCormick, Richard A., *To Save or Let Die: The Dilemma of Modern Medicine* JAMA 229:172 (1974); Weber, Leonard J.; *Who Shall Live?* 105 (Paulist Press, N.Y. 1976); Duff, Raymond S., *Counseling Families and Deciding Care of Severely Defective Children: A Way of Coping with 'Medical Vietnam',* 67 Pediatrics 315-320, (March 1981).

3. Ramsey, Paul, *The Patient as Person,* 38 (Yale University Press, 1970); Robertson, *Involuntary Euthanasia of Defective Newborns: A Legal Analysis,* 27 Stan.L.Rev. 213-269 (1975); Horan, *Euthanasia, Medical Treatment and the Mongoloid Child: Death as a Treatment of Choice;* Baylor L.Rev. 76-86 (Winter 1975); Fost, *Counseling Families Who Have a Child with a Severe Congenital Anomaly,* 67 Pediatrics 321-324 (March 1981).

4. Byrn, *Compulsory Lifesaving Treatment for the Competent Adult,* 44 Fordham L.Rev. 62 (1975).

5. Kamisar, *Some Non-Religious Views Against Proposed Mercy Killing Legislations* 42 Minn.L.Rev. 969-1042 (May 1958).

6. *People* v. *Conley,* 49 Cal.Rptr. 815, 411 P.2d 911 (1976).

7. Horan, Dennis J., "Euthanasia as a Form of Medical Management," in *Death, Dying and Euthanasia,* ed. by Horan, D. J. and Mall, David, Aletheia Books, University Publications of America, Inc., Frederick, Maryland, 1980, pp. 196-221.

8. Cal. Health and Safety Code Secs. 7185-7195 (1977).

9. Arkansas, Idaho, Nevada, Texas, North Carolina, New Mexico, Oregon; Ark. Stat. Ann Sec. 82-3801-3804 (1977); N.C. Gen. Stat. Sec. 90-320-322 (1977); Idaho Code, Sec. 39-4501 to 4508 (1977); Nev. Rev. Stat. Sec. 449.540-690 (1977); Tex. Health Code Ann. Act. 4590h (1977); An Act Relating to Medical Treatment of Terminally Ill Patients, 33rd Leg. 1st Sess. Ch. 287 1977, New Mexico Laws; Or. Rev. Stat. Sec. 97.050 *et seq.*

10. As of July 15, 1981.

11. Texas has dropped the provision that two weeks must elapse after diagnosis of the terminal treatment before a directive can take effect. The 5 year limitation has also been removed. North Carolina has changed the brain death section and clarified a section that deals with incompetency. It now allows a notary public to witness such wills.

12. Horan, D. and Marzen, T., *Death with Dignity and the Living Will,* 5 Notre Dame J. of Leg., 81-88 (1978); Horan, D. "Right-to-Die Laws: Creating, Not Clarifying Problems" in *Hospital Progress* Vol. 59, No. 6, pp. 62-65, 78 (June 1978).

13. Because of its brevity we are here setting the Arkansas Act out in its entirety:

BE IT ENACTED BY THE GENERAL ASSEMBLY OF THE STATE OF ARKANSAS

SECTION 1. Every person shall have the right to die with dignity and to refuse and deny the use or application by any person of artificial, extraordinary, extreme or radical medical or surgical means or procedures calculated to prolong his life. Alternatively, every person shall have the right to request that such extraordinary means be utilized to prolong life to the extent possible.

SECTION 2. Any person, with the same formalities as are required by the laws of this State for the execution of a will, may execute a document exercising such right and refusing and denying the use or application by any person of artificial, extraordinary, extreme or radical medical or surgical means or procedures calculated to prolong his life. In the alternative, any person may request in writing that all means be utilized to prolong life.

SECTION 3. If any person is a minor or an adult who is physically or mentally unable to execute or is otherwise incapacitated from executing either document, it may be executed in the same form on his behalf:

(a) By either parent of the minor;

(b) By his spouse;

(c) If his spouse is unwilling or unable to act, by his child aged eighteen or over;

(d) If he has no spouse or child aged eighteen or over, by either of his parents;

(f) If he has no parent living, by his nearest living relative; or

(g) If he is mentally incompetent, by his legally appointed guardian. Provided, that a form executed in compliance with this Section must contain a signed statement by two physicians that extraordinary means would have to be utilized to prolong life.

SECTION 4. Any person, hospital or other medical institution which acts or refrains from acting in reliance on and in compliance with such document shall be immune from liability otherwise arising out of such failure to use or apply artificial, extraordinary, extreme or radical medical or surgical means or procedures calculated to prolong such person's life.

SECTION 5. All laws and parts of laws in conflict with this Act are hereby repealed.

14. Grisez, Germain, "Suicide and Euthanasia," in *Death, Dying, and Euthanasia, supra,* note 75 at 742-817.

15. This is so since the competent adult's right to reject medical treatment has been universally recognized by the courts. Byrn, *Compulsory Lifesaving Treatment for the Competent Adult,* 44 Fordham L.Rev. Rev. 62 (Oct. 1975).

16. We wish to distinguish at this point medical treatment from food and sustenance and other care. The words "medical treatment" and/or "treatment" as used in this chapter always refer to specific modalities of medical care such as, for example, surgery or a respirator. Termination of medical treatment does not mean termination of medical care. Even after the specific modality of treatment has been terminated, other means of medical care, as appropriate, continue. Obviously, sustenance and amelioration of pain continue, as does the general obligation to continue to see that another human being receives care until such time as all medical care becomes useless, as only prolonging an inevitable and imminent natural death.

17. *In re Quinlan,* 70 N.J. 10, 355 A.2d 647 (1976), *cert. denied sub. nom. Gorger* v. *New Jersey,* 429 U.S. 992 (1976).

18. 70 N.J. at 11.

19. See sections of Quinlan opinion marked "Declaratory Relief" and "conclusion".

20. Horan, Dennis J. and Halligan, Patrick D., "Informed Consent", in *Defense of Medical Malpractice,* 4-1 through 4-74 (Ill.Inst. for CLE, 1980).

21. This is so since the action for lack of informed consent presumes that that procedure is done without negligence. Where negligence in the performance of the medical services is present, plaintiff's counsel will always rely on proving that negligence, since to do so enhances both his chances for recovery and the size of his recovery.

22. *Superintendent of Belcher Town School v. Joseph Saikewicz* 373 Mass. 728, 370 N.E.2d 417 (1977).

23. 370 N.E.2d at 420.

24. *In the Matter of Shirley Dinnerstein,* 380 N.E.2d 134 (Mass.App.Ct. 1978).

25. *In the Matter of Earle N. Spring,* 405 N.E.2d 115 (Mass. 1980).

26. 370 N.E.2d at 431.

27. *Matter of Shirley Dinnerstein,* 380 N.E.2d 134 (Mass. App. Ct. 1978).

28. 380 N.E.2d at 137-138.

29. *Supra,* note 25.

30. 405 N.E.2d at 118.

31. *Id.* at. 120.

32. *Id.*

33. *Id.*

34. *Id.* at 121.

35. *Id.* at 122.

36. *Id.*

37. *Id.*

38. In the Matter of Father Philip K. Eichner, S.M., on behalf of Brother Joseph Charles Fox, Nassau County New York, Supreme Court, 73 A.D.2d 431, decided March 27, 1980, Slip Opinion at 1-73.

39. *Id.* at 46-47.

40. In the Matter of John Storar, State of New York Court of Appeals, decided March 31, 1981, Slip opinion.

41. *Id.* at 10.

42. *Id.* at 12.

43. *Id.* at 14-15.

44. *Id.* at 16.

45. *Id.* at 17.

46. *See, e.g.* Annas, George J. *Help from the Dead: The Cases of Brother Fox and John Storar,* The Hastings Center Report, 19-20 (June 1981). George Annas is a director of the Society for the Right to Die.

47. Curran, William J., *Court Involvement in Right-to-Die Cases: Judicial Inquiry in New York,* 305 N.Eng.J. of Med., No. 2, 75, 76 (July 9, 1981).

48. *Id.* at 76.

49. 421 A.2d 1334 (Del.Sup. 1980).

50. *Id.* at 1346. *Cf. Satz* v. *Perlmutter,* 379 S.2d 359 (Fla. Sup. Ct. 1980) (suggesting enactment of a comprehensive legislative scheme to deal with the termination of treatment problem.)

51. *Id.* at 1349.

52. *Id.*

53. *Custody of A Minor,* 375 Mass. 733, 379 N.E.2d 1053 (Mass. 1978).

54. *Maine Medical Center v. Houle,* No. 74-145 Superior Court, Cumberland, Maine, decided February 14, 1974. See also, *In the Matter of Kevin Sampson,* 317 N.Y.S.2d 641 S.Ct.N.Y. 1972); *In the Matter of Webberlist,* 360 N.Y.S.2d 873 (S.Ct.N.Y. 1974).

55. *In the Application of Cicero,* 421 N.Y.S.2d 965 (S.Ct.N.Y. 1979).

56. *Satz v. Perlmutter,* 379 So.2d 359 (Fla. 1980).

57. 429 U.S. 589 (1977).

58. *Id.* at 599-600.

59. 410 U.S. 113 (1973).

60. *Harris* v. *McRae,* 100 S.Ct. 2671, 2686, 448 U.S. 297, (1980).

61. *Whalen* v. *Roe,* 429 U.S. 600 (1977).

62. Gorby, *West German Abortion Decision: A Contrast to Roe v. Wade,* 9 J. Marsh. J. of Prac. and Pro. 551, 559-60 (Spring 1976).

Chapter 12

Contemporary American Opinion on Euthanasia

William J. Monahan, Ph. D.

Introduction

Public opinion pollers have set for themselves the difficult task of identifying, with quantitative precision, the opinions of the American people on a variety of issues. As indicators of contemporary American thinking on prolonging life, the results of public opinion polls on euthanasia will be presented in this paper. The question of euthanasia was first raised in such polls in 1936 and continues to be asked, though with variations in wording. The results of these polls are unambiguous: the proportion of Americans favoring euthanasia has grown steadily to over half the population. This chapter will present and discuss briefly that growth in support and then present some qualifying factors which should be taken into account regarding this sobering phenomenon.

1) Opinions on Euthanasia

From 1936 to 1978, public opinion in favor of euthanasia has grown to over half the population, following a sharp drop in support in the years immediately following World War II.

Although the wording of questions has varied through the years since the Gallup Poll first queried about euthanasia in 1936, the opinion poll results are unequivocal in showing increasing public support for some form of the direct taking of human life in extreme medical situations. Results of the Gallup Poll and other opinion polls trace this general development of support in Table 1 as follows:

TABLE 1
EUTHANASIA

	1936	1939	1947	1950	1973	1977	1978
Favor euthanasia	46%	46%	37%	36%	53%	59%	58%
Do not favor euthanasia	54%	54%	54%	64%*	40%	36%	38%
No opinion (or don't know/ not ascertained)	—	—	9%	—	7%	5%	4%
	100%	100%	100%	100%	100%	100%	100%

Sources
1936, 1939, 1947and 1950: George H. Gallup, *THE GALLUP POLL: PUBLIC OPINION, 1935-1971.* American Institute of Public Opinion. New York: Random House, 1972. Three Volumes. Vol. 1: *1936*, p. 46; *1939*, p. 151; *1947*, p. 656; Vol. 2: *1950*, p. 887.

1973: George H. Gallup, *THE GALLUP POLL: PUBLIC OPINION, 1972-1977.* American Institute of Public Opinion. Wilmington, Delaware: Scholarly Resources, Inc. Two Volumes. Vol. 1: *1973*, p. 143-144.

1977 and 1978: James A. Davis, *General Social Surveys, 1972-1978: Cumulative Data.* Chicago: National Opinion Research Center, 1978, pp. 139-140. Cited in paper by Raymond J. Adamek, "Some Major Polls on Euthanasia and Suicide," Department of Sociology and Anthropology, Kent State University, Kent, Ohio, p. 2.

*The categories, "No and No opinion," were combined in reporting the 1950 survey results.

As a fortunate starting point, the wording of the Gallup Poll question on euthanasia was the same the first two times the pollsters posed it. The 1936 and 1939 questions were as follows:

"Do you favor mercy deaths under government supervision for hopeless invalids?"

This question clearly deals with direct, active euthanasia. The respondents were stable in their opposition to it: a majority of 54% being opposed in both survey years. Although persons opposed to euthanasia can take comfort in the fact that a numerical majority opposed this procedure, it is nonetheless evident that a sizable proportion of respondents favored euthanasia some forty-five years ago.

The Gallup Poll next raised the question of euthanasia in 1947. The question was as follows:

"When a person has a disease that cannot be cured, do you think doctors should be allowed by law to end the patient's life by some painless means if the patient and his family request it?"

The question had grown since the 1936 and 1939 versions and embodied a more personal, if not persuasive, tone. Notably, the question refers to agents of euthanasia, "doctors," whereas the earlier versions referred to, "government supervision." The 1947 question explicitly refers to the support of the law, a factor implied in the earlier questions, and spells out "painless means" and the consent of the patient and his/her family. Most notable of all is the fact that the category of those subject to euthanasia had expanded from "hopeless invalids" in the 1936 and 1939 versions to "a person who has a disease that cannot be cured." The continuation of the question later refers to the "patient's life."

Respondents opposed this elaborated question in the same proportions as they had in 1936 and 1939, namely, 54%. A smaller proportion gave direct support to it, 37%, while 9% fell into the newly-introduced category of "no opinion." Opposition to euthanasia had remained steady and even increased, if we consider the reduction in the proportion of those who directly favored it.

What explains this enhanced opposition to euthanasia? We can only offer conjecture. First, the people of America close on the heels of World War II may have simply seen enough of the direct taking of life. On the other hand, the wording of this question appropriately brings

182

the issue out of the abstract realm of "governmental supervision" and speaks of "doctors . . . patient's life . . . his family . . ." The question has grown more real and immediate. Most respondents backed off from it; 37% supported it.

Opposition and support held steady in almost exactly the same proportions when the Gallup Poll used the exact 1947 wording again in 1950. As Table 1 indicates, 36% supported euthanasia and 64% opposed it or had no opinion.

A review of the index of the Gallup Poll indicates that they did not raise the euthanasia question again until 1973. A significant shift in opinion occurred in the interim. The pollsters again used the exact wording of the 1947 and 1950 questions, i.e.:

"When a person has a disease that cannot be cured, do you think doctors should be allowed by law to end the patient's life by some painless means if the patient and his family request it?"

For the first time, a numerical majority favored euthanasia. As Table 1 shows, 53% responded affirmatively to this question, 40% negatively, and 7% had no opinion. The sizable minority of respondents consistently in favor of euthanasia had grown to a majority.

The most immediate interpretation of this increased support for euthanasia is that people had simply changed their thinking about the value of human life in the two-plus decades since 1950. In corroboration of that statement, we can look at the Gallup Polls on abortion. The polls taken in 1969 and 1974 show an increase from 40 to 47% of those who favor abortion during the first trimester. The obvious intervening factor here was the Supreme Court decision of January, 1973, permitting abortion within the first trimester. Such approbation would serve as a catalyst for those for whom legality serves as a criterion for morality. No such judicial approval of euthanasia took place, nonetheless, support for euthanasia also increased. A significant increase in support of abortion occurred within a part of the period in which support for euthanasia increased. Recent American history has seen an erosion of respect for life within medical settings, for it is precisely there where abortions are carried out and where euthanasia would be practiced. (Needless to say, the value of life has deteriorated in other settings. The reported rates of violent crimes have doubled in post-World War II America. One gets the sense of a great assault on life in this country.)

Returning to the issue of euthanasia, we can refer to recent data prepared by Raymond J. Adamek which indicates that acceptance of euthanasia by over half the population is well-established. In 1977 and 1978, the National Opinion Research Center posed the same question used by the Gallup Polls on euthanasia in 1947, 1950 and 1973.

> "When a person has a disease that cannot be cured, do you think doctors should be allowed by law to end the patient's life by some painless means if the patient and his family request it?"

In 1977, 59% of the respondents answered "yes," and in 1978, 58% likewise answered affirmatively, as shown in Table 1.

Within the same period of the mid-seventies, pollster Louis Harris inquired about the issue of simply allowing people to die as distinguished from the direct taking of a patient's life. Adamek has also prepared material on the results of two such questions raised by *The Harris Survey*.

> "All doctors take an oath saying they will maintain, restore and prolong human life in their treatment of patients. It is now argued by some people that in many cases people with terminal diseases (those which can only end in death) have their lives prolonged unnecessarily, which makes them endure much pain and suffering for no real reason. (sic) Do you think a patient with a terminal disease ought to be able to tell his doctor to let him die rather than extend his life when no cure is in sight, or do you think this is wrong?"

	1973	1977
Ought to be allowed	62%	71%
Think is wrong	28%	18%
Not sure	10%	11%
	100%	100%

It is difficult to interpret the above question in moral terms. Does the final sentence, the question proper, refer to "passive euthanasia," in the sense of withdrawing the ethically ordinary means for support of life or does it refer to the elimination of ethically extraordinary measures to sustain life? Some clarification would be necessary before a statement could be made about the American people's opinions on these two very distinct steps in dealing with the terminally ill. Despite this ambiguity, opinion is strongly in favor of some generally passive means of not prolonging the life of the terminally ill. The following question is more clearly one of withdrawing extraordinary means to support life.

"There have been cases where a patient is terminally ill, in a coma and not conscious, with no cure in sight. Do you think that the family of such a patient ought to be able to tell doctors to remove all life support services and let the patient die, or do you think this is wrong?"

	1973	1977
Ought to be allowed	—	66%
Think is wrong	—	19%
Not sure	—	15%
		100%

Support for these passive measures of allowing the terminally ill to die is considerably stronger than for direct measures or euthanasia. Nonetheless, there remains a sizable pocket of people who oppose passive measures and who would presumably benefit from some information on their moral obligations to terminally ill patients.

Interestingly enough, Harris also asked about the direct taking of a terminally ill patient's life in language that was bolder than that used by Gallup. Harris' results (below) show lower levels of support for euthanasia than found by Gallup and the National Opinion Research Center for the same years.

"Do you think the patient who is terminally ill, with no cure in sight, ought to have the right to tell his doctor to put him out of his misery, or do you think this is wrong?"

	1973	1977
Ought to be allowed	37%	49%
Think is wrong	53%	38%
Not sure	10%	13%
	100%	100%

Harris' results place support for euthanasia at below the 50% mark, but do confirm a trend of increasing acceptance of the idea of the direct taking of a patient's life.

To conclude this part of the consideration of opinion polls regarding euthanasia, we can say the following:
1) At least half of the American people support the idea of direct mercy killing or euthanasia;

185

2) This support is growing;

3) At least two-thirds of the American people support some form of withdrawal of life-support systems from the terminally ill;

4) The remaining one-third of the population would benefit from some education regarding the morality of extraordinary measures of preserving life.

2) Some Qualifications on These Opinions

Opinions do not take shape in a personal or social vacuum, as all would readily agree. The straightforward reporting of opinions favorable or unfavorable to euthanasia without any discussion of qualifying factors leaves one wondering about the influence of such factors as sex, age, education and family situations on the respondents' views of euthanasia. But before entering into this discussion of the influence of personal and social characteristics, it is worth noting that even a change in the wording of the questions reduced the responses in favor of euthanasia.

Personal Responsibility

In 1975, the Gallup Poll raised the following question:

"Do you think a person has the moral right to end his or her life when this person has a disease that is incurable?"

Respondents replied in these proportions:

Yes	40%
No	53%
No Opinion	7%
	100%

These results stand in rather sharp contrast to the responses found in the 1973 poll in which 53% of the respondents favored euthanasia (see Table 1). In 1973, the question was posed in general terms:

"When a person has a disease that cannot be cured, do you think doctors should be allowed by law to end the patient's life by some painless means if the patient and his family request it?"

Thus, when the question of euthanasia becomes one of establishing a personal, moral right to end one's life in the face of an incurable disease, respondents are more reluctant to answer in favor of this right than they are to favor granting legal authority to a doctor to do so in consultation with the patient and his/her family. This suggests that the respondents saw a kind of moral safety in numbers, whereas they were less willing to assert an individual right to euthanasia.

In the same poll, the Gallup interviewers heightened the question by adding the factor of great pain. Respondents replied in almost exactly the same proportion in terms of unwillingness to grant a personal moral right to end one's life.

"Do you think a person has the moral right to end his or her life when this person is suffering great pain and has no hope for improvement?"

Yes 41%
No 51%
No Opinion 8%

100%

Family Relationships

When the issue becomes one of being a burden to one's family, rather than great pain and incurability of disease, respondents were even more unwilling to concede a personal, moral right to euthanasia.

"Do you think a person has the moral right to end his or her life when this person is an extremely heavy burden on his or her family?"

Yes 20%
No 72%
No Opinion 8%

100%

The above data indicate that most respondents do not see being a burden to one's family as justification for taking one's life. This suggests an affirmation of family relationships in the face of serious illness. The invocation of family ties seems to elicit a sense of support and a choice of life, rather than being a reason for ending life.

Age

In the Gallup Polls for 1939 through 1973, discussed above, persons 50 and older were consistently those least favorable to euthanasia. From 1939 to 1973, the support of this age group for euthanasia did not increase significantly, overall. Those favoring euthanasia were 41% in 1939, 30% in 1950 and 44% in 1973. In the same period, general support for euthanasia grew slightly more significantly. (The influence of age was not available in the data reported from other sources for 1977 and 1978.)

Summary of Selected Characteristics

Raymond J. Adamek, cited above, has prepared a table of Selected Characteristics of persons who responded "yes" to the same question on euthanasia asked in Gallup Polls of 1950 and 1973.

"When a person has a disease that cannot be cured, do you think doctors should be allowed by law to end the patient's life by some painless means if the patient and his family request it?"

Percent Saying "Yes," 1950 and 1973,
by Selected Characteristics

	1950	1973
Total Sample	36	53
Men	38	53
Women	34	53
College	42	61
High School	39	54
Grade School	31	39
Under 30 Years	39	67
30-49 Years	37	51
50 & Over	30	44

Men formerly showed stronger support for euthanasia, but support was equal between the sexes in 1973. The favoring of euthanasia increases with education and decreases with age, when these factors are considered by themselves. Support for euthanasia has grown in all the categories considered, with the rate of growth being least among those with only a grade school education. The college-educated are the strongest single bloc in support of euthanasia.

Technical Considerations

A statistical critique of the way in which the Gallup Poll and other public opinion polls are conducted would be beyond the scope of this paper and the competence of the author. Suffice it to say that the Gallup Poll and the other major opinion polls have established a solid record of accuracy in estimating national opinion through the use of small and highly-defined samples. Although the 1980 presidential elections proved troublesome for the public opinion pollsters, such polls in the long run have a good record. In 1978, the Gallup Poll reported that it enjoyed an "Average Deviation for 22 National Elections" of 2.2 percentage points and an "Average Deviation for 15 National Elections since 1950, inclusive," of 1.4 percentage points.

For the purposes of our consideration of national attitudes toward prolonging life decisions, it is appropriate to assume the statistical accuracy of the percentages reported for particular responses and examine the meaning of people's responses. We can ask what do people's responses to a particular question mean in terms of subsequent behavior?

A basic problem of opinion surveys is the instability of the connection between the expression of an opinion and the taking of action consistent with that opinion. One might safely say that the more emotional the issue, the more unstable the connection between the expression of opinion and action consistent with that opinion. Opinions are expressed in the emotionally-sanitized situation of an interview. The respondent feels no expectation of acting on his/her words and, through the assurance of anonymity, is even relieved of responsibility for having uttered them.

Action necessarily involves responsibility, the certainty of consequences for oneself and others. Action also implies the presence of other people and their direct or indirect reactions to what one does. All of this usually results in feelings on the part of the one acting, particularly where the matter is serious. One could hardly imagine a more serious or emotion-fraught situation than making a decision to act directly to end one's own life or the life of another, frequently a loved one. The public opinion interview could hardly capture the effect of such emotions on one's decision to prolong life. Thus, stated opinions about prolonging life would have to be qualified by the lack of emotion in the interview setting. When confronted with such a decision in real life, many of those expressing an opinion in favor of euthanasia are likely to be unwilling to act on this opinion.

Nonetheless, whatever the slippage between opinion and action, a steadily increasing proportion of Americans, now well over half, favors euthanasia. Such widespread support, if only at the level of opinions, creates an ambience in which more determined efforts must be made to apply Christian criteria in making decisions to prolong life.

— o —

The author makes grateful acknowledgement to Jean Heithaus, Saint Louis University, and Firooz K. Hekmat, Missouri Institute of Psychiatry, for their assistance in preparing this chapter.

Bibliography

Raymond J. Adamek, "Some Major Polls on Euthanasia and Suicide," Department of Sociology and Anthropology, Kent State University, Kent, Ohiio.

James A. Davis, *General Social Surveys, 1972-1978: Cumulative Data* (Chicago: National Opinion Research Center, 1978). Cited in Paper by Raymond J. Adamek, "Some Major Polls on Euthanasia and Suicide," Department of Sociology and Anthropology, Kent State University, Kent, Ohio.

George H. Gallup, *The Gallup Poll: Public Opinion, 1935-1971* American Institute of Public Opinion. (New York: Random House, 1972.) Three Volumes.

George H. Gallup, *The Gallup Poll: Public Opinion, 1972-1977* American Institute of Public Opinion .(Wilmington, Delaware: Scholarly Resources, Inc.) Two Volumes.

George H. Gallup, *The Gallup Poll: Public Opinion, 1978* American Institute of Public Opinion. (Wilmington, Delaware: Scholarly Resources, Inc.) One Volume.

Part III

Clinical and Pastoral Applications

Introduction

The previous eight chapters, in Part II, have described moral responsibility in prolonging life as involving two elements. These are: 1) a prudential *judgment* to estimate what are reasonable and available medical treatments and procedures, and, 2) a morally obligatory *decision* to employ such procedures, while other possible treatments or procedures remain morally optional for the individual. The prudential *judgment* must take into account both the medical prognosis and non-medical factors such as the burden which a treatment presents. The *decision* derives its obligatory aspect from each person's responsible stewardship of the gift of human life.

This approach occupies a middle ground between two extremes. According to one extreme, moral responsibility would routinely mandate every possible medical treatment or procedure. According to the other extreme, each individual makes a completely arbitrary choice of which, if any, medical treatments and procedures will be employed. Thus, this middle approach situates itself between the extremes of medical-moral scrupulosity, on the one hand, and medical-moral laxity, on the other.

But this middle approach demands more study, consultation, and serious moral deliberation than either of the two extremes. As a result, the remaining eight chapters of this resource book turn to clinical and pastoral applications of this middle approach. Each chapter reflects one of the seminars at the three Institutes from which this volume originated.

In chapters 13 to 15, Father Donald G. McCarthy, Director of Education of the Pope John Center in St. Louis, discusses three kinds of cases which frequently occasion prolonging life decisions. He applies the ethical reflections of chapters 8 and 9 to these cases with particular discussion of the various perspectives of patients, their families, and the health care team and pastoral advisors.

In chapter 16, Father Albert S. Moraczewski, O.P., Vice-President for Research of the Pope John Center, studies cases of a related but different nature — cases where a person desires to die, but is not terminally ill. Here the conscience of the person may well be so burdened with suffering and fear that the sense of moral responsibility toward life itself has been overshadowed or smothered.

In the final four chapters, the same two authors present practical applications of the prolonging life principles of this volume to the roles and responsibilities of the four groups of professional persons most directly involved: administrators of health care facilities, physicians, nurses, and pastoral care persons. Pastoral care persons who are involved in prolonging life decisions often include parish clergy, so the final chapter will interest them particularly. These four chapters originated with discussions held in St. Louis, Tampa, and Phoenix with groups of such professional persons and reflect their own concerns and contributions.

These eight chapters of Part III exemplify genuinely prudential judgments about life-prolonging treatments and procedures. Without such judgments, decisions cannot be correctly made which will reflect the middle approach between moral scrupulosity and laxity.

Chapter 13

Care of Persons in the Final Stage of Terminal Illness or Irreversibly Comatose

The Reverend Donald G. McCarthy, Ph. D.

Introduction

This chapter focuses on the care of persons who are either irreversibly comatose or in the final stage of terminal illness. The former group are unable to be consulted about their care, and the latter group comprises persons usually too drained of life and energy to participate very actively in prolonging life decisions. The persons who represent these patients, normally close family members, must make decisions in their behalf.

The model for health care decisions suggested in this volume is that of responsible stewardship of human life. Hence both the health care professionals and these helpless patients and their representatives are challenged to guide their decisions by the general norm of responsible stewardship based on reverence for the priceless gift of human life.

Because the persons discussed in this chapter are in a medically hopeless condition, responsible stewardship, as understood here, does not necessarily entail scientific efforts to further prolong life, though it surely does mandate maximum comfort and palliative therapy and it likewise strenuously forbids interventions to shorten or terminate life.

The successful development of life-support technology has led to the difficulties discussed above in chapters three and four: the possible maintenance of a dead person in a condition of simulated life. If the artificial support of heart and lung activity has masked the actual death of a patient, responsible stewardship of human life no longer enters into decision-making efforts. As already indicated, a legal and medical consensus has developed which would certify death upon the total and irreversible cessation of all brain functions, including that of the brain stem.

If competent physicians have carefully verified this condition, they may pronounce that death has occurred, even in the face of apparent circulatory and respiratory activity which is artificially supported. Since they are acting upon a medical examination for which they must accept professional responsibility and liability, they do not need consent of a patient's representative to pronounce that death has occurred.

On the other hand, family members and even nursing staff who witness the artificially supported circulatory and respiratory activity of the patient, now pronounced dead, deserve an explanation why the diagnosis has been made. In one of the seminars on this subject a physician suggested that a temporary 3-5 minute withdrawal of the life support can be used to show the family that spontaneous life has ended. In cases where a patient qualifies for this determination of death by brain criteria rather suddenly because of trauma or accident, the family may be particularly unbelieving of the diagnosis. In such cases the diagnosis may appropriately be postponed for a reasonable period of time until the family can realize what has happened. In the face of continuing non-acceptance by the family, the physician in charge may choose to seek further consultation with hospital administration and even legal counsel before pronouncing death and removing life support equipment.

However, this chapter concerns the appropriate care of persons who are not yet dead. If they are irreversibly comatose one might classify them as "virtually dead" or "practically dead," but such terminology only confuses the situation. Some physicians would prefer to have a method of classifying even these persons as dead in order to withdraw life-support equipment without fear of liability for neglect or negligent homicide.

The tradition of stewardship of life followed in this volume insists on continuing to recognize irreversibly comatose persons as *living persons* who must not be killed or falsely declared dead by new criteria of death. However, this same tradition recognizes limits to the responsibility to prolong life so that it *does* permit withdrawal of life-support in given situations, even though death may then occur. Some persons assume that, if death occurs, the act of withdrawal must be classified as an act of killing, despite the careful discussion presented in this volume. The Karen Quinlan case, decided by the New Jersey Supreme Court in 1976, recognized the legitimacy of withdrawing life-support for the irreversibly comatose even though death might follow.

Within the tradition of stewardship and reverence for human life the withdrawal of life-support procedures is morally acceptable in terms of two considerations:

1) the ethically extraordinary and therefore optional nature of the medical procedure in this case, and
2) the consent of the patient or patient's representative to forego the ethically extraordinary treatment.

The remainder of this chapter will first reflect upon the situations of irreversibly comatose persons and persons in the final stage of terminal illness, and then offer some relevant concerns from the perspectives of physicians, nursing staff, and pastoral care or social service counselors.

Irreversibly Comatose Persons

As described in chapter 9 by Fr. Connery, if a medical treatment becomes an unreasonable burden, it may be omitted without moral fault. On this basis the use of a respirator may be discontinued when physicians have reached medical certainty that a comatose condition is irreversible. Since one can conclude with certainty that the respirator no longer constitutes ethically ordinary and obligatory treatment, the physician should not be considered morally obligated to provide it. Yet, out of respect for the patient's rights, the decision to withdraw it should be made in consultation with the patient's representative. Whether the patient should be expected to have made an anticipatory statement of intention to forego such procedures in such events has been a matter of some legal discussions. Morally, it seems sufficient that the patient's representatives make a decision conforming as far as possible to their understanding of the patient's probable wishes. It cannot be simply presumed that in all cases an ethically extraordinary procedure would always be omitted, but in the case of irreversible coma that presumption becomes very strong.

One might even question whether artificial feeding need be continued for an irreversibly comatose person. Moralists have admitted the plausibility of this position, but it has not been tested in the courts, and the instinctive urge not to cease nourishing a living human being resists this option. One might more easily accept the option of not initiating artificial feeding for an irreversibly comatose person, but, in practice, artificial feeding is often necessary for a long period of care before the comatose condition can be medically determined to be irreversible.

In cases of a coma which accompanies the final stage of a terminal illness such as cancer, the irreversibility of the coma may not be definitively determined, but the irreversibility of the terminal illness may be so determined. Hence the prolonging of such a comatose condition can be discussed as the final stage of terminal illness.

Persons in Final Stage of Terminal Illness

Obviously no precise point can be determined as the threshold of the final stage of terminal illness. In general, the term as used here means that point in terminal illness when an attending physician can observe clear signs of impending death within a matter of a few days.

The case of Dr. R. was cited in one of our seminars. Dr. R. had practiced in St. Z. Hospital for 30 years and was now a patient there, dying of cancer. He had been put on a respirator by his friend, the attending physician. After he became comatose his wife and his son, a practicing lawyer, requested that the respirator be removed. The physician refused, even after the administrator of the hospital seconded the request. Dr. R. survived another week and then expired while still on the respirator.

Since the respirator was prolonging a comatose and terminal condition it could readily be judged ethically extraordinary and removable in Dr. R's case. The consent to remove it came from the wife and son who can be assumed to conform their decision to their understanding of the patient's probable wishes. Unless the attending physician was convinced that they misjudged the patient's own wishes, it seems the physician acted improperly and in a manner of medical scrupulosity.

Another kind of case involving a respirator is that of Mr. M., suffering from chronic pulmonary insufficiency because of Black Lung disease. The repirator here became an important instrument of comfort by assisting breathing long before Mr. M. reached the final stage of terminal illness. When Mr. M. was put on the respirator it was a useful form of medical treatment. It did not constitute a burden but a relief from the burden of labored breathing. Hence one could not readily describe the respirator as ethically extraordinary for Mr. M. on such grounds. This case did not reach a point at which Mr. M. lapsed into deep coma so there was never a consideration of withdrawing the respirator.

Looking at cases like that of Mr. M., one does find that respirator therapy significantly prolongs people's lives at great expense to their reimbursement agency or even their own personal resources. On this ground, one may suggest that such therapy can be considered ethically extraordinary. However, since reimbursement programs are often designed to cover such large expenses, those who benefit need not hesitate to accept the expensive treatment. If reimbursement does not cover the therapy in cases like Mr. M.'s, the financial concern could legitimately dictate less expensive treatment. Mr. M.'s family, for example, would not be strictly obligated to go into serious debt for his treatment, though this may readily happen because of their sincere love and concern for a dying family member.

The final stage of terminal illness remains totally individual according to each person's previous health and strength and other imponderable factors. Hospice staff workers have seen patients hang onto life until the return of a family member from out of town or until an observance of a 50th wedding anniversary. Thus it seems that sometimes, even without significant medical intervention, persons may themselves prolong the final stage of terminal illness until they are ready to "let go" of life.

Another case presented in one of our seminars described Mr. H., a 75-year-old man who lived alone without near relatives, who fell and broke his fibula. He was brought into the hospital, an unidentified mass was noticed in his abdomen, and he contracted pneumonia. He indicated to the nurses that he didn't want to live, but they and the physicians were hesitant to abandon treatment.

Ethically speaking, initial treatment of the pneumonia and the broken fibula would seem to be ordinary means of prolonging life, offering reasonable hope of benefit to Mr. H. without excess pain, expense, or other hardship. Hence physicians would presume to provide ordinary treatment unless clearly forbidden by a competent patient's well-considered refusal of treatment. In Mr. H.'s case, one might anticipate some subsequent hesitation by the physicians regarding treatment of the abdominal mass, and the possible consideration of surgery as ethically extraordinary if the mass were malignant with evidence of possible metastasis.

In fact, decisions about cancer treatment often hinge on the degree of expected hope of benefit. Oncologists who recommend radiation and chemotherapy must try to estimate and inform patients of the expected benefit and side effects of treatment. A patient may decide in good conscience that a treatment does not offer sufficient hope of benefit or involves excess suffering or other hardship.

On the other hand, Mrs. T. was a 72 year old woman living in a nursing home. When the physician discovered a small but malignant tumor on her breast he recommended immediate removal and felt sure he could remove it completely. Mrs. T.'s daughter persuaded her to refuse the surgery, possibly because of her own fear of hospitals. Mrs. T. died a rather painful death within a few months. By objective standards the surgical removal of the tumor might well have been an ordinary and ethically obligatory means of prolonging life.

The roles of physicians, nursing staff, and pastoral care and social service counselors in the care of persons who are in the final stage of terminal illness or irreversibly comatose call for sensitivity, patience, and sustained efforts to communicate honestly with both patients and their families.

The Role of Physicians

A physician at one of our seminars commented that throughout medical school he had never been taught how to care for the dying or communicate with them. The last decade has seen enormous progress in this area, thanks especially to the pioneering work of Dr. Elizabeth Kubler-Ross. This progress comes none too soon as the need of such communication continues to grow with the advance of medical expertise. If physicians are to allow patients the option of foregoing unnecessary treatments to prolong life, they must be able to discuss with them calmly and comfortably death itself and the final stages of life. It has become axiomatic that physicians who deny death or cannot face their own mortality cannot comfortably communicate with dying patients.

Another major responsibility of physicians is pain management. The fear of addiction from analgesics should be forgotten in the final stage of terminal illness. Catholic medical ethics has always admitted the use of sufficient medication to relieve pain even though such a dosage may shorten life. Thus, Directive #29 of the *Ethical and Religious Directives for Catholic Health Facilities* states:

> "It is not euthanasia to give a dying person sedatives and analgesics for the alleviation of pain, when such a measure is judged necessary, even though they may deprive the patient of the use of reason, or shorten his life."

The *Declaration on Euthanasia*, issued in June, 1980, by the Sacred Congregation for the Doctrine of the Faith, confirmed this teaching. Obviously, one should seek to avoid life-shortening pain medication, but, when it becomes medically appropriate, death need in no way be intended or sought, even if the risk of it is involved. Shortening life can be seen as the unintended evil effect which follows the intended good effect of relieving pain. The distinctness of these two effects can be emphasized by pointing out that in some circumstances the use of proper pain medication produces another, equally unintended and secondary but desirable effect, the lengthening of life.

The increasing popularity of the British hospice movement of care for the dying in the United States has heightened interest in Brompton's mixture, a popular liquid pain medication used in Britain.[1] However, many American physicians prefer their own recipes for pain medication and prefer to vary the recipe according to side effects and individual circumstances. They generally concur in the appropriateness of the hospice practice of providing pain medication according to a patient's needs, rather than by a strict formula of set time intervals.

Medications like Brompton's mixture can be provided to dying patients in their homes. Attending physicians often prefer to put a family member in charge of administering them to avoid confusion if the patient has lost alertness. The hospice movement supports patients and families when a patient comes home to die and, generally, about half of hospice patients are able to die in their own home.

Physicians themselves often admit that the most difficult period in caring for a dying patient occurs when they have no more therapeutic treatment to offer. Acute care hospitals understandably hesitate to continue hospitalization for such patients and are happy to recommend skilled care nursing facilities or hospice programs.

Several physicians in our seminar spoke frankly of their difficulty in keeping abreast of all aspects of the care of their dying patients. Only the nurses who maintain continual presence at the bedside can do so. The nurse caring for the patient during the daytime shift will most likely see the physicians and the important family members and provide whatever medical interventions have been ordered. Hence this nurse becomes the central figure in the difficult task of maintaining communication between patients, physicians, nursing staff, family members, and counselors in pastoral care or social services.

Role of Nursing Staff

A nurse at one of our seminars described the case of Mrs. D. She was given a cancer diagnosis at age 55 and had surgery three times in the next four years. Then the next operation revealed metastasis and she received hospital radiation therapy. Subsequently, she refused further chemotherapy and IV's which would prolong her increasing discomfort. She made a beautiful preparation for death with the continual support of her family, friends, and physicians, and with a deep faith in God. But, apparently, over the long months of hospitalization none of the nursing staff were taken into her confidence. Possibly they saw how well she was handling her condition and communicated to her non-verbally that they had other patients more in need of their personal attention.

Generally, nurses find dying patients more inclined to share their anxieties and uncertainties with them than with physicians, particularly the specialists brought in for technical consultations and services. One gynecological oncologist at our seminar indicated that only a very few patients question him about their chances of remission, whereas 95% of them discuss this with his nurse-clinician. However, this nurse-clinician specializes in listening to patients and helping them verbalize their feelings. In fact, she feels that traditional rules about not sitting on patients' beds and not becoming involved in patients' emotional crises must be broken in the cases of terminal illness. The oft-cited fact that some patients communicate more openly with housekeeping staff than either physicians or nurses hints that presence and sympathetic listening are more indispensable to good communication than professional qualification.

However, nurses play the key role in the art of administering pain medication. Alert nurses can obviate the anxiety of suffering patients who fear their pain will return before the next scheduled dosage. Studies on pain have indicated that the psychological component magnifies enormously the actual physical discomfort.[2] Nurses need the confidence of physicians and a close working relationship with them to practice skillfully the art of pain relief.

Only the nurse on duty observes the final stage of terminal illness continuously as it unfolds. Only this nurse can relay to the physician a professional description of the patient's condition. Only this nurse, too, can provide patients and families with a continual professional understanding of the symptoms and signs created by terminal illness.

An increasingly common complaint among nurses arises from frustrating situations like that of Dr. R., cited earlier in this chapter. The attending physician who adamantly refused to withdraw the respirator prolonging Dr. R's final stage of terminal illness seldom visited the patient more than once a day. The resentful family members spent long hours at the bedside. The nurse on duty shared their resentment.

In the face of such tense situations nurses sometimes see their most important role as patient and family advocates to the absent physician instead of physician representatives to the patient and family. Nurses do not claim the right to substitute for physicians in making medical decisions. But they very naturally claim the right to confront physicians with their failures to consult patients and families and to give legitimate consideration to their rights to forego medical treatment which merely prolongs dying.

Furthermore, as treatment options proliferate with medical advances and as subspecialties multiply, the team concept of health care becomes more and more essential. Nurses must have a leadership role in these teams as the team members who maintain the continual care for suffering persons. At one of our seminars a physician himself advised colorfully, "There are times when the nurse simply must corner the physician and alert him to what's really happening!"

This physician also pointed out how often communications break down between the family and the physician. The physician may feel guilty for having failed, and thus may find discussion with the family difficult and embarrassing. The physician's medical school training does not allow for failure; death becomes a paradox. An intelligent nurse recognizes this situation and can be a bridge between the physician and the family at this critical time.

Role of Pastoral Care and Social Service Counselors

Religious concerns emerge as a top priority in the care of persons in the final stage of terminal illness. Pastoral care persons cannot give a symbolic pat on the head and reassurance that "everything will be all right." The kind of sympathetic listening that earns the patient's confidence and which nurses should cultivate becomes totaly essential to pastoral care staffs. Whereas the awesome event of death can be readily shunted aside by many hospital patients, it has become an absorbing preoccupation with dying patients. Physicians and nurses generally welcome the presence of pastoral care persons who have the time and the expertise to assist dying patients. The five stages of dying outlined by Dr. Kubler-Ross conclude with depression and then acceptance. Religious faith and reconciliation with God and with the whole circle of relatives and acquaintances assist tremendously when patients are vacillating between depression and acceptance. Prayerful pastoral care persons assist that process which includes the Sacrament of Reconciliation in the Catholic tradition.

During that critical final stage of terminal illness patients need round-the-clock attention. Hospices offer such a constant availability with twenty-four hour phone contact for patients in their homes. Pastoral care persons are called to approximate such availability because critical spiritual needs also occur around the clock.

Ministry to the comatose and nearly comatose patient presents special challenges. One pastoral care minister in our seminar pointed to the helplessness experienced when there was no previous pastoral contact with the patient. However, the generally agreed-upon fact that the sense of hearing persists, even after the apparent onset of coma, encourages pastoral care persons and nursing staff to continue communicating in a loud voice. One nurse pointed out that she regularly reassures the apparently unconscious patient about the family's love and the provisions made for elderly spouses and the handling of temporalities such as the hospital bill itself.

The role of pastoral care counselors and social service workers in behalf of the dying and comatose tends to support the vision of health care as a caring covenant between the patient and the professional health care team. These counselors meet needs which go far beyond contractual obligations for the physical well-being or comfort of dying persons.

Social service counselors in acute care hospitals become experts in helping patients and families untangle the myriad reimbursement regulations. Furthermore, they accumulate invaluable information about alternatives for patients who must be dismissed because no further therapeutic treatment is indicated. Hospitals win the hearts of the people they serve by retaining cheerful and cooperative social service counselors.

Conclusion

Within the tradition of responsible stewardship of human life one finds an acceptance of the reality and inevitability of death. The theological roots of this tradition are found intertwined with a firm belief in life after death. Death cannot be seen as an absolute evil or a final defeat amid the suffering and contradictions of human life.

Hence in caring for the persons described in this chapter we have proposed a primary concern for the comfort and spiritual well-being of the patient. If these goals are met, patients, families, and care-givers can accept death without scruple and without pursuing technological victories at the price of prolonging human suffering.

Notes

1. A. Jann Davis, "Brompton's Cocktail: Making Good-byes Possible." *American Journal of Nursing,* Vol. 78, No. 4 (April, 1978), pp. 610-12. Cf. Florence S. Wald, "Terminal Care and Nursing Education," *ibid.,* Vol. 79, No. 10 (October, 1979), pp. 1762-64.
2. C. J. Glynn, "Factors that Influence the Perception of Intractable Pain," *Medical Times,* Vol. 108, No. 3 (March, 1980), p. 108 (11s-26s). Cf. Ada K. Jacox, "Assessing Pain," *American Journal of Nursing,* Vol. 79, No. 5 (May, 1979), pp. 895-900.

Chapter 14

Care of Persons with Irreversibly Deteriorating Health

The Reverend Donald G. McCarthy, Ph.D.

Introduction

Medical humorists sometimes remark that all of us are born terminally ill, it is just a matter of time until we die. Similarly, one might say that everyone experiences irreversibly deteriorating health, or that each day we die a little.

This chapter, however, discusses the care of persons who experience progressively deteriorating health because of some identifiable physical ailment(s). One may cite, for example, chronic illnesses like cancer and heart disease, or arteriosclerotic disease, arthritis, diabetes, neuromuscular diseases, strokes, or cerebral disease with dementia. These persons, unlike those discussed in the previous chapter, are not irreversibly comatose or in the final stage of terminal illness. But all these persons share a common sense of diminished well-being without hope of return to normal health.

Yet the stewardship of life approach, described in this volume, considers the moral dignity and rights of such persons as equal to those in robust health. Ethicists and theologians following this approach refuse to diminish the duty of such persons to use life-prolonging procedures and the duty of health professionals to provide them, simply on the basis of the deteriorating health or diminished quality of life of these persons. In other words, the life-prolonging procedures do not automatically become proportionally more extraordinary as the quality of continued life diminishes. The benefit of continued human experience should not be calculated on a mathematical scale.

On the other hand, even though medical treatments offer a reasonable hope of benefit for such persons, the burden of undertaking them *has* traditionally been the primary norm for determining if the procedures are ethically ordinary and obligatory. The burden which the patient experiences from a medical procedure may be physical pain or hardship, emotional and psychological repugnance, excess expense for self or family, or some other hardship. (See chapter 9 of this volume.)

In our seminars, these estimates of the burden of medical treatment were cited repeatedly. Because of widespread reimbursement coverage in the United States, the financial burden of medical care does not figure prominently in some cases. Yet most reimbursement programs include regulatory limits and a certain proportion of the United States population has practically no coverage. Furthermore, the allocation of huge sums of money from reimbursement systems for treatment of exceptional cases tends to inflate the whole system. The question of limiting such exorbitant financial burdens cannot realistically be ignored in designing such systems.

The seminars which discussed caring for person with irreversibly deteriorating health focused chiefly on various aspects of the decision-making process and the increasing development of support groups for both patients and staff members, with some additional concerns for persons undergoing rehabilitative therapy.

The Patient as Decision-Maker

Many of these patients are mentally competent to make decisions about their care. They have a right to give informed consent to medical treatment, even though medical language must be translated to language they can understand.[1] The right to refuse treatment correlates, in the stewardship of life approach, with a responsibility to consent to reasonable burdens and ethically ordinary treatments. But the patient cannot participate in weighing such burdens until they have been explained as simply and honestly as possible. Health care professionals who fail to give such explanations implicitly deny a patient's right to consent and manipulate the patient into following their own judgment.

Father Connery, in one of our seminars, cited the case of Mrs. B., a 70 year old woman with deteriorating health, who had been receiving hemodialysis. The procedure was particularly difficult for her with blood clotting and difficulties in the use of the necessary shunt. She indicated her desire to forego hemodialysis. In their concern for a truly informed consent her physicians set up an interview at a time when her system would be most free of toxicity which might cloud her judgment. After a frank and open discussion, they accepted her decision to cease hemodialysis. She had judged that this procedure was ethically extraordinary because of the burden it presented and she was able to exercise her prerogative of an informed decision-maker.

An opposite decision was made by Richard K., a 22-year old man receiving extensive treatment for second and third degree burns. Over a period of time he constantly protested the painful procedures his physicians were performing upon him in an almost mechanical routine with very little explanation of what they were doing and why. Finally, they listened to Richard's protests and sat down to discuss with him the option of foregoing further treatment. To their surprise, he then indicated his desire to continue treatment. It might be said Richard was finally able to give informed consent. Perhaps the physicians presumed their treatment was ethically ordinary, but, even so, they owed it to Richard to obtain his consent.

Health care professionals have a clinical knowledge of the therapies like chemotherapy, hemodialysis, pacemakers, and surgical procedures which they provide, but patients have their own estimate of the burdens posed by such therapies. Patients, however, need help from both health professionals and pastoral counselors in deciding when the burden of treatment should be considered sufficiently grave to forego it with consequent shortening of life. In the context of a moral responsibility for the gift of life, patients should pray over such decisions and seek advice from others who have faced similar challenges. The Vatican *Declaration on Euthanasia* spoke to such patients when it said: "Life is a gift of God, and on the other hand death is unavoidable; it is necessary therefore that we, without in any way hastening the hour of death, should be able to accept it with full responsibility and dignity." (See Appendix I, p. 290.)

Role of the Health Care Team

As patients puzzle over their decisions about undergoing the various therapies available to them, they take counsel from numerous members of the health care team. The attending physician cannot and should not seek to curtail such consultation. Yet the other physicians and health care professionals must respect the primary role of the attending physician and never undermine it or deliberately weaken the patient's confidence in that physician. Other team members may know the patient's situation better than that physician. If so, the physician *needs* their insights. If the physician does not encourage this, the others should legitimately insist on "button-holing" that physician privately. Those physicians who welcome the team concept must be prepared for opinions differing from their own. One physician at our seminar spoke of encouraging team members to be assertive, but not aggressive, since the latter trait often betrays hostility and creates communication barriers.

On the other hand, the attending physician, after frankly discussing all the facts and clinical aspects of a case with other team members, may be persuaded in conscience that a proposed treatment is ethically ordinary and obligatory, in the face of strong disagreement from other team members. Such a physician may not simply shift responsibility to the team, but must continue to counsel the patient to accept treatment. Should the patient continue to refuse treatment upon the advice of other team members, the physician may eventually judge it necessary to withdraw as attending physician.

However, from the nurse's perspective, one of our seminar leaders criticized the "Eichmann Syndrome", referring to blind obedience to unethical procedures. Another participant pointed out the usefulness of the written patient care plan which makes clear the rationale of treatment being provided each patient. These observations highlight the continuing need to improve interpersonal communications and an atmosphere of cooperative concern among health care professionals for the primary goal of each patient's well-being. Hospital inservice programs can clarify the principles of moral responsibility outlined in this volume and can assist team members to define their own roles. Workshops in interpersonal communications can facilitate teamwork and the appropriate means for team members to communicate their feelings and judgments.

Consulting the Patient's Family

Family members should assist patients in their decision-making and try to interpret their wishes when they are not fully competent. Therefore, they deserve the time and attention necessary to be made fully aware of their particular patient's condition. In one of our seminars, the rather bizarre case of 69 year old Mr. A. was described. Mr. A. came home from the hospital in a semi-senile and confused condition. The physician saw him monthly for nine months in his office, leaving the wife in the waiting room each time. The only information given the wife was a general diagnosis of arteriosclerosis until the physician finally proposed readmitting the patient to the hospital for prostate tests. The physician had then decided, unilaterally, that upon discharge the patient should be transferred to a nursing home!

Family members, as well as patients, often have difficulty comprehending medical diagnoses and terminology. Various kinds of human dynamics influence their attitudes toward patients, as, for example, that of a wife who resents her husband's alcoholism and considers the cirrhosis of the liver a well-deserved retribution. Health professionals often have the opportunity to assist in healing and reconciling family relationships while treating medical conditions.

The Process of Health Deterioration

In one of our seminars, the case of Sally, a 14-year-old girl diagnosed with terminal cancer, was presented. During a period of two years, her health progressively worsened despite experimental use of new drugs, one of them costing $1,000 a gram. This teenager wanted to know all about her condition, and her parents respected her autonomy as fully as possible. She chose chemotherapy when it was offered and then eventually chose to discontinue it when told how unsuccessful it was.

She returned to her home and family at that point, preferring a few weeks with them to continued hospitalization. Actually, she survived from January until August, preparing not only herself but everyone around her for her impending death. Three days before her death she spoke happily about her coming meeting with Jesus, and joked that she would ask Him what really caused her cancer.

Although, in Sally's case, her deterioration of health moved along a fairly obvious path, certain key elements of her experience should be common to all the patients discussed in this chapter. She was fully aware of her condition, she participated actively in decisions about her treatment, she prepared herself spiritually for her death, she retained her sense of self-worth even as she became more and more incapacitated, and she actually taught those around her a deeper appreciation of the value of life and the human acceptance of death.

Hence the special challenge to health professionals caring for persons with irreversibly deteriorating health emerges particularly from the drawn-out process of gradual debilitation. Although crisis periods may occur during the process, love, patience and joyful courage are the essential virtues in caring for these persons. The moral issues of choosing or foregoing certain treatments or procedures may reappear repeatedly during this period of extended care, as they did for Sally as the cancer got progressively worse. Our seminars touched on the variety of support groups that develop both for these patients and their care-givers.

Support Groups

The need for intimacy and interpersonal communication, deeply buried within the human psyche, manifests itself whenever persons experience stress and strain. Persons who carry the gnawing disease of malignant cancer within their bodies find a powerful bond uniting them. Persons residing in nursing homes and experiencing together the gradual deterioration of physical health and alertness are drawn together by their common situation. And health care professionals who together share such burdens vicariously experience a bonding sense of their mutual responsibility toward their patients.

Pastoral care directors in many health care facilities have sparked support groups which foster these mutual bonds. For persons with chronic illness one facility has a group entitled "Born Free" which meets monthly and also involves nursing staff, social workers, physicians, therapists, and, of course, pastoral care persons. At the same facility, another group of cancer patients, entitled "Open Door," meets regularly. In another hospital, the staff from each floor meet weekly with a pastoral care person to share experiences and relieve some of the sense of emotional "burn out" which plagues the most sensitive and dedicated health care professionals. In yet another hospital, the pastoral care department sponsors a monthly physician-clergy luncheon for one hour with brief presentations by a physician and a clergy representative on a theme of "Religion and Medicine."

The Judeo-Christian heritage of love for neighbor, especially neighbors who are hurting, motivates these efforts to assist suffering persons and help them cope gracefully with the crosses they carry. One hospital uses volunteers to alert parishes about the discharge of patients so that the parish may reach out to those persons at home. Prayer groups offer magnificent support to persons in deteriorating health. One religious sister with multiple sclerosis has been "adopted" by a neighborhood prayer group. Perhaps the most direct and human role of all such support groups lies in their continual reassurance to persons in declining health and vigor that their value and self-worth remains intact and unmarred. Persons in need of rehabilitative programs struggle particularly intensely with their own self-image.

Patients in Rehabilitative Programs

Persons who have suffered a permanent and severe handicap, such as a stroke or a broken neck, are not terminally ill and the deterioration of their health is irreversible but often stable over an indefinite period. Such individuals experience a reaction to their condition parallel to those with terminal illness. Their attitudes tend to progress through denial, anger, bargaining, and depression before acceptance of their condition.

An ethical analysis of life-prolonging decisions for such patients often reveals that the major burden they face is not medical treatment but their handicapped condition itself. In fact, although the medical treatment offered them may present a financial burden, it generally relieves to some degree the physical burden of their handicap.

Yet physicians who direct rehabilitative programs for these persons often encounter resistance because of their patients' depression and despair. In one seminar, the case of Mrs. J. was presented. She is a 31-year-old woman who experienced a progressive deterioration of the central nervous system confining her to a wheelchair. Her alcoholic husband divorced her and she lost all will to live. The rehabilitative physician found her in a darkened room with her thin and emaciated body curled into a fetal position, symbolizing her withdrawal from the human community. With six months of loving care and therapy, she regained her sense of self-worth and her will to live. She learned to walk again with the aid of a cane.

Another case was that of Harry C., a young man who broke his neck in a fall from a tree at the age of 12. For five years he was bed-fast without rehabilitative assistance. Then he was enrolled in a program which, among other skills, taught him oil painting. He has done beautiful nature scenes and achieved great fame. He paints trees and houses and people in mid-air because a grounding for them would represent gravity, his enemy! Harry is now 25 years old. When asked about the first five years he spent without progress or therapy after his accident, he replies, "No one told me that it wasn't all right to just do nothing."

Hence, the key ethical concern of rehabilitation therapy seems to be to motivate patients in their will to live and their desire to succeed in therapeutic efforts. If they refuse therapy because of their depression, their refusal may be construed as a refusal of life-prolonging procedures, but these should be deemed, more appropriately, "life-enriching" procedures. The urgent need to motivate patients and to involve family members in their care suggests that rehabilitative programs must heal the spirit as well as the body.

Conclusion

This chapter has surveyed prolonging life decisions which people make in the face of irreversibly deteriorating health. The moral obligation to use medical treatments and procedures depends primarily on the burden they pose the patient. The obligation on physicians, however, to make such therapies available to the patient should be considered one of justice because of professional duty. However, where reimbursement is not available, the obligation in justice gives way to one in charity. Much the same can be said of hospitals and nursing homes. The Christian ideal of offering charity care has been restricted by reimbursement audits and financial regulations to the point where administrators need great creativity to find means of caring for the indigent.

Yet, the religious dimension of health care reminds all in that profession of the faith values which explain the very origin of religiously-sponsored health care facilities. A physician doing rehabilitative care summarized this faith motivation at one of our seminars.

"The success of our work depends not only on what we do, but how we do it. If we care for people in Christ's name, our work has a telling effect which we don't even understand. If we polled 100 people, I suspect that all would agree that to seek out the most abandoned people in one of the poorest nations of the world is an irrational way to approach health care. Yet Mother Teresa of Calcutta is doing just that and has touched the whole world in her work!"

Note

1. Kathleen Krekeler R.N., Ph.D., "Introduction to Patient Education", in Barbara Shelden Czerwinski, *Manual of Patient Education for Cardiopulmonary Dysfunctions* (St. Louis, C. V. Mosby Co. 1980). Cf. also "Declaration of Helsinki", *Opinions and Reports of the Judicial Council*, American Medical Association (Chicago, IL, 1971) pp. 74-75.

Chapter 15

Care of Severely Defective Newborn Babies

The Reverend Donald G. McCarthy, Ph. D.

Introduction

Whereas the last chapter discussed care of persons usually advanced in years, this discussion concerns newborn babies. The recognition of the needs of the newborn in making the transition from intra-uterine to extra-uterine life led to the sub-speciality of Neonatal-Perinatal Medicine. Sophisticated medical technology developed simultaneously. Both medically and ethically difficult decisions arise in caring for an ill neonate. The ethical difficulties are greater than those encountered in caring for adults because: 1) newborn babies have not had, and do not have, any way of indicating their own preferences, and 2) their medical prognosis remains more obscure than that of adults because of the resiliency of the young developing human being and the difficulties in differentiating and being certain of the pathologic processes of an infant.

As a consequence of babies' inability to communicate, ethicists are forced to acknowledge that the only suitable criterion for considering omission of procedures which ethical principles might judge to be extraordinary must be "the best interests" of the baby. Ordinarily, the proxy persons most properly expected to speak in behalf of those "best interests" are the parents of the baby. Note that if a procedure were judged *ethically ordinary* the health care team, while still needing consent from the parents to offer care, could presume implied consent in emergency. If a procedure is judged *ethically extraordinary* after competent medical and ethical consultation, and is then to be omitted at the discretion of the parents and according to their judgment of the "best interests" of the baby, the health care team should accept that decision. However, as we will discuss in this chapter, it seems clear that the instances where life-prolonging procedures for newborn infants are genuinely extraordinary in an ethical sense are infrequent.

In our seminars, the second fact, the obscure medical prognosis for newborn babies, often emerged in case examples. For instance, one physician described the unusual case of baby Beth who manifested some indications of brain death, including a flat electroencephalogram. Although removal of the ventilator supporting her respiration was seriously contemplated over a period of time, it was not removed. She lived to breathe on her own, and today, five years later, is walking and talking in reasonably normal health like any other kindergarten child.

While artificial support of respiration often fails for newborn babies because of inadequate lung formation and the technical difficulty of adapting the respirator to such tiny patients, the prognosis of failure cannot easily be foreseen. The marvelous capacity of babies to respond to treatment led one physician to comment that for the first several years of life a newborn child's appearances can be radically deceiving: the ones who look the most hopeless can improve remarkably. On the other hand, some babies who seem normal can begin to manifest hidden defects during the age range of 2-5 years.

Significantly, the 1980 "Standards and Guidelines for Cardiopulmonary Resuscitation (CPR) and Emergency Cardiac Care (ECC)," published in the August 1, 1980, issue of the *Journal of the American Medical Association* do not specifically discuss omitting resuscitation or life support for infants. Yet the issue of using or not using life-prolonging procedures for defective newborn babies has surfaced repeatedly in recent years. Since much of the reluctance to use life-prolonging procedures for defective newborn babies hinges on the expectations of a future handicapped existence, this theme of diminished quality of life surfaced in the seminars on caring for these babies.

This chapter will first offer an ethical critique of the use of quality of life considerations in decisions about infants and then, in the second section, review the notion of ethically extraordinary means of prolonging life as appropriately applied to defective newborn babies. The third and final section will discuss the parents' role in decision-making about defective newborn babies.

1) Quality of Life Considerations

Handicapped persons are met with some ambivalence in society at large. On the one hand, special efforts are made to accept them and appreciate their dignity and rights. The federal legislation to insure equal treatment of handicapped persons in the United States has contributed immeasurably to these efforts, even though some impractical applications must be modified. Religious belief, and specifically Christian belief, wholeheartedly supports the morally equal dignity and rights of all members of the human family.

On the other hand, society and the public media tend to assume that handicapped persons are abnormal as persons. Furthermore, persons of normal health and quality of life readily judge that life is not worth living in a handicapped condition. This unspoken conviction surely influences the discussions about prolonging the lives of newborn babies.

Yet, persons blessed with normal health have no evidence for making such judgments about others. In one of our seminars it was noted, for example, that studies do not show a higher incidence of suicide among handicapped persons, as if *they* would consider themselves better off dead.

Several cases of handicapped adults were described. Carol is a thirty year old college teacher with a Ph.D. in biology, despite her handicap associated with a spina bifida condition and her use of crutches. Dan is a victim of cerebral palsy who is constantly bent over nearly double and presents a most distressing appearance. Yet, he is a talented writer and editor of a newsletter for handicapped persons. After joining a new parish, he wrote a touching open letter to the congregation to thank them for their warm acceptance.

Undoubtedly the ambivalence which society manifests toward

215

handicapped persons reflects the unresolved questions in the public at large about the meaning and value of human life itself. Those who view the universe as without purpose and human lives as products of a blind process of evolutionary interaction may be less disposed to attribute fully equal dignity and meaning to the handicapped than those who believe in God. Yet, even the rational principles of justice which society seeks to implement do not support such discriminatory dispositions. Current discussions of allowing defective infants to die because of their handicapped condition shroud a basic discrimination under the cloak of compassion and non-violence.

Several participants in our seminars pointed out that religious values have contributed enormously to assuring full justice and rights for the handicapped. One theologian noted that, beginning with the Edict of Toleration by Constantine, the Church began to enhance the inviolability of the lives of slaves and the unborn in the new Christian civilization which arose to replace the pagan Roman Empire.

Pope John XXIII pointed to the role of religion in supporting morality in a particularly striking passage of his famous encyclical, *Mater et Magistra*, in 1961:

> "However, the guiding principles of morality and virtue can be based only on God; apart from Him, they necessarily collapse. For man is composed not merely of body, but of soul as well, and is endowed with reason and freedom. Now such a composite being absolutely requires a moral law rooted in religion, which, far better than any external force or advantage, can contribute to the resolution of problems affecting the lives of individual citizens or groups of citizens, or with a bearing upon single States or all States together." (#208)

The Holy Father's reference to "problems affecting the lives of individual citizens or groups of citizens" can be applied directly to handicapped persons. Human reason and fundamental justice should protect these persons. Yet compromises seem almost inevitable without the vision and strength which faith provides. The theological doctrine of the fall of the human family from grace, with its consequent clouding of the intellect and weakening of the will, seems to help explain the ambiguities which a purely secular society manifests toward weak and helpless persons.

Hence, this volume, which discusses moral responsibility for prolonging life decisions from the perspective of the Judeo-Christian

216

religious tradition and, specifically, of Catholic teaching, cannot support a policy in any way discriminatory toward the defective newborn, the most voiceless members of a minority group, the handicapped. The fact that medical treatments cannot overcome expectations of a quality of life diminished through mental or physical handicap does not constitute such treatments ethically extraordinary or lacking in reasonable hope of benefit. Father Connery stated this succinctly in chapter 9 above:

"Handicaps in themselves have never been considered reasons either for taking a life or neglecting ordinary means that would effectively preserve it." (p. 136).

The affirmation of this tradition has become doubly important in the United States today because of the practice of abortion of unborn human beings since the 1973 Supreme Court decisions. Abortions can now be performed throughout pregnancy. Those which are performed when amniocentesis reveals a genetic defect have taken on a certain respectability for many people — a plausible explanation can be advanced in terms of precluding a lifetime of misery and hardship. This same rationale is used by those who would omit life-prolonging procedures in order to allow defective newborn infants to die instead of surviving with a diminished quality of life.

The stewardship of life tradition supported in our seminars rejects the inherent injustice and discrimination of using quality of life considerations to determine who shall live. However, the discussion cannot end here. Situations still arise where life-prolonging measures can be considered ethically extraordinary within the tradition of equal justice and respect for all human lives. We will review these considerations.

2) Ethically Extraordinary Means

The ethical principles outlined in chapter 9 by Father Connery also apply to defective newborn babies. They hinge on the judgments made about benefit and burden in using life-prolonging procedures. We will consider benefit first.

Theologians have applied the *benefit* consideration in terms of the basic therapeutic outcome as either useful or useless. They considered this primarily in terms of a dying patient: a life-prolonging procedure which merely prolongs the dying process is considered practically useless. This can surely apply to anencephalic infants who cannot

217

survive more than a short time. Hence it would not be ethically necessary to use a respirator for such an infant, although ordinary procedures like clearing the infant's air ways and providing warmth and nourishment are appropriate.

Other instances arise where the prognosis of survival allows for a period of months or even a year or two. Here the criterion of useless benefit becomes less clear. Those who wish to measure benefit in terms of the conscious life experience of the baby itself may tend to minimize benefit since there will be such a minimal development of human relationships before death occurs. Yet the prognosis will often be clouded and the degree of conscious experience difficult to estimate. More important is the fact that the baby is a living human being who does respond to care and affection and can develop relationships long before he or she begins to walk or talk.

From the previous discussion of quality of life considerations and their prejudicial use in decisions for the handicapped, it is clear that the reduced benefit of a life-prolonging procedure when it cannot overcome a handicapped condition does not thereby constitute a procedure extraordinary. Hence, the famous case where a Down's syndrome child's duodenal atresia was not surgically remedied cannot be excused on grounds of insufficient benefit. The child would have enjoyed conscious human experience — the precious gift which flows from the very nature of human personhood and which distinguishes humans from all other animals.

The other criterion of an ethically extraordinary procedure, the *burden* it entails, can also be applied to the treatment of defective newborn babies. Note that the burden must be the burden of a medical treatment, not the burden of a handicapped existence. As Fr. Connery noted in chapter 9, theologians do not recognize the burden of a handicapped existence itself as a reason for omitting life-prolonging procedures. If they did, the outcome would be that only people with a normal quality of life would have the full right and duty to prolong their lives. Society would, in a sense, unburden itself of the burden of medical treatment for the handicapped.

However, the burden which *medical treatment* imposes can be seen in a different light, as Fr. Connery noted. Here a patient, or a parent acting as a proxy for a newborn child, must decide if a treatment or procedure represents an excess burden. This burden can be considered excessive in terms of the hardship it imposes on the patient or even on others who must provide it.

Yet this theoretical norm provided by theologians can easily be abused in the case of infants. The projection of whether a series of surgical operations, the placement of a shunt, or the use of a ventilator for an extended period of time represents an excess burden to a newborn child will easily reflect the decision-maker's own estimate of the value of a human life.

In our seminars one of the theologians insisted strongly on what he called the "purity of heart" of the decision-makers. This means a morally upright disposition which would clearly exclude the omission of medical procedures with the intention of hastening death — a form of moral and legal homicide. Beyond that, this purity of heart demands a reverence for the gift of life, a valuing of life rooted in its inherent transcendance and mystery. Hence, the ethical reasoning and moral casuistry about excessive burdens must respond with particular sensitivity to the mystery and the marvel of human life in its infant form. Unfortunately, the mentality which justifies abortion of the unborn does not readily support this respect for lives of defective newborn babies.

A baby born with a spina bifida condition presents a case where life-prolonging procedures may involve multiple medical interventions. One cannot readily state that such babies are dying and that for this reason the life-prolonging procedures are ethically optional. Yet, in our seminars, several cases were cited of spina bifida babies left untreated.

For example, a physician in one seminar described Elizabeth, an 8½ pound baby girl born with a low lumbar meningomyelocele. He estimated she had a 60 percent chance of normal mental function. She did not have hydrocephalus at birth but would probably develop it and need surgical insertion of a shunt within a month or two. She could possibly develop infections requiring further treatment. She would remain incontinent in bowel activity and would require a urinary diversion procedure at some point. She could end up with chronic renal disease, multiple orthopedic procedures, and spend the rest of her life in a wheelchair. Elizabeth's parents were unwilling to consent to medical treatment. She died between two and three weeks after birth with meningitis.

A priest at another seminar described another spina bifida baby. This baby, Joseph, had been brought to a large city hospital from a rural area. Despite this transfer to a facility offering the advantage of more advanced neonatal care, the baby was not only not receiving treatment but was being allowed to die by receiving only a so-called "low calorie" IV of glucose and water. The ethical principles discussed in this chapter cannot justify the failure to provide nourishment to a spina bifida infant. With the advance of medical care and knowledge of this condition, one can hardly say that these infants, as a group, are dying and thus argue that nourishment is a useless procedure. Nor can one readily propose that feeding a baby constitutes an excess burden. The recent Document of the Holy See for the International Year of Disabled Persons addressed this very question:

> Furthermore, the deliberate failure to provide assistance, or any act which leads to the suppression of the newborn disabled person, represents a breach not only of medical ethics but also of the fundamental and inalienable right to life. One cannot, at whim, dispose of human life, by claiming an arbitrary power over it. Medicine loses its title of nobility when, instead of attacking disease, it attacks life; in fact prevention should be against the illness, not against life. One can never claim that one wishes to bring comfort to a family, by suppressing one of its members. The respect, the dedication, the time and means required for the care of handicapped persons, even of those whose mental faculties are gravely affected, is the price that a society should generously pay in order to remain truly human.[1]

It is true that the decisions about the possible excess burden of providing surgical and rehabilitative treatments for Elizabeth and Joseph can take into account the burden such treatments place on the family as well as the infants. But society at large has a responsibility to assist families like the families of Elizabeth and Joseph. The Vatican document mentioned above states this principle:

> It is necessary therefore for families to be given great understanding and sympathy by the community and to receive from associations and public powers adequate assistance from the beginning of the discovery of the disability of one of their members.

Undoubtedly, there can be honest differences of opinion regarding the proxy judgments to be made about the burdens of life-prolonging

220

and life-enhancing treatments for defective newborn babies. In their penetrating study of this issue, Germain Grisez and Joseph Boyle appeal to the criterion of what a competent reasonable person would desire in similar circumstances:

> The basic requirement of justice with respect to care for non-competent persons is easy enough to state: The noncompetent person ought not to be denied that care which any reasonable person who was competent probably would desire in similar circumstances, and the noncompetent person ought not to be given care which any reasonable person would refuse in a like case.[2]

These two authors present this criterion in their discussion of "Justice and Care for the Incompetent." Since the law exists to insure justice, one may expect the courts to become involved in these cases. For example, one case of a spina bifida baby was decided in the Dade County, Florida, Circuit Court on June 24, 1981. The parents had wished to forego treatment and the Variety Children's Hospital brought the case to court for resolution. Judge Ralph Ferguson ordered that treatment be provided.[3]

The ethical principles presented in this volume clearly prohibit omissions of medical treatment for defective babies like Elizabeth and Joseph with the intention of their dying. To omit all treatment in the hopes of death resulting should be understood as a form of killing and prohibited. On the other hand, it is morally permissible to omit specific procedures on the grounds of the burden they impose on the child or even on the family.[4] Hence the spina bifida babies have occasioned serious ethical and legal controversies. Paul Ramsey, the well-known Christian ethicist at Princeton, reviewed these questions incisively in his 1978 volume, *Ethics at the Edges of Life.*[5]

Ramsey makes clear that decisions about omitting medical treatment for spina bifida babies must not be based on their prospects of a diminished quality of life or the unwillingness of their parents to raise a handicapped child. Even the rationale of foregoing certain procedures on the grounds of the burden they might impose on the spina bifida child usually does not advance the best interests of the child. For the children who survive without rehabilitative treatment, and many of them do, carry a permanent burden of hardship which the temporary burden of treatment could have alleviated. Hence the screening practice of the British physician, Dr. John Lorber, which uses an index of anticipated quality of life to designate which spina bifida children will be treated, should be abandoned. A medical indications criterion, such as that advocated by Dr. R. B. Zachary, more adequately protects the rights of these babies.[6]

Since parents carry the legal and moral responsibility of caring for their defective newborn children, they are obligated to provide what have been called in this volume the ethically ordinary means of preserving their lives. Parents may not arbitrarily decide that a form of treatment is ethically extraordinary and optional. If that decision is made on sufficient medical and moral grounds, the parents must then still decide, as proxy representatives of their child, whether that treatment is in their child's best interests. Participants in our seminars frequently discussed the anxieties and emotional turmoil parents face in these important decisions.

3) Parents' Role in Decision-Making

Despite the callousness toward the unborn which abortion manifests in society today, parents still instinctively experience a deep sense of concern and responsibility for their newborns who are defective. One of the physicians in our seminars illustrated this with the case of the infant Roger. This child had been delivered by Cesarean section and manifested Down's syndrome. The mother had gone home from the hospital and Roger remained in the nursery awaiting surgical correction of duodenal atresia. Roger was actually being wheeled to the operating room when a phone message from the mother refused consent for the surgery. The attending physician was not about to abandon Roger. He put him on IVs for a week until he could persuade the mother to come and visit Roger. She brought her two other children with her. One of them said quite simply to the mother, "Gee, Mom, we have to do something." The corrective surgery was performed.

That same physician told of another case, in a large city hospital, of baby Arnold whose parents resided 75 miles away. Upon the advice of the surgeon they were going to forego necessary surgery on the intestine, partially because the child showed signs of neurological deficiencies. The family refused to visit the baby. Eventually the attending physician drove the 75 miles to visit the family with pictures of Arnold. He then described the necessary treatment for Arnold and the

222

parents decided in favor of it. In fact, they said they would never have refused consent in the first place if they had properly understood what would be entailed.

Several resource persons in our seminars insisted strongly that parents who make decisions about life-prolonging treatments should first see and hold their child. They should appreciate the child as a living human person before any attention is focused on the baby's defect and decisions to be made. This approach should not be considered prejudicial to "objective" thinking, since it reflects the very basis of the parents' role — their intimate and life-long relationship with their child.

Paul Ramsey cites a case in which a respirator was stopped and a tiny baby allowed to die.[7] The mother, herself only partially recovered from a Cesarean section, wanted to hold her baby to "give him love and comfort so he won't die alone." Assisted by the father and the staff she was present when the respirator was stopped. The parents held and rocked their baby for 45 minutes when his heart stopped beating. The mother gave the baby to the nurse with the comment, "Please handle him tenderly." Ramsey speculates that this may have been a child born dying. In that case, the withdrawal of the respirator would not constitute involuntary euthanasia or the removal of ethically ordinary and obligatory medical treatment.

Theologically speaking, one may describe as redemptive the influence a defective child can have upon parents and siblings. The child's helplessness invites heroic love and sacrifice. Countless instances are recounted of such children bringing a family closer together through the simplicity and innocence that often accompanies their helplessness. One priest recounted the simple statement of a retarded child to her unmarried and distraught mother: "I'm a gift because I give you someone to love."

Needless to say, redemptive graces do not eliminate pain and hardship. Families do break up under the burden of handicapped children, more often due to the emotional than the financial burden. The pastoral approach to such families offers supportive counseling, reference to community resources, and, most important in the religious tradition, an invitation to accept the grace that a handicapped child offers.

Conclusion

This chapter began by citing the two facts that newborn babies have no way of expressing their own decisions for medical treatment and that the prognosis of that treatment is frequently obscure. Despite the complexities reviewed in this chapter certain parameters of the ethical decision-making were made clear. Parents are the primary proxy representatives to give consent to treatment in behalf of their babies, just as they bear moral responsibility for their care and education. But parents are not free to abandon defective newborn babies. If the babies are not dying, medical treatment most often offers them genuine hope of benefit even if it cannot totally overcome their defects and provide a "normal" quality of life. The burden of undergoing medical treatment is usually not excessive for newborn babies although families may encounter excessive financial burdens. Hence, while cases may arise where parents are morally justified in refusing some treatments for their defective newborn babies, this may not be an arbitrary choice or one made simply to escape the lifelong responsibility of a handicapped child.

A statement on seriously deformed newborns from the *Current Opinions of the Judicial Council of the American Medical Association* of 1981 does not adequately protect their interests. It is included here, not as a recommended statement, but as an example of present trends in our society:

> QUALITY OF LIFE. In the making of decisions for the treatment of seriously deformed newborns or persons who are severely deteriorated victims of injury, illness, or advanced age, quality of life is a factor to be considered in determining what is best for the individual.
>
> In caring for defective infants, the advice and judgment of the physician should be readily available, but the decision whether to treat a severely defective infant and exert maximal efforts to sustain life should be the choice of the parents. The parents should be told the options, expected benefits, risks, and limits of any proposed care; how the potential for human relationships is affected by the infant's condition; and relevant information and answers to their questions. (2.10)

With regard to the first paragraph above, it should be noted that in this chapter we have insisted that a prognosis of continued poor quality of life does not render medical treatment ethically optional.

With regard to the second paragraph, it must be noted that physicians should respect the choice of parents in foregoing treatment which is not ethically and legally obligatory. If the treatment is ethically and legally *obligatory* (ethically ordinary means of preserving life), the physicians should seek to change the parent's minds. Failing that, the physician clearly has a moral obligation to withdraw from the case or seek legal redress.

Paul Ramsey's comments on the above opinions expressed by the American Medical Association might be surmised from his discussion arguing that, if physicians play God, they must play God as God plays God:

> If physicians are going to play God under the pretense of providing relief for the human condition, let us hope they play God as God plays God. Our God is no respecter of persons of good quality. Nor does he curtail his care for us because our parents are poor or have unhappy marriages, or because we are most in need of help. Again, a true humanism also leads to an "equality of life" standard.[8]

This chapter has highlighted a serious problem in the making of decisions on behalf of defective newborn babies on a quality of life standard rather than the equality of life which Paul Ramsey mentions. Another clergyman-ethicist, John Fletcher, has summarized well this issue and his summary will conclude our chapter:

> If we choose to be shaped by Judeo-Christian visions of the "createdness" of life within which every creature bears the image of God, we ought to care for the defective newborn as if our relation with the creator depended on the outcome. If we choose to be shaped by visions of the inherent dignity of each member of the human family, no matter what his or her predicament, we ought to care for this defenseless person as if the basis of our own dignity depended on the outcome. Care cannot fall short of universal equality.[9]

Notes

1. Washington, D.C., NC News, Mar 16, 1981.
2. Germain Grisez and Joseph Boyle Jr., *Life and Death with Liberty and Justice* (Notre Dame, IN: University of Notre Dame Press, 1979). pp. 260-61.
3. *Miami Herald,* June 24, 1981.
4. See Leonard Weber, *Who Shall Live?* (New York: Paulist Press, 1976), pp. 73-103.
5. New Haven: Yale University Press, 1978, pp. 189-227.
6. John Lorber, "Results of Treatment of Myelomeningocele: An Analysis of 524 Unselected Cases With Special Reference to Possible Selection for Treatment," *Developmental Medicine Child Neurology* 13 (1971): pp. 279-303. R. B. Zachary, "Life with Spina Bifida", *British Medical Journal*, Dec. 3, 1977, pp. 1460-62.
7. *Op. cit.,* p. 191.
8. *Op. cit.,* p. 203.
9. "Abortion, Euthanasia, and Care of Defective Newborns," *New England Journal of Medicine* 292 (January 9, 1975): pp. 75-78.

Chapter 16

Care of Persons Desiring to Die, Yet Not Terminally Ill

The Reverend Albert S. Moraczewski, O.P., Ph.D.

Introduction

One of the most difficult situations which faces a care giver — be it physician, nurse, or pastoral care person — is the person who wants to die but is not, at the time, terminally ill. For a variety of reasons, such individuals find their current life intolerable and seek to exit this world as soon as possible. Desiring to help the individual, the ministering person experiences much frustration in attempts to foster hope and stave off suicidal attempts. Not always convinced that the patient really means or knows what he is saying, the care giver is at a loss as to the course of action to follow and wonders whether or not it is ethical to accede to the patient's wishes (e.g., to withhold therapy), and whether forcing the patient to continue existing would be ethically mandatory.

During the seminar upon which this chapter is based, it became apparent that there were different perspectives from which the patient was being viewed. The physician, the nurse, and the pastoral care person each saw the patient and his problem in a somewhat different manner. However, all sought to understand how and why the patient had such a strong desire to die. All were desirous to provide the best care for such a patient. And all desired that what they did for the patient would be ethically acceptable.

This chapter will present some of the major considerations raised in our seminar which was held six times. For convenience of presentation, the chapter will be divided into three major parts, plus a short concluding section. Part I will present some dimensions of the problem. A reflection on the principal ethical issues which may arise when a person seeks to die will constitute Part II. Part III will discuss the issue from three different points of view: the physician's, the nurse's and the pastoral care person's perspective. To bring together the highlights of the three parts, by way of synthesis, will be the goal of the concluding section.

Dimensions of the Problem

One may be tempted to think that it is only, or primarily, the elderly who wish to die. Yet, not at all uncommon is the suicide of an adolescent or young adult. Situations such as the following selections abound.

1) A young nurse, Helen, had not reported for duty at her scheduled time. Concerned friends went to her apartment and found her in a coma having overdosed on barbituates. She was immediately taken to the emergency room where she was successfully revived. She is now furious that she was not allowed to complete her suicide.

2) A 22-year-old man, Tom, in a depressed state, sought the help of a general practitioner, who apparently did not assess the situation accurately. That evening Tom shot himself in the mouth. Although after extensive surgery he is still living, he cannot speak and is completely paralyzed. He insists that he does not want to live.

3) A British film entitled "Whose Life is it Anyway?" presented

very well the case of a sculpturer, a young man in the prime of his life, who became a quadraplegic as a result of an accident. Apart from the paralysis, he has full control of his senses, but sees no future at all in his life which had been built entirely around his sculpturing. After careful consideration, he concludes that there is no point to living and, therefore, the ongoing, life-sustaining therapy which he was receiving should be terminated and he be allowed to die.

Cases such as the last one mentioned above have given impetus to movements advocating legal suicide. A British organization named EXIT is probably the leader in the field. They have prepared a do-it-yourself manual on how to commit suicide rationally and effectively, with a minimum of mess for others to clean up. Whether or not decisions made weeks, months, or years prior to the actual suicide would automatically render that suicide *rational* remains a contested question. And a suicide being rational does not make it ethically good.

As earlier chapters of this volume have indicated, the right of self-determination is critical. "The law has never required a competent patient to undergo a medical treatment for his own good against his own wishes. . . . The crime of treating such a patient against instructions is assault and battery."[1] If, therefore, psychiatric examination reveals that a patient who expresses a wish to die is mentally competent, the patient cannot be compelled to undergo medical treatment which he refuses. For the incompetent patient, however, not only "a reason to refuse treatment" is necessary, but "a *good* reason." The agent's refusal of treatment for the patient must be close to, but not necessarily the judgment that society would have made. "A treatment is expendable if it is within reason to see it as useless, or to see in it any significant patient-centered moral objections, including severe physical or mental burden."[2] In some situations, it may be necessary for the individuals in charge of a patient's treatment to institute appropriate legal proceedings for the determination of mental competency before the law. A judge can make the final *legal* determination regarding an individual's competency.

Moral Reflection

The moral analysis presented here will proceed from the point of view, in general, of the Judeo-Christian tradition and, in particular, of official Catholic teaching. For the believing Jew as with the Christian, the universe and all its content — material and spiritual — were created by the one God. All life comes from God, but human life has a special place because to humans was given a dominion over the remainder of the world. Such a delegation involved a responsibility: humans are accountable to God, not only for their own individual lives, but for the lives of others. The story in *Genesis* of Abel and Cain emphasized that we *are* our brother's keepers.

Life is a good to be cherished, protected and promoted. Death and its suffering were not part of God's original design, as it were, but were the result of sin. While all humans have to die, death is not seen as annihilation or destruction of the human person. Rather, through the redemption brought about by Jesus Christ's loving sacrificial death, the human person has the opportunity to enjoy eternal happiness with God. Death, then, is not merely the disintegration of the present body-soul unit, but is also the transformation of the individual *person* from one mode of existence (temporal) to another which is transcendental and eternal.

Because humans are persons, they have a spiritual, i.e. non-material, dimension as well as the more obvious physical one. Humans are a *unity,* albeit a psychosomatic unity. While, on the other hand, persons by virtue of their spiritual nature transcend the limitations of the material world (consider the flights of human conceptual power), at the same time, they are influenced and limited by their materiality.

Consequently, while a person is morally responsible because of his immateriality and radical freedom of choice, that very freedom is subject to various limitations because of the material conditions in which he exists. Or, in other words, moral responsibility is proportionate to the degree of freedom actually prevailing at the moment. Freedom can be impaired to varying degrees by such factors as misinformation, lack of appropriate knowledge, and various altered states of consciousness (coma, sleep, drug states, hypnosis, disease, certain brain injuries, abnormal metabolic states, depression), as well as prejudice, anger, lust and fear.

The individual who is not terminally ill, but wishes to die may or may not be depressed. If that person is depressed, then the freedom of the person stating such a desire or taking steps leading to a potential act of self-destruction which might follow may well be partially impaired.

230

Consequently, the *culpability* of those acts would be proportionately diminished. At the same time, one should not forget that life is a precious gift from God which we may not unjustly destroy. *Objectively,* for an individual to take his life is a violation of God's love and the proper love the person should have for himself. We should choose life rather than death.

However, what is our obligation to prevent suicide? Objectively, suicide is morally evil. Although the patient's state of mind and reduced freedom of will — when present — lessen or remove the person's *culpability,* they never make suicide objectively a morally good act. Physicians, nurses and others may not voluntarily cooperate with that act. But what about the patient who refuses to eat? Is the physician justified in ordering, and the nurse carrying out, forced feeding by intubation? For the short term, intravenous feeding and intubation might be advisable. Before trying such extreme measures, it may be advisable to permit family or friends to prepare and bring the patient's favorite foods. Properly presented, such a meal could well overcome the opposition to eating (institutional food).

But once it is evident that the patient really does not want to be fed by any means, and steadfastly and vigorously resists attempts at forced feeding, then it would seem to be dehumanizing continously to feed the individual by force. No one can or may *force* another against his will to act virtuously. Efforts to prevent another from terminating his life generally are obligatory unless the requisite preventive measures are seen to be potentially more harmful to that person, say, by hardening his determination and generating a *hatred* of others and of God. Under such circumstances, there would be no moral requirement for those who have the care of the patient to feed forcefully the individual, unless there were genuine hope, based on some evidence, that the patient's opposition to eating was only temporary.

A somewhat similar issue is that of the individual who at the moment is not actually dying, but who needs constant medical assistance in order to keep living, and finds this too great a burden to bear. Examples of this condition would be those persons who require life-supporting measures such as chronic hemodialysis (kidney machine), mechanical ventilator for respiratory support, and frequent, repeated surgery for tumors. Such a patient may demand that these life-prolongation efforts be terminated.

231

Clearly, no one, no staff member, can cooperate with a patient who wishes to take matters in his own hand and actively terminate his own life. At the same time, a physician or nurse is not obliged to use every possible means to maintain life in a person who would otherwise die. As criteria two questions can be asked (discussed more fully in Chapter 9):

1) Is the means (medical procedure) of no benefit to the patient?
2) Does this means lay a burden on the patient (or others) which is too great to carry?

If the answer is "yes" to either question, then the means can be judged generally to be non-obligatory.

Specific Professional Concerns

a) The Physician and the Patient Seeking to Die*

Most patients in a hospital setting, who express a desire to die, either verbally or by action, are in one of the following four situations. They are:

1) choosing death in order to escape pain
2) severely depressed
3) suicidal because of non-organic psychosis with associated poor reality testing
4) demented or delirious because of an organic psychosis

It is of note that these four situations are ones in which medico-legally the physician may prevail against the will of the patient (with regard to treatment refusal) *if* the next of kin or the guardian concurs.

Since the majority of expressions of desire to die in hospitalized patients occur in situations in which the patients can often be treated successfully (to alleviate pain, relieve depression, or ameliorate psychosis), it is obvious that the first responsibility of an ethical physician is to be sure of an adequate medical/surgical diagnosis. A psychiatric consultant will often see patients, however, in whom delirium is not recognized and therefore the patient's behaviors or emotions are not understood.

Perhaps a more striking example of a need for adequate diagnosis is that recorded in a paper by Hudson, entitled "Death, Dying, and the Zealous Phase"[3] in which a man in his 60's has had a stroke. During the months that led to his full recovery of mental and physical functions, there had been frequent discussions among the patient, his wife, and the

---

*This section was structured around the initial presentation made by Alice Dean Kitchen, M.D.

physician about their joint desire that, if the patient were to have another stroke, no extraordinary life-prolonging measures would be used. The physician recounts the story that, subsequently, he received a call from the emergency room reporting that the gentleman in question had been brought in in a comatose condition and that the wife wished to talk to him. The wife reminded the physician of their desire to avoid extraordinary measures for prolongation of life. The physician wisely, however, told her that he could not make that decision without seeing the patient and being sure that the diagnosis was adequately made. This was quite fortunate, for examination revealed the patient to have a subdural hematoma, which was correctable by neurosurgery; after the operation, the patient fully recovered.

A second responsibility of the physician, after an adequate medical-surgical diagnosis, is the obtaining of a psychiatric consultation (which should usually be requested) in order to evaluate fully a person desiring to die, yet not terminally ill. As alluded to above, this is necessary for the assessment of several possible causes for such behaviors. Probably the most basic assessment has to do with the person's cognitive ability. Is there such impairment of cognition (perception, comprehension, memory and judgment) that the person does not in fact understand his or her situation and so is incapable of making a rational judgment? An answer to this question will provide a guide to the selection of management options.

A search should be made for evidences of depression. Any psychosis needs to be identified, as well as any extremes of affect or emotion which may result in such limited reality testing that the person feels that he could kill himself but would not die.[4]

In dealing with depression, it is well to recall that it is not a monolithic condition. Depressions exist along a continuum of which one end is neurotic depression and the other is the depression rooted in a biochemical imbalance. The latter cannot be treated with mere talk, although such may help the reactive depression secondary to the biochemically induced depression. The patient experiences the latter as something which comes over him as a cloud, and over which he has no control. He feels worse in the morning and relatively better in the afternoon, but, when profound, this depression results in relative immobilization of the individual.

The third responsibility of the physician is to institute the appropriate medical or psychiatric treatment for any of the above conditions which can be remedied. Delirium can usually be reversed by medical treatment and the competency of the patient restored. Depression can usually be treated successfully, so that suicidal thoughts and intentions may disappear. The elderly, for example, frequently respond to anti-depressants, although depression is not part of the aging process itself. Psychosis can usually be treated; many psychotic people can be restored to a state of mental competence. Yet it should be noted that a person can be judged competent for one activity, e.g., to make a will, and be judged at the same time, not competent for another, e.g., to make decisions or judgments regarding accepting or refusing treatment.

b) The Nurse and the Patient Seeking to Die*

To consider the topic of those who desire to die involves dealing with "suicide," and raises a host of troubling questions for the Christian nurse involved. The nurse, for example, is frequently the one in whom the patient confides regarding the desire for death. How should she respond? We also cannot ignore that there is growing interest in the proposition that suicide can be "rational." Perhaps the issue that suicide prevention may have unethical aspects and that there should be limitation on interference with suicide attempts needs to be raised.

However, what nurses are most accustomed to seeing in the hospital is the depressed or hopeless person who desires to die, whether due to physical illness and pain, or the culmination of many personal problems resulting in instability or crisis, or because of a chronic depressive state. Many elderly suffer from a sense of hopelessness and have difficulty coping with major changes in their life — e.g. loss of spouse and children, loss of independence, loss of meaning to their lives. The desire to die in these various states is frequently ambivalent. Many times the person sees death, not as a desirable end in itself, but as a way to interrupt or end severe anxiety or pain.

A special case, perhaps, are the elderly religious who have a deep faith and a great personal love of Jesus Christ. Having long been faithful pilgrims on the road to heaven, they are increasingly anxious to complete it as they get closer to their eternal destiny. Such persons — Sisters or otherwise — are not escaping from their current situation; instead they are "running" eagerly to the goal of life. Rather than fearing death, having lived their whole adult lives with a constant awareness of God's

*This section regarding the nurse's viewpoint is structured around the presentation made by Ms. Marti Templin, R.N., B.A.N.

presence and His love for them, they wish to embrace it as soon as possible. Indeed, some get angry and upset when another Sister in the same infirmary dies first. One Sister complained bitterly that a particular Sister had always beat her in life (she was her religious Superior for many years) and now at death beat her again by dying first!

It has been pointed out[5] that it is difficult to "respect the freedom of choice for self, when the self is fragmented." In these situations, when the patient is an obviously disturbed or upset person, the obligation to prevent suicide seems more clear cut than in a situation where the individual clearly values suicide as a brave act.

The nurse should realize that it is possible to encounter patients whose values differ from the nurses' own in this area which can create difficulties in functioning as an advocate for the patient. Myra Levine talks[6] about creating "a climate of moral respect essential to a climate of therapeutic effectiveness — the most basic premise being that the value system of the patient will be recognized, defended and even cherished."

As a nurse intent upon accepting a person as he is and where he is (and generally nurses highly value this caring principle), there have been many times when a nurse has been deeply moved by a patient's conviction that life for him is not worth living. The dilemma, when faced with a person who desires to die in these circumstances, seems to be: How does the nurse go about treating the decisions and desires expressed by the patient with respect while still attempting to alter them?

Creating a climate of moral respect *is* a major obligation on the part of the nurse. At the same time, it is wise for the nurse to keep in mind the following factors regarding suicide:

1) most people who express a desire to die have underlying ambivalent feelings;
2) suicide is *not* the norm in our culture and generally represents a desperate solution to problems on the part of the patient;
3) there seems to be a great deal of impulsiveness involved in the decision, i.e., even though a person is convinced of his argument, he may not be a week later;
4) the causes of suicide (precipitating factors) although uncertain, seem to be related to loneliness, hopelessness, and isolation.

All of these factors can be ameliorated by a caring attitude on the part of others, so it is definitely worth a try to intervene in such situations. In problematic situations, to assess the strengths or assets of a given patient along with the weaknesses or problems is desirable. In difficult situations, it is all too easy to see only the problems and get caught up in the patient's helplessness. Resisting that trap, the nurse can help the elderly be realistic and accept old age with its limitations, and learn to live their life to the fullest according to their available physical, mental and spiritual resources. One religious wisely pointed out that the elderly, who age at individual rates, represent "a lifetime of unique experiences wrapped up in a cloak of wrinkles."[7]

Nurses also need to be aware of what constitutes an ethical dilemma. Sometimes nurses are upset by things which do not truly pose a dilemma. For example, a patient may value life but need help finding alternatives other than suicide. In this instance, the need is for problem-solving. However, if the patient truly sees suicide as an acceptable alternative, this may pose more of a dilemma for the Christian nurse whose beliefs identify this action as a sin.

In chapter 10, Father Reilly's comments regarding the necessity for dialogue among health care providers should not be passed over lightly. The nurse is frequently employed in a bureaucratic setting and is frequently caught in the middle of an ethical dilemma. The need to discuss honestly such matters is imperative and not simply a luxury.

Some suggestions for dealing with suicidal patients may be of help:

1) Maintain an open dialogue. If a patient has chosen a particular person as a confidant, he or she should not "pass the buck." The need of the patient may be to see the willingness of another to be involved.
2) Provide a nonjudgmental environment with the opportunity for discussion.
3) Encourage the patient to share his feelings with those capable of providing support, or ask his permission to serve as a liaison.
4) Do not make promises which cannot be kept, i.e. do not promise to keep secret suicidal intentions.
5) Help the patient to bear painful feelings with your support and to discuss the meaning in this suffering.
6) Be truthful with the patient about your own beliefs and concerns.

Along with these specific approaches the nurse knows the factors to be considered regarding the safety of the environment, identification of persons at high risk for suicide, and the standard crisis intervention steps to be taken.

236

There are always gray areas when we begin talking about human rights. The desire to die, when not terminally ill, is directly related to the principle of autonomy and the right to self-determination and deserves careful consideration. Yet such self-determination does not include the right to self-extinction. Suicide is contrary to the basic needs (rights) related to life.

c) The Pastoral Care Person and the Patient Seeking to Die

As with the physician and the nurse, the pastoral care person dealing with a nonterminally ill patient who wishes to die is faced with a challenge. How is one to help such an individual, and how is one to deal pastorally with the patient's desire to end it all, and with its possible realization?

The pastoral care giver needs to approach the individual who seeks to die with an appreciation of the moral status of that desire to die, as briefly outlined above. A fundamental objective of the care giver is to assist the patient to make good decisions, decisions that contribute to the person's growth, maturation and sanctification. Part of that process will be to provide the individual with the appropriate information — as prudentially judged — which will present him with a better perspective of his present situation. Depending on the religious circumstance, the pastoral person may wish to remind the individual about God's loving care and mercy, about the life, death and resurrection of Jesus, as well as suggesting relevant Biblical passages.

Careful and tactful inquiry will reveal the individual's basic life orientation, strengths and weaknesses, future plans (or lack thereof), sources of present frustrations, irritations, disappointments, and anger. From such data, the pastoral care giver can begin to evaluate any stated reasons for the desire to die.

Having accomplished the above, the care giver can now seek for an area of strength and build on it. The objective is to rekindle hope in a realistic manner. It would be unwise simply to assert that, "the doctors are going to cure you and soon you will be home with your family," if that is not reality. If, on the other hand, that is indeed the situation, then the desire to return home and be once again in the midst of one's loving family can be an area of strength which can be used to foster the individual's hope.

Often times, there is no loving home to which to return and the only prospect for the individual is a "bleak" existence in a long-term-care facility or hospital until death comes to release the individual from a miserably experienced life. Faced with that kind of situation, the pastoral care person is challenged to elicit hope in that individual. That effort is directed to making the present existence more attractive to the person than its total absence, death.

One approach is to suggest a goal attainable by the patient so as to provide some kind of victory, insignificant as it may appear to be a vigorous and healthy peson. Such might be the writing or calling of a friend long forgotten, or completing some small task in the hospital. Small as it might be, the flame of a single match in the midst of total darkness throws considerable light. Another tactic would be to manipulate, as it were, the environment by urging family and friends to be more supportive, to keep the patient informed about daily events at home and in the neighborhood, to include the patient more often in decisions involving the family, and to seek his advice and wisdom in various matters.

Some patients claim that their life has been, and is now, meaningless. One approach is to encourage the individual to tell his life's story. Encouraged by the listener's patience, occasional affirmative remarks, and a nonjudgmental manner, the patient will speak about his past with increasing readiness. At suitable points, the care giver can point out the importance and significance of events in the individual's past. Thus, gradually, the patient can be led to see that his life has had meaning and that now that meaning perdures because of the impact his life has had on others. In addition, when appropriate, the pastoral care person can underline the importance of the present as a witness to others — family, friends, staff — of their cherished values, whatever these may be. For a religiously-oriented person, such might be to love and to trust God, for a more secular person, those values may be friendship or family or integrity, or some other values.

The most powerful instrument for bringing such a change in attitude is the care giver's own personhood. He or she can be a visible sign of God's love. How that person relates and interacts with the individual who seeks to die will determine whether or not God's love is concretely experienced. As one patient said to the chaplain: "Don't preach to me about God's love for me. First, show me by your actions that *you* truly love me, then I'll decide about God's love."

A particularly difficult situation is represented by a young man, Jim, who is in his early twenties, after experiencing at age 18 a motorcycle accident which left him as a quadraplegic. Having been very athletic and self-sufficient, he now finds himself completely dependent on others, even to urinate. Jim oscillates between anger and depression, and very much wants to die. Since he is not at all religious, religion is one resource not currently available to Jim.

Dealing with Jim when he is depressed likely would not be successful; a better chance of success would be to approach Jim when he was angry. He is more likely to be more accepting, and to act towards using and maximizing what little resources he has. In view of his previous athletic interests and ambitions, his ambition needs to be re-directed to new goals, such as learning to paint by holding the brush in the mouth — assuming he could still move his head. An example of constructive adaptation to a crippling disease is Father Paschal, who, very soon after ordination to the priesthood, was stricken by a severe muscular disease which left him essentially bedridden. He conceived, initiated and developed an extensive telephone ministry which consisted in calling other persons confined to their homes and sharing with them his deep faith and hope.

Perhaps more than the medical and nursing profession, the pastoral care person has to depend on the authenticity of his or her love of the patient to meet the challenge. While the physician and nurse have tangible skills they use to carry out their ministry, which also, of course, can be done with tender loving care, the pastoral care person is almost bereft of publicly recognized tangible and identifiable skills, and must depend more fully on a person-to-person impact. The authenticity and depth of love, the vitality of the pastoral care person's spiritual life, the strength of true hope, all are tested sharply in the strength of true hope, all are tested sharply in the close, helping encounter with a person seeking to die.

Concluding Synthesis

The physician, nurse and pastoral care peson face the same patient but see him through somewhat different glasses, as it were. Clearly, a cooperative approach to the patient generally will more likely result in a better management of the patient. It is less likely that the patient would successfully manipulate all three care givers and play one off against the other. Furthermore, the combined insights and skills will better utilize the special contributions of each.

Any close collaboration will depend, of course, on the personalities and desires of the physician, nurse and pastoral care person. Essential to a successful outcome is a willingness to submit one's pride of place and opinion to the test of "peer review." But these various conditions having been met, the team can proceed.

There are, it would seem, three principal concerns:
1) Why does this patient wish to die?
2) What can be done to remove that reason for wishing to die?
3) And how does one instill and support a desire to live?

In determining the reason for the patient's desire to die, the physician, and especially the psychiatrist, has a deep grasp of the kinds of psychological factors which can lead to such a desire. The nurse with an appreciation of this patient's personal situation and to whom the patient may confide (as perhaps a less formidable person than the physician) his fears, anxieties and desires, is able to contribute those concerns to an overall view of the patient. To this view, the pastoral care person offers the insights of religion and the spiritual status of the patient as still another dimension. In addition, the pastoral care person can often reflect on the ethical dimensions of the patient's situation and desires, as well as providing some guidance to the physician and nurse regarding any ethical concerns they may have relative to the management of this patient.

Having determined — to the extent possible — the dynamics of the patient's desire for death, the question of what to do about it assumes center stage. Here the physician's special skills and, when applicable, his armamentarium of drugs and other medical procedures can be brought into play. The application of medical art and the use of appropriate technological resources can be reinforced by the nurse in her dealings with the patient. But the nurse, with a compassionate and accepting manner, can do much to make the patient feel respected and wanted — both qualities necessary to sustain hope.

Building on whatever *spiritual* resources the patient may have, the pastoral care person helps the patient to view his present unpleasant state against the larger background of Faith. Acutely mindful that, in spiritual matters, authenticity is of paramount importance, the pastoral care giver approaches the patient, not with a plastic smile or with a superficial veneer of friendliness, but seeks to communicate the hope and the love of God by his or her very being. A prayerful and prayer-directed approach is perfectly appropriate and expected.

If, in spite of all the efforts of the physician, nurse and pastoral care person, the patient insists that life-sustaining therapy be terminated, or the patient steadfastly refuses to eat and vigorously resists forced feeding, the issue of suicide becomes acute. As briefly discussed above, suicide, *objectively* speaking, is morally evil, even if, *subjectively,* the culpability is reduced because the person's freedom of the will has been impaired by physiological or psychological factors.

But what about the nonterminally ill patient or person who wishes to die? In that situation, the issue generally is not the nonuse of a life-saving *therapeutic* measure. Rather, it is a question of ordinary food and drink. Basically a person is obligated to take necessary food and water. Yet when the *taking* of nourishment with technical assistance — such as *continuous* forced feeding by intubation — becomes so burdensome to the patient, then it would seem that the obligation of the staff to provide food to the patient is eliminated. As discussed above, this response presumes that all other appropriate means to alter the patient's attitude and actions have been exhausted.

In concert, the physician, nurse, and pastoral care person can do much to alleviate the terrible loneliness of the person who seeks to die. Having initiated the process of cutting himself off from ordinary human communion by the desire to die, the patient needs the caring support of physicians, nurses, and pastoral care persons to help him with reasons for living.

Notes

1. Veatch, Robert M., "Caring for the Dying Person — Ethical Issues at Stake," in David Bahm's *Dying and Death: A Clinical Guide for Caregivers,* Williams & Wilkin, 1977.
2. *Ibid.*
3. *Annals of Internal Medicine,* pages 696-702, 1978.
4. Olin, Harry S., "Death Without Dying: The Third Wish in Suicide," *American Journal of Psychotherapy*, 32:270-5, April 1978.
5. Levine, Myra, "Nursing Ethics and the Ethical Nurse," *American Journal of Nursing,* 77:845-47, May 1977.
6. *Ibid.*
7. Gasek, George, "How to Handle the Crotchety Elderly Patient," *Nursing 80,* March, 1980, p. 48.

Chapter 17

The Responsibilities
of Administrators

The Reverend Donald G. McCarthy, Ph. D.

Previous chapters have examined many facets of prolonging life decisions and many kinds of such decisions. Where such decisions are made within hospitals and long term care facilities, the person in charge of the operation of the facility, the administrator, carries a moral and legal responsibility for them. This chapter will consider the administrator as servant, as policy formulator, as educator, and as Church liaison.

The Administrator as Servant

In his remarks to administrators at one of our seminars, Father Lawrence Reilly spoke of them as Christ figures, reflecting the Father's love to those they lead, and drawing them closer to the Father through the common mission they share. Since person-centered health care must serve people in their need, the administrator becomes the chief servant, in the image of Jesus Who said, "The Son of Man has not come to be served but to serve" (Mk 10:45).

In the face of the common complaint that health care institutions are becoming excessively preoccupied with impersonal delivery of expert specialized services, the administrator has the responsibility to assure that quality services are delivered to the people in their facilities, while maintaining proper concern for the staff who deliver them. Each administrator personifies the prevailing attitude and atmosphere of his or her facility. Those who manage to spend part of each day meeting with department heads and moving about their buildings in face to face communication with staff and patients, or residents, in the case of long term care facilities, set an example of personal service. Those who usually remain inaccessible in their offices and board rooms set an example of impersonal leadership.

Some years ago, Bishop Albert Ottenweiler of Steubenville, Ohio, gave a famous speech to the National Conference of Catholic Bishops in which he used the "funnel" metaphor. He described the multitude of movements and agencies wishing to reach the people of modern parishes who send the pastor endless bulletins, announcements, questionnaires, appeals for funds, and summons for important meetings. The pastor, already heavily burdened with parish responsibilities, feels as though all these extraneous requests are pouring into a funnel somewhere above him and come out the bottom in a constant stream right on top of his head.

The servant-administrators of modern hospitals and nursing homes experience a similar funnel syndrome. Besides the internal responsibilities of day to day management of their facilities, they feel the pressure of a constant stream of additional concerns — the legal and legislative developments that affect their facilities, the economic and inflationary trends that cause fiscal headaches, the paperwork and staggering complexity of government regulations and reimbursement practices, and the constant growth of specialization and sophistication in health care itself. Small wonder that Fr. Reilly, in the remarks mentioned above, stressed the need of administrators having a deep and strong prayer life to support and strengthen them!

The appropriate way to handle the funnel syndrome, of course, involves a distribution of the many concerns facing the administrator among many members of the leadership team in each institution. This, in turn, presumes a shared sense of mission and a shared responsibility for living the ideals and striving toward the goals of the facility. The working document for self-renewal of Catholic health care facilities, the *Evaluative Criteria for Catholic Health Care Facilities,* published in 1980 by the Catholic Health Association, clearly and convincingly presents eight principles, supported by numerous guidelines, which spell out these fundamental ideals. As the administrative leadership of Catholic facilities involves an ever increasing number of lay men and women, an intense study of these ideals, all rooted in the Gospel vision of life, health, and service, is becoming ever more crucial.

The prolonging life issues presented in this volume typify the complex responsibilities of administrators. Often an administrator must personally face sensitive problems in which conflicts growing out of the situation of individual patients or residents, as well as conflicts arising from different physicians', nurses', and families' views of patients' needs, must be resolved.

For instance, in one of our seminars an administrator described the case of *Florence E.,* a 96 year old woman, brought to her acute care hospital in a coma. Her blood pressure, temperature, and urinary output were normal. The cause of her coma was undetermined, though it could have been related to a cardiovascular accident. She was receiving intravenous nourishment. After Florence had been receiving IV's for several weeks, the nurses found increasing difficulty in locating veins and her arms were badly bruised by their efforts.

The nursing supervisor approached the administrator about Florence's case because the nurses had been complaining that continuing the IV's was unnecessary and impractical. They pointed out that Florence's family had requested only comfort measures. The administrator was expected to settle this problem involving moral, legal and professional complications.

The first thing she discovered was a lack of communication between Florence's attending physician and the nursing staff. When she spoke to the physician, he frankly acknowledged the difficulties the IV's were causing the nurses. He made clear, though, that he felt an obligation to provide minimal nourishment so that Florence would not die of starvation or suffer from dehydration. He promised to discuss the situation more fully with the nurses and keep closer contact with them.

The moral responsibility of providing ordinary and ethically obligatory medical treatment led to the doctor's use of IV nourishment. To judge the IV ethically extraordinary, one must establish either that it is useless or an excessive burden on the patient. The physician was not convinced that it was useless, since the patient was not actually dying, and her coma may not have been irreversible. The burden on the patient was difficult to estimate since she was unconscious and noncompetent. The administrator respected the physician's ethical and professional concern, and made no attempt to change his mind. Two weeks later, Florence expired without ever regaining consciousness.

In this case, the administrator acted as arbiter to help resolve a dispute within her own institution. She and the attending physician discussed openly the difficult question of withdrawing artificial provision of nourishment which is also discussed briefly in chapter 20 of this volume. Through the mediating role of the administrator, everyone involved in the care of Florence came to a fuller appreciation of their own painful sharing in the mysterious life crisis of this aged patient.

Administrators cannot expect simple answers to resolve complex dilemmas like the one created by Florence's condition. The Judeo-Christian view of the universe accepts the reality of an almost unlimited variety of human illnesses which sometimes leave health care professionals pondering whether they are prolonging living or prolonging dying. In Florence's case, reverence for life and the provision of basic life-support, even of a 96-year-old woman who could hardly be considered a "productive" member of society, produced much uneasiness and ambivalence among the nursing staff. Yet the concern for this elderly woman offers a prophetic witness value in a society which tends to devalue elderly persons, particularly when their care becomes burdensome.

The decision about continuing the IV for Florence had to be made by her attending physician in the light of his own conscience since he felt the IV was ethically ordinary and obligatory. Administrators must be prepared for situations where physicians' consciences are not nearly as sensitive as that of Florence's physician. While administrators cannot themselves make decisions in place of physicians or patients, they can establish basic institutional policies to be upheld by physicians and patients within their institutions.

The Administrator as Policy-Formulator

The *Ethical and Religious Directives for Catholic Health Facilities,* revised and approved in 1971 by the National Conference of Catholic Bishops as the national code, subject to the approval of the bishop for use in each diocese, provide several key directives for prolonging life issues in Catholic facilities. For instance, directive #28 excludes mercy killing and the failure to supply ordinary means of prolonging life, while pointing out that neither the physician nor the patient is obliged to the use of extraordinary means. Directive #29 permits use of necessary pain medication, even though it may deprive the patient of the use of reason or shorten his or her life. Directive #1 insists on the consent of the patient or his guardians, at least implied or reasonably presumed, for all permissible procedures. Directive #8 specifies the physician's duty to inform patients if their condition is critical, or have some other responsible person impart this information, unless it is clear that the dying patient is already well-prepared for death as regards both spiritual and temporal affairs.

Each health care facility under Catholic sponsorship has, in the sum total of the 43 Directives, including the four mentioned above, a competent and authentic statement of some key ethical and religious principles for health care to guide its own policy and procedure manuals. The specific policies formulated in each institution for medical and nursing staffs will vary greatly according to individual needs and preferences. However, two major concerns in the prolonging life issues addressed in this volume should be carefully treated in institutional policies. These are the matters of consent of patients or patients' representatives for treatment, and the responsible determination of when medical procedures are ethically extraordinary and hence nonobligatory within the stewardship of life ethical tradition.

With regard to *consent* policies, most facilities have a general consent form signed upon admission which covers all ordinary medical procedures. In the light of prolonging life issues, a policy statement should somehow make clear that this consent does not cover whatever procedures may become ethically extraordinary. For an extraordinary procedure, a specific consent of the patient or patient's representative seems necessary, either to provide or to forego such procedures. Normally, a special consent form is required for surgery and for some test procedures which may well be extraordinary. But, to be consistent with the principles presented here, consent should be obtained for any ethically extraordinary procedures. In given circumstances, this may include hemodialysis, use of a respirator, calling an emergency code for resuscitation, implanting a heart pacemaker, transfer to an Intensive Care Unit, or transfer from a nursing home to an acute care hospital.

Need such consent be obtained in writing and in a legally acceptable form? This may be advisable, although many lawyers feel that a general consent to medical treatment provides a sufficient legal consent for most of the examples mentioned above. Undoubtedly, some physicians handle these kinds of situations without much concern for explicit consent. If they judge that medical benefits can be attained by these means, they often implicitly presume they are ethically ordinary, and no further patient consent is necessary. Yet the next chapter, on "Responsibilities of Physicians," points out the possibility that nonmedical considerations, like the expense or burden of a given treatment, might render it ethically extraordinary and optional in the case of individual patients.

From the very nature of the patient-physician relationship discussed earlier in this volume by Dr. Boyle in chapter 6, physicians are always expected to inform their patients about their medical condition and their proposed treatments. Hence, it is inappropriate for a physician to inaugurate any treatment without informing the patient and thereby obtaining an implicit consent, simply by offering an opportunity of refusal of the treatment. And the very submission of a patient to a physician's care supports the assumption of consent to ordinary medical treatment.

However, the discussion in this volume about ethically extraordinary means of prolonging life has highlighted the patient's moral right to refuse ethically extraordinary treatment. Therefore, physicians are encouraged to obtain explicit patient consent for procedures that may be judged ethically extraordinary. Administrators of health care facilities can support this recommendation in policy statements for their facility.

For example, a statement like this could be included in an institutional policy regarding consent practices:

> The consent of patients for treatment in this facility included with admission requirements extends to all standard medical treatments. However, it is understood that in given circumstances such treatments may offer minimal hope of benefit or represent an excess burden or expense to the patient. In such circumstances, explicit consent to such treatment should be obtained from the patient or patient's representative and this should be noted in the patient's chart.

This recommendation arises more from the ethical ideal of full recognition of the patient's own right and responsibility to choose or forego ethically extraordinary procedures than from legal concerns.

Admittedly, the effort to obtain consent from patients' representatives poses many practical difficulties. In our seminars with administrators, instances were cited in which the person who assumed responsibility for a patient was not the next of kin. For example, Sharon P. admitted her aunt to the hospital and assumed responsibility for her. Subsequently, her cousin, Ken, the aunt's only son, returned on a brief visit from a distant state, thus posing a conflict about who really represented the patient.

Physicians attending patients have the responsibility to clarify such ambiguous situations. In this case, the son, from out of state, may well assert his legal right as next of kin to represent his mother, if there is no legally binding document which excludes him. Of course, he would also assume legal and financial responsibilities, if he replaced his cousin, Sharon. The policies of health care facilities cannot resolve such individual difficulties, but they can encourage maximum efforts to locate the next of kin of patients, and notify them of the admission of their relatives.

The *second* major concern for administrators, in questions of life-prolonging decisions, centers on the often difficult question of whether a given treatment or procedure should be considered *ethically extraordinary*. As already indicated by Fr. Connery in chapter 9 above, the burden a treatment imposes on a particular patient may be sufficiently serious to render the treatment ethically optional. The fact that this involves an individual and subjective judgment will be discussed in the next chapter on "Responsibilities of Physicians." It remains the task of patients or their representatives, in consultation with physicians, to determine if a procedure or treatment should be considered ethically extraordinary.

Health care facilities can hardly determine by policy statements which medical procedures are ethically extraordinary and nonobligatory. Within the facility, an effort should be made to clarify the general meaning of this distinction. A medical-moral committee can serve as an advisory committee to examine difficult cases and to prepare statements for general guidance. A book like this one can serve as a resource for those concerned with the distinction.

However, one practical application of this distinction which is receiving increasing attention in hospitals and even in nursing homes comes from the decision not to call a code or emergency resuscitation procedure. According to the ethical principles presented in this volume, a no-code order should be based on a *judgment* and a *decision*. By *judgment* is meant the conclusion that for a given patient the calling of a code is an ethically extraordinary and nonobligatory procedure for prolonging life. The *decision*, following upon this judgment, directs that the code will be omitted.

The most obvious cases where a resuscitation procedure can be judged ethically extraordinary are those where a patient is genuinely dying and the procedure merely prolongs the dying process. By analogy, one might extend this judgment to the irreversibly comatose patient, considering the procedure a useless burden. By extension of the same analogy, one might consider the resuscitation a useless burden in the case of a person of advanced age and generally deteriorating health who is terminally ill from an accumulation of physical causes.

When a competent patient makes the judgment in consultation with an attending physician that the resuscitation is not obligatory and chooses against it, the ethical requirements of the omission have been most satisfactorily fulfilled. Unfortunately, many patients for whom the procedure is nonobligatory are not able to make a competent judgment and decision. The ethical principles outlined in this volume permit a patient's representative to make this *judgment* with medical advice and to make the *decision* to omit in behalf of the patient.

However, the legal and professional responsibilities of attending physicians expose them to civil or criminal charges of neglect if they order the omission of a code without adequate medical basis and patient, or patient representative, consultation. One hospital's policy in this regard distinguishes between competent and noncompetent patients, and those who are terminally ill and nonterminally ill. The patient's consent is required for the competent patients. For the noncompetent who is terminally ill, the physician may write the order after consultation with the patient's legal guardian, if any, or with the patient's family. For the noncompetent who is not terminally ill, this hospital, influenced by court decisions within its own state, only permits writing the order after court direction or authorization.

In the light of the *judgment* and *decision* involved in a "no code" order, the physician's notation on the patient's order sheet should indicate the medical basis for the judgment that a code is not to be called, and should record the consent of the patient or patient's representative who have approved the decision not to resuscitate. Physicians have understandably hesitated to write such orders, fearing that such orders might be understood as a kind of medical neglect. Yet, writing down the reasons for the order and the consent obtained will offer legal protection. It seems clear that occasions can arise when resuscitation would violate a patient's rights and represent a form of medical over-treatment.

The "Standards and Guidelines for Cardiopulmonary Resuscitation and Emergency Cardiac Care," published by the *Journal of the American Medical Association* on August 1, 1980, direct that physicians write the order not to resuscitate on the physician's order sheet when this decision has been reached for a hospitalized patient.[1] Since this decision comes under the responsibility of the attending physician, it cannot be made by nursing personnel, and merely verbal orders from the physician are not legally satisfactory. Some hospitals have made explicit in medical policy statements the fact that every patient shall receive cardiopulmonary resuscitation in the event of sudden respiratory or cardiac arrest, unless an order not to resuscitate is *written* on the physician's order sheet. Nurses and resuscitation team members are understandably anxious to see physicians write this order, when appropriate, to preclude their being obligated to perform a procedure which is contrary to a patient's best interest. Hence, hospitals have a legitimate interest in encouraging physicians to discuss the possible judgment that resuscitation is not morally obligatory, and the decision to omit it, with patients or patients' representatives in those cases where performing resuscitation may be inappropriate.

Nursing homes and long term care facilities also must face the issue of resuscitation. The same basic concerns about a *judgment* and a *decision* apply. Even though the equipment for emergency resuscitation may be unavailable, nurses who have learned the technique are expected to initiate the emergency procedures of CPR manually and mouth-to-mouth. Nursing home administrators who foresee situations where resuscitation might be inappropriate should bring this to the attention of the attending physicians of those residents.

Resuscitation procedures have been discussed here as an example of a life-prolonging procedure which may be ethically extraordinary and nonobligatory. The same basic pattern of a *judgment* and a *decision* applies to other situations which may arise. As a result of the *Karen*

Quinlan case, many hospitals are developing administrative policies regarding the withdrawal of life-support equipment. The categories of competent and noncompetent patients and of terminally ill and non-terminally ill patients can be used here also.

The most obvious situation for withdrawal of life-support equipment arises with a patient in the final stage of terminal illness or irreversibly comatose, as discussed above in chapter 13. If that patient is noncompetent, as is usually the case, the role of the patient's representative becomes crucial. That representative must concur both in the judgment that the life support procedure is ethically nonobligatory, and in the actual decision to withdraw it. Furthermore, the decision to withdraw it must be based either on the patient's own previously expressed and reasonable wish, or a judgment of the patient's own best interest. These are the ethical prerequisites according to the principles presented in this volume.

The legal requirements for withdrawal of life-support are influenced by the legislation and court precedents in the different states. Hence, any facility's policy in this matter must be drawn up according to the considered judgment of legal advisors of that state. Several sample hospital policies about orders not to resuscitate and the withdrawal of life-support equipment are presented in Appendix II of this volume. This chapter will conclude with some practical recommendations for administrators as education-facilitators and Church-liaison persons.

The Administrator as Education-Facilitator

This volume has focused particularly on *moral* responsibility in prolonging life decisions. Since health care facilities are moral persons pledged to the care of patients or residents, these facilities have a moral as well as a legal responsibility for prolonging the lives of these persons. Because this responsibility obligates them to provide ethically ordinary means and to offer the option of ethically extraordinary means, the facilities do need medical-moral policies similar to those discussed above. Individual decisions can then be made within the framework of such policies. But no administrator wishes to write policies about such complex questions singlehandedly.

Hence, medical-moral committees, discussed more fully below in chapter 20, can be used by the administrator in formulating institutional policies. Medical-moral committees usually include representative physicians, nurses, therapists, social workers, administrators, pastoral care workers, ethical and legal advisors, and, sometimes, patient or patient-family representatives. Medical-moral committees can only function properly if the members diligently study the moral and legal status of the issues they address. Hence, such a committee must always give first priority to the self-education of its own members.

Such a committee may assist a facility with prolonging life decisions in three different ways. *First* of all, it can lessen the burden on administrators and diminish the impact of the funnel syndrome mentioned early in this chapter, by drafting proposed policies which can then be given appropriate authorization within the facility. *Secondly*, the members of this committee can help initiate the proper educational programs for other staff members of their own particular skill or role regarding these policies and their rationale. *Thirdly*, the committees can serve as advisors in difficult individual situations like the case of Florence E. above. Their role must remain advisory — they may never assume the actual decision-making which belongs to the patient or patient representatives and attending physicians.

In one of our seminars with administrators, a story was told of a medical-moral committee in a Catholic long-term-care facility. The committee was formed because of three difficult medical-moral issues about prolonging life within the facility. The three issues were those of: 1) decisions about whether or not to transfer residents to acute care hospitals, 2) the problem of decisions about emergency resuscitation, and, 3) the issues relating to artificial feeding similar to the case of Florence E. above. After a year's work together, two hours a month, this committee had still not formulated any written policies and had even begun to feel that no further written policies were necessary. But the committee members had become much more confident of the appropriate way to approach the three issues of concern and were able to function much better in their leadership role within the facility. They were prepared to meet difficult situations, and provide understanding and support to the administrator because of their work together.

This educational process for members of medical-moral committees should somehow be broadened to reach the other physicians, nurses, therapists, social workers, administrators, and pastoral care persons who staff each health care facility. The representatives of these professions on the medical-moral committee need help in finding ways of accomplishing this. If an inservice educational program exists in the

252

facility, medical-moral education should by all means be included.[2] As mentioned below in chapter 20, the pastoral care staff members usually have the background and initiative to assist in these programs. The scope of this education goes far beyond prolonging life issues. It should include a basic study of the philosophy and theology of health care, patients' rights and responsibilities, ethical principles of confidentiality, personal dignity and professional integrity, social justice and employee rights and responsibilities, and all the ethical issues flowing from responsible stewardship of human life, health, and procreation.

Religiously-sponsored health care facilities have a special privilege and responsibility to create a spirit of mission and service in accord with the religious ideals which they represent. A basic theological analogy which is particularly helpful to persons of the Judeo-Christian tradition is that of *covenant*, an agreement between persons based upon mutual trust and fidelity. The Old Testament of the Bible portrays God's original covenant with His people while the New Testament records the new covenant Jesus established by His life, death, and resurrection. When a Jewish or Christian health care facility admits a patient or resident, it does so in the spirit of covenant, reflecting the love and fidelity of the religious covenant. The facility says implicitly, "We will bring the Father's tender loving care to you and you will be our people." Staff and employees of a health care facility can prepare annual celebrations to renew their role in the health care covenant, perhaps on a religious feast day like St. Luke's day in October, or on the anniversary of the founding of the facility. They might even sign a book of the covenant when first employed, and renew that signing annually.

The Administrator as a Church Liaison Person

Catholic health care facilities should be considered ecclesial communities belonging to the Church of their particular diocese or archdiocese. They serve the people of God under the leadership and support of their local Bishop. In our seminars with administrators, it became apparent that the chief contact many facilities have with their Bishops arises when difficult and even explosive medical-moral issues must be faced, especially the traditional Catholic prohibition of performing tubal ligations in Catholic facilities. A consensus emerged that ways must be found to strengthen the relationship of Catholic health care facilities with the local Church and the local Bishop. Events such as the covenant renewal mentioned above could provide joyful occasions to bring the Bishop and local pastors to hospitals and nursing homes. Religious feast days, communal celebration of anointing, Confirmation, and even Lenten penance services might provide other occasions in the Catholic liturgical tradition. The Bishop would often be honored to speak at annual meetings of the medical staff, as well as fundraising events sponsored by the facility or the volunteer auxiliary.

In the spirit of communication to the public, many health care facilities prepare annual reports of their services and activities. If the facility wishes to emphasize its ecclesial commitment, this report might be presented annually to the Bishop and selected clergy, religious, and lay leaders of the Church, in a program featuring audiovisual documentation and the participation of department heads and other leaders in the facility. Bishops are becoming more aware of the challenges of health care ministry and the tremendous problems and potential of health care facilities. Efforts from within the ranks of administrators can only enhance this awareness and strengthen the relationship with the local Church and Bishop.

Conclusion

This chapter began with reflections on the administrators as servants. In their role, they need not pretend to be either ethicists or lawyers. Administrators can reduce most of their problems to one fundamental need — to build a strong commitment of their entire staff to focus on their patients or residents as persons. This will assure proper patient consent and responsible deliberation in the life-prolonging decisions discussed in this volume.

This fundamental need flows directly from the teaching of Jesus, appealing to administrators to recognize all their patients and residents as members of His family and to realize His norm of entering the kingdom: "I was ill and you comforted me." (Mt. 25:36)

Notes

1. *Journal of the American Medical Association*, 244:507, 1980.
2. See *Evaluative Criteria for Catholic Health Care Facilities*, (St. Louis, MO, Catholic Health Association, 1980), pp. 33-37.

Chapter 18

The Responsibilities
of Physicians

The Reverend Donald G. McCarthy, Ph. D.

Introduction

Some physicians, in recent years, have felt themselves trapped by their own amazing capacity to prolong human lives through life-support equipment and procedures. They remember the ancient Hippocratic oath to "use treatment to help the sick according to my ability and judgment, but never with a view to injury and wrongdoing." They hesitate to withdraw life-support equipment and allow death to occur, because this seems dangerously close to the "injury and wrongdoing" forbidden by the oath.

Some physicians have felt that broadening the criteria for determining death might relieve some of this tension. Obviously, once a patient has been declared dead, the physician is relieved of the onus of providing life-support equipment or procedures. To declare an irreversibly comatose person dead may seem acceptable since that person is not ever going to regain consciousness or function in a human way. Experienced physicians can cite numerous circumstances where their patient is "practically dead," "as good as dead," or "virtually dead."

Logic and ethics, however, strongly oppose classifying the near-dead as dead. To treat a living human being as dead legitimizes, not only removal of life-support, but lethal acts such as removal of the heart or draining of the blood in preparation for embalming. The discussion in chapters 3 and 4 of this volume argued that determination of death by brain criteria must identify as dead only those individuals who are truly and certainly dead, not half-dead or nearly dead.

This means that physicians cannot escape the trap of indefinitely maintaining life-support procedures by devising a determination that death has occurred when it has not. It means that physicians must either practice a kind of medical scrupulosity by never omitting or withdrawing life-support, or participate in a decision-making process to identify when treatments or procedures are ethically or legally nonobligatory.

Although patients and their families are free to choose physicians and they sometimes dismiss them, as long as a physician is the attending physician of any given patient, that physician holds moral and legal responsibility for the treatment of that patient. Dr. Boyle pointed out, in chapter 6 above, that the physician who is responsible for a noncompetent patient faces special difficulties because someone other than the patient authorizes treatment or nontreatment.

This chapter considers the responsibilities of physicians who must both follow their own consciences and yet provide only authorized treatment according to the principles of free and informed consent. The three sections will present: 1) A review of the ethical norms, 2) Some cases of physician responsibility, and 3) Practical moral and legal conclusions.

A Review of the Ethical Norms

The Vatican *Declaration on Euthanasia* made clear that the distinction between an ethically ordinary and obligatory means of prolonging life and an ethically extraordinary and optional means involves more then purely medical considerations:

> It will be possible to make a correct judgment as to the means by studying the type of treatment to be used, its degree of complexity

256

or risk, its cost and the possibilities of using it, and comparing these elements with the result that can be expected, taking into account the state of the sick person and his or her physical and moral resources.[1]

Clearly, the physician who takes into account the *cost* of a life-prolonging treatment, the *possibilities* of using it, and the sick person's *moral resources*, as mentioned here, has gone beyond purely medical and scientific judgments. A physician may or may not know a patient and family very well, hence including these nonmedical considerations may or may not seem practical and feasible. Yet, even the physician who knows the patient well should realize that the patient's *own estimate* of these factors must be respected and may differ from the physician's.

How should the physician handle these nonmedical considerations? The physician should surely begin any discussion with patients or families by presenting the relevant *medical* considerations. It may be that a procedure is practically useless from a medical perspective. The physician should explain why this leads to an ethical judgment that this procedure is ethically extraordinary and nonobligatory. Should the patient or family still request the procedure, the physician should comply, providing there are financial resources to provide it. It is understandable that reimbursement programs may be designed to exclude coverage of such treatments. This is ethically acceptable providing the exclusion is nondiscriminatory. Hospitals which have only limited funds for nonreimbursement treatment might legitimately refuse to provide this kind of practically useless treatment without reimbursement.

On the other hand, the treatment under consideration will much more frequently offer some true medical benefits, either as a standard medical treatment or at least as a common treatment of choice. The physician should explain this to the patient or family because this medical judgment favors the ethical conclusion that the procedure may also be ethically ordinary and obligatory. *At this point*, responsible physicians proceed differently. Some ignore the nonmedical considerations and wait for consent or nonconsent. Others suggest that nonmedical factors may have a bearing on the decision without offering much elaboration. Others find ways of discussing the nonmedical factors, sometimes by offering their own opinions or how they would weigh such factors.

As a matter of fact, the *same* physician may sometimes ignore, sometimes briefly allude to, and sometimes fully discuss nonmedical factors like cost and burden to the patient or family, depending on how significant the physician considers these factors in a given case. Since cases do differ so substantially in the complex world of modern medicine, this may be an appropriate policy for a physician. But a comment can be made about each of the three ways a physician may handle nonmedical factors.

First, if the physician ignores these factors, this should be based only on a sufficient knowledge of the patient and family to assure that these really would be irrelevant concerns in their own judgment.

Secondly, if the physician only alludes to these factors without elaborating on them, this must be done in such a way as to leave this subject open for further clarification. A physician should not merely allude to such factors in passing without leaving an opening for further discussion, unless convinced that these factors are really irrelevant in the judgment of patient and family.

Thirdly, if the physician does explicitly discuss the nonmedical factors, this must be done objectively enough not to manipulate the opinion of the patient or family. A physician speaks from a position of authority, and can easily sway some patients or families to either consider or not consider the nonmedical factors in their decision-making. However, the physician should be willing to express and explain his or her own opinion.

Admittedly, many physicians prefer to limit their discussions of proposed treatments to purely medical aspects of the treatment, and simply attempt to portray accurately the medical advantages and disadvantages. Patients expect and deserve this kind of thorough clarification. Obviously, the limited medical advantages of a treatment may render it ethically extraordinary or optional. The physician will be best prepared to make this kind of judgment. But the *nonmedical* factors may also render a treatment ethically extraordinary, despite the medical outcome which would seem to render it ordinary. Sensitive physicians must be prepared to deal with these nonmedical factors also.

This volume has consistently reflected the ethical tradition which admits that nonmedical factors like burden and expense can render a medical treatment ethically optional. Some who read this volume may be tempted to interpret this position as total subjectivism, as if the consideration of nonmedical factors would undermine objectivity and reduce prolonging life decisions to the arbitrary whim of patients or families.

The possibility of such arbitrariness cannot be ignored, but the possibility of abuse does not vitiate the principle itself. Ethicists would designate the concrete judgment that a medical treatment for a given patient is ethically extraordinary and nonobligatory as a prudential, rather than an empirical judgment. Prudential judgments require both wisdom and experience. They also can often be the subject of disagreement among sincere and upright people, even though prudence depends on general principles which are reasonable and rational.

A volume like this one offers background principles for such prudential judgments. It teaches the priceless value of even the most debilitated human life and opposes the moral evil of destroying innocent lives, even for reasons of mercy. It also teaches the affirmative obligation to care for human life and make reasonable efforts to prolong it.

When does a life-prolonging procedure become unreasonable? Fr. Connery responded in chapter 9 that this happens when the burden of providing it is excessive or when the procedure is useless because the patient will soon die anyway. In the seminars with physicians, it became clear that no specific empirical or scientific norm of excessive burden can be set down for all cases. Instead, it was clear that the ethical method of casuistry must be used — comparing one case with another, drawing analogies and relevant points of agreement. Moral theologians would insist, as pointed out above in chapter 15, that those who make casuistic judgments act with "purity of heart," a reverence for the gift of life rooted in its inherent transcendance and mystery.

Physicians who care for hundreds of patients with similar problems and with similar decisions to make spontaneously develop some casuistic skill, providing they have been properly instructed themselves. In that sense, they can be seen as value educators and medico-moral catechists for their patients and families. Such physicians teach patients and families to make reasonable and informed decisions about life-prolonging procedures; they would be the last to suggest that these decisions can be made at the mere whim or arbitrary choice of a patient.

The discussions in chapter 15 about severely defective newborn babies insisted that the moral casuistry in determining if a medical procedure is ethically extraordinary must not be used in a way which discriminates against those persons who suffer a diminished quality of life. In other words, physicians, patients, and families must not suppose that a treatment becomes ethically extraordinary simply because it cannot lift such a person to a more normal quality of life. As Fr. Connery pointed out in chapter 9, handicapped people are ethically obliged and privileged to receive the same basic standard of medical care as others in the population. It is true that, in certain cases, a handicapped person may find a medical procedure more burdensome than someone else, and this might lead to the judgment that the procedure has become ethically extraordinary and nonobligatory because of that additional burden.

This highly theoretical review of the ethical norms for life-prolonging decisions from the physician's perspective has emphasized the importance of studying individual cases and applying the theoretical principles accordingly. Several cases discussed at our physicians' seminars are presented here.

Some Cases of Physicians' Responsibility

The first case concerns Frederick F., a 58 year old truck driver, with a carcinoma of the bowel metastasized to the lymph nodes and liver. The oncologist presented Frederick with the medical facts and a prognosis of inevitable death. Chemotherapy could prolong life an additional 3-6 months. The medical advantages and disadvantages were presented as accurately as possible. The nonmedical factors which could figure in the decision about chemotherapy included the expense, since Frederick had no private health insurance coverage, and the burden on his wife who herself was both arthritic and diabetic. Frederick had an ample life insurance policy and was spiritually prepared to accept death.

Most physicians would instinctively recognize that the inevitable terminal outcome of Frederick's carcinoma lessens any moral or professional responsibility to use the chemotherapy. The nonmedical factors in Frederick's own situation seemed likewise to support the judgment that the chemotherapy was not an ethically ordinary or obligatory medical treatment. Frederick and his physician established this judgment in the course of an office visit and decided to forego the chemotherapy.

Yet, there is no ethical obligation to forego an ethically optional treatment. Frederick actually changed his mind after a discussion with his wife and his daughter who was pregnant with her fourth child. He requested the chemotherapy after all — that decision remained entirely in his hands. He did live seven more months.

If, on the other hand, Frederick's physician had a 95 percent hope of remission of a non-metastasized cancer, the picture would have changed radically. In fact, the physician might then be convinced that chemotherapy is ethically obligatory, and to omit it a form of medical and moral negligence. Should Frederick refuse the treatment for fear of side effects or because his wife is divorcing him and he has no will to live, the physician may face a genuine conscience question. Should the physician continue to treat Frederick in a less than adequate manner — would this not violate the physician's conscience? It seems possible that a conscientious physician might tell Frederick that he would appreciate his finding a different physician since he would be refusing ethically ordinary treatment.

A second case concerns baby Jonathan, born with congenital lung and heart defects. Dr. N., the attending physician, had informed the young parents of the hopeless condition of Jonathan. Corrective surgery was impossible. The financial burden for the neonatal intensive care was mounting overwhelmingly and Jonathan's parents had only minimal insurance coverage. An informal consensus developed among Jonathan's parents, the nursing staff, the pastoral care advisor, and the other staff physicians that life-support equipment was no longer ethically obligatory for Jonathan. But Dr. N. could not accept that judgment. In her daily conversations with the family she pleaded for more time, hoping that either Jonathan would show unforeseen improvement or expire naturally. Jonathan lived three weeks after his parents and their pastoral advisor first requested the removal of the life-support equipment, and died without its being removed.

In this case, Dr. N. either could not accept the judgment that life-support equipment had become ethically extraordinary or she may have feared the legal repercussions of removing the equipment. Unfortunately, three weeks seems a long period of indecision and, from the facts as presented, Dr. N. seems to have acted wrongly. Jonathan's parents could surely have substituted another attending physician for Dr. N. The hospital administrator and lawyer could have been consulted to assure proper legal procedures, if the physicians agreed to withdraw the life-support equipment.

While respect for newborn human persons and the mysterious survival power of infants surely justifies giving newborn infants the benefit of medical-moral doubt, as discussed above in chapter 15, in this case the conscience of Dr. N. seemed excessively strict to the other professional persons involved. It seems they were convinced an ethically extraordinary treatment was involved.

The third case, on the other hand, involved a problem with

parents' consent. Paul T., a thirteen year old boy, was brought to the hospital with irreversible brain damage from an accidental gunshot wound in the head. After two days in I.C.U., the neurosurgeon in charge was ready to agree with the request of Paul's mother to withdraw life-support equipment. Papers were prepared for the parents' signature to relieve the physician and hospital of any liability for removing the equipment. However, when the hospital attorney discovered that the father was Paul's stepfather and his real father's whereabouts were unknown, he advised delay to search for Paul's father. Two days later, Paul expired while still on the life-support equipment. Here there was little question that the life-support procedures were ethically extraordinary and nonobligatory, but legal cautions dictated delay. The case is cited to highlight the dual ethical-legal aspects of prolonging life decisions.

A fourth case involves the written order to forego cardiopulmonary resuscitation. Dr. E. found Stella J. a difficult patient. She was a 74 year old unmarried woman who lived with her two sisters, also unmarried. Dr. E. put Stella in the hospital after a stroke, but she was extremely irritable and uncooperative. When she was released, he suggested physical therapy at her home. She and her sisters disliked the physical therapist and the vigorous exercises she recommended. Stella then complained of chest pains and Dr. E. put her back in the hospital after a house call indicated a weakened heart condition.

A heart specialist examined Stella and informed her that her condition was critical. Stella told Dr. E. she didn't like the hospital, knew she was incurable, and didn't want anyone pounding on her chest or anything like that. Dr. E. made a brief notation in the chart, "this patient should not have a code." The very next night she expired.

After the funeral, Stella's two sisters began complaining about the medical treatment she had received. They consulted a lawyer, and he wrote the hospital to request the medical records. The two sisters were already upset with the physical therapist for suggesting such vigorous exercises, and with the heart specialist for so frankly informing Stella of her critical heart condition.

When Stella's sisters found the "no code" order on her chart, they became vehemently critical of Dr. E. and threatened a damage suit. He tried to explain that his order on the chart reflected Stella's own request, but he had not documented her request on the chart, and had not informed the two sisters as he might have. No suit was actually filed but Dr. E. has become much more cautious about writing no-code orders!

In this case, Dr. E. apparently was satisfied that CPR would be ethically extraordinary in Stella's case. He assumed this was also her judgment and she was disposed to forego such a procedure. But the facts that Stella had not made her disposition known to her sisters and that the doctor had not documented her own attitude in the chart created much confusion and consternation. It would have been better if Dr. E. had discussed the omission of CPR more thoroughly with Stella, and had shared this decision with her sisters who were responsible for her care.

These four cases have exemplified some real instances of applying the ethical norms reviewed in the previous section. This chapter will conclude with some practical moral and legal conclusions.

Moral and Legal Conclusions

Throughout this volume, ethical or moral principles have been presented which reflect the stewardship of life tradition that is supported by the Judeo-Christian religious ethic and the moral theology of the Catholic Church. People who accept these ethical principles should form their moral consciences accordingly. The normative principles of civil law do not necessarily correspond completely to these ethical principles, as in the question of abortion in the United States today. Mercy killing does remain contrary to the civil law, but, supposing it ever became legalized, it would still be contrary to these ethical principles.

Because ethics and the law function in the separate spheres of moral and legal responsibility, this chapter will conclude with separate moral and legal conclusions for physicians in the questions of prolonging life.

Three specific conclusions reflect the *moral* principles in this volume:

1) Physicians who assume responsibility for patients have a moral obligation in conscience to provide all ethically ordinary means of prolonging life and to obtain the free and informed consent of the patients for these procedures. Furthermore, they should make known to the patient their option of choosing or refusing ethically extraordinary means of prolonging life. If patients refuse ethically ordinary means, the physician should consider

263

the possibility of arranging to withdraw from their care, although there may be justifying reasons not to do so.

2) Because nonmedical factors, like burden or expense, can render a treatment ethically extraordinary, physicians must be willing to consider these factors and allow them to be weighed in the judgment of what treatment is morally obligatory.

3) In caring for noncompetent patients, physicians must obtain consent from appropriate patient representatives, normally the persons who have assumed responsibility for the patient. As described in chapter 9 above, these representatives have the moral obligation to consent to ethically ordinary procedures and to decide as the patient would decide about ethically extraordinary procedures, or, if the patient's wishes are unknown, to decide in their best interests.

Three specific conclusions reflect the *legal* obligations of physicians as presented in this volume:

1) The law generally expects an informed consent from patients or, if necessary, their representatives, for all medical treatment. This consent, given in a general form in writing upon admission to a hospital, is normally sought specifically for surgical procedures and certain tests. It may not be legally necessary, but still morally necessary, to give specific consent for treatments which become ethically extraordinary, such as indefinite use of a respirator, or dialysis treatments, or the calling of an emergency resuscitation code.

2) The law generally recognizes the right of competent patients to refuse treatment, even procedures which are considered ethically ordinary means of prolonging life. This legal right has been limited in cases where the rights of others are involved, as in the case of pregnant women who might refuse blood transfusions. This legal right does not absolve the physician of the moral responsibility of providing ordinary means as mentioned in the first of the moral recommendations above.

3) The law exercises great caution regarding refusal of treatment for noncompetent patients. The *Quinlan* case in New Jersey set a precedent allowing guardians of irreversibly comatose persons to consent to the removal of life-support. The situation

in each state of the United States will vary somewhat according to court precedents and state legislation. It seems morally imperative that the law should prevent the omission of ethically ordinary means of prolonging life for noncompetent persons and should seek to prohibit discriminatory practices in which otherwise ordinary means are considered extraordinary in the case of handicapped persons or those with a diminished quality of life.

From these six conclusions, it can be seen that the moral and legal responsibilities of physicians do not perfectly coincide. The law tolerates refusal of ordinary means of prolonging life by a competent patient, but the moral principles presented in this volume oppose this as a moral equivalent of suicide. On the other hand, some legal decisions have reserved to the courts decision-making for noncompetent persons which our moral principles would attribute directly to the patient representative, with the court's role limited to correcting abuses.[2]

Hence it can be said, in summary, that physicians have dual responsibilities. As professional persons responsible for their skill and their knowledge, they have a moral conscience guiding their actions in behalf of the life and health of their patients. As citizens of states founded for the protection of life and the security of the citizenry, they have legal responsibilities subject to judicial review. This dual role amply supports the respect and honor in which society holds the medical profession. *Noblesse oblige!*

Notes

1. See Appendix I of this volume, p. 000.
2. See chapter 11 above.

Chapter 19

Responsibilities of Nurses

The Reverend Albert S. Moraczewski, O. P., Ph. D.

Introduction

The changing role of nurses as it is evolving has resulted in some conflict between themselves and other health-care providers. Nurses need to formulate their new self-identity in a manner which is both intelligible to themselves and to others, and which would serve to minimize conflicts between groups. One general question which is emerging with increasing frequency is whether the nurse is more an advocate than a mediator or vise versa.

The role of *advocate* means that the person is more aggressive, takes initiative in bridging gaps of communication between the patient and others, and, if necessary, defends the rights of the patient. On the other hand, *mediator* is a person who tries to interpret the physician's instructions to the patient. In addition, the mediator attempts to be aware of the patient's specific particular needs and bring these to the attention of the appropriate persons. Hence, it would seem that the nurse is primarily a mediator — he or she often mediates between the patient and the physician, and between the patient and the family.

There are other mediators, however, such as the social worker and the pastoral care person. It is true, of course, that the social workers mediate on the larger scale among patients, families and the external agencies, and so their role need not be in conflict with the nurse's role if each understand their proper situation. Conflicts which have arisen between nurse and physician, and between the nurse and other health-care providers would probably be lessened if the focus were truly on the patient himself. The nurse's primary task is to respond appropriately to the needs of the patient.

In light of these general considerations, we shall examine several ethical issues which the nurse may be likely to face today.

Some Ethical Issues

In the area of ethics, several responsibilities of nurses may be identified:

1. To recognize and identify ethical dimensions in nursing practice.
2. To support basic human rights and work tirelessly to preserve these rights.
3. To foster the practice of informed consent as it applies to health care and human experimentation.
4. To recognize the dilemma of control over life and death, the patient-family-physician and nurse controversies.
5. To obtain necessary guidance from organized religion, from professional organizations of nurses, and from law.

These five responsibilities will serve as the basis for the subsequent, very brief discussion.

1. In the addition to the acquisition and practice of appropriate nursing skills, nurses have the important responsibility of being aware of, and sensitive to, the ethical issues which daily confront them. Many issues can be overlooked because of the pressure of work and the blunting of emotions which can result from routine. Promotion of, and attendance at, continuing education programs in nursing ethics can do much to alert nurses to ethical issues which surround them. Some

267

hospitals have inaugurated "Ethics Rounds," or alternatively have introduced ethical concerns, during the specific Rounds of the various services. When opportune, participating at such Rounds will help to sharpen the nurse's awareness of the various ethical issues which surround patient care.

2. Human rights of the patient are, of course, another responsibility of the nurse in her special care of the patient. The *Code For Nurses*[1] lists 11 points, the first one of which emphasizes that the nurse is to provide "services with respect for human dignity . . . and the uniqueness of the client . . ." Nurses, and especially nurse supervisors, need to be aware of differences among human beings and, additionally, to be accepting of those differences.

The *Code for Nurses* points out that, whenever possible, the patients should be involved in the planning of their own health care. As persons, patients have the basic right, and responsibility, to make decisions regarding their health and life. Because of the special vulnerability of the patient, there is a particular need for the nurse to support and promote the patient's right with regard to self-determination. Since basic human rights are consequent upon personhood, social and economic status, sex, age, race; personal and cultural differences as well as the nature of the health problems of the patient should not alter the quality of the nursing care. While prejudices can influence attitudes and behavior markedly, nurses — as well as other health care providers — are challenged to exercise their professional skills in a manner which fully respects the fundamental human dignity of patients.

3. While the obtaining of informed consent is specially important for volunteer subjects involved in human experimentation, it is also important for patients receiving treatment and for the nurse as another responsibility to the patient. Because the individual has the ultimate responsibility for his own life and health-care, he has the right (and obligation) to make decisions which have a bearing on life or health. An individual who is ill seeks the help of "experts" to assist in carrying out his responsibility for self health care. The expert can only do what the patient *permits* him to do. The expert health provider may not assume a *carte blanche* merely because the individual sought out his knowledge and skills. Informed consent must be sought at the appropriate times. The specifics of this process are determined by the particular circumstances of the patient and the health provider. The nurse, as having concern in a special manner for the patient as person, can be of assistance

268

in this matter. In order for the patient to make a responsible decision regarding health care, he needs to know in suitable detail his diagnosis and prognosis, together with alternative courses of treatment with their respective consequences. This latter requirement applies to nontreatment as well. All this information, of course, needs to be communicated in a manner intelligible to the patient. Such a communication process requires tact and sensitivity to the patient's condition and state of mind. No doubt the fulfillment of these requirements may often be a difficult task. But the nurse here can be of special help to the patient in comprehending and dealing with what the physician has told him about his condition and proposed treatment.

4. Because the patient's life and health are often in the balance, communication among the concerned parties — patient, physician, nurse, family, social worker, clergy, etc. — is paramount if controversies which are to the detriment of the patient are to be avoided. Here, too, the nurse's role gives her another responsibility of mediator.

One of the specific areas of concern for the nurses today is the matter of overtreatment, undertreatment, or inadequate treatment. Conflicts, whenever possible, should be settled with the lowest level of authority. Without encroaching on the rights and responsibilities of the physician, the nurse seeks to understand the nature of the complaint and endeavors to resolve it in an appropriate manner with the least amount of disturbance.

It happens sometimes that the nurse will be approached by the patient or family with regards to the treatment wondering whether it is any good, wondering whether it is appropriate, and perhaps asking whether it should be stopped. The nurse's role is a sensitive one, while on the one hand she should not tear down the authority of the physicians, on the other hand she has to protect the well-being of the patient. Under those circumstances, the nurse may remind the family and/or patient that, after discussing it with their own physician, they can have recourse to a second opinion regarding their particular situation.

Occasionally, there are emergency situations in which there is no time for consultation, no time to refer to a higher authority. These may be situations in which the nurse's conscience is involved, in which something is being done or not done in opposition to her or his conscience. It is necessary, in these conditions, that the nurse acts according to her best analysis and sensitivity.

Since such conflictual situations can have significant repercussions on the health or life of the patient as well as on the reputation of the nurse, physician and hospital, a carefully worked out institutional policy would be advisable. Guidelines for hospital staff in dealing with patient complaints about treatment or with crises of conscience could be helpful in averting seriously harmful consequences.

5. Perhaps more than before, people have been encouraged to develop a personal value system which helps sort things out. But it is also an important responsibility for the nurse to engage in self-study and be familiar with the relevant ethical developments made in these areas so that she or he can respond to the needs of people in an intelligent and informed manner. Recent publications carry a number of helpful articles on nursing ethics.[2]

The nurse needs some external religious guides and inner strength in order to deal well with the myriad needs of patients. Ethical guidelines and the sacraments of the Church are available to Catholic nurses. Nurses with other religious beliefs and ethical convictions also often have resources in their respective traditions. In either event, knowledge of what the various religious groups expect from their adherents would be very helpful to nurses in their dealing with patients with a variety of religious backgrounds.

While nurses have multiple responsibilities to the patient, they also have a responsibility to themselves and to one another. Nurses should be aware of their own needs. In particular, the nurse should be aware of the consequences of conflicts and concerns which can lead to the burnout often seen among nurses. Doona[3] lists some of the sources of nursing breakdown: failure of professional vigilance, failure in supporting each other from emotional burnout; failure to match patients and nurse in assignments; and failure to unite with peers to affect direction of health care. Some help with management of burnout may be obtained from an article by Mullins and Barstow.[4]

Provision should be made for a structural process that would allow ventilation of emotions. It is very difficult for people who work under constant stress not to have some sort of an outlet in terms of persons who can listen and accept them, and help them deal with their emotions that may have arisen.

Illustrative Cases

Several cases will serve to illustrate some of the situations the nurse may encounter.

An elderly lady was institutionalized for a long time and now wishes to die, and to die without tubes and wires protruding from her. What can the nurse say or do under these circumstances? May an elderly person who wishes to die and contracts pneumonia refuse the antibiotic therapy for the pneumonia? Is the use of an antibiotic an ethically extraordinary means.

When faced with a concrete situation, a nurse, or physician, needs to ask, first of all, is the patient refusing ethically *extraordinary* therapy? If so, then the nurse and the physician are ethically free to respect the patient's decision should he elect to decline therapy. They would recognize, of course, that there may be a legal issue which would have to be resolved, but the topic under consideration is the ethical order at this point.

In determining whether the means to sustain life are to be considered ethically extraordinary or ethically ordinary, we have two questions to ask: 1) is there a reasonable hope of benefit from the utilization of these means, and 2) do the means place a great burden on the patient and others? One ought to note that in applying these distinctions of ethically ordinary and ethically extraordinary means of sustaining life that there will be variations in individual cases; that is, for one person a particular means may be ethically ordinary and, for another, those same means may be ethically extraordinary because of particular circumstances and mindset of that individual (See chapter 9 for a fuller discussion of this principle).

In the case of legitimately withholding treatment, in that instance the person is allowing a concurrent pathological process to continue and come to its natural conclusion — which could be death. This situation should be distinguished very carefully from the actual taking of a person's life, that is, actually *causing* death as, for example, by injecting a high dose of barbiturate or morphine so as to bring about a person's death.

Yet, it may not be evident, for example, that withholding an antibiotic from an aged and senile person, who has contracted pneumonia, is morally acceptable. While it is likely that a cure of pneumonia will take place, but is that a *benefit* for that individual in the circumstance in which they are? Namely, if they are already so aged and senile that they are barely functioning, then we might say that the cure of the disease is not sufficient, that is to say, it does not cure the fundamental problem of the person, namely, advanced age with certain degenerative diseases concurrently present. So from that perspective, we might want to call the means ethically *extraordinary* because no true benefit results from the utilization of the antibiotic in this particular case. In this situation, the death of the person, when it does occur, results from the pneumonia. The withholding of the antibiotic only permitted the existing disease to follow its natural course.

Most nurses have been trained in acute care and are accustomed to respond to a person's medical need as fully as possible and to use all available resources in these elderly patients. Yet, the patient's real need may be *not* to be subjected to the awesome technological array which the nurse and physician could muster. Rather, the need may be for the nurse just to stand there, as it were, but be truly caring and allow the person to die. It was Paul Ramsey who wisely wrote (*Patient as Person*), "we may not always cure but we can always care." The nurse, or whoever deals with a patient in an incurable or terminal condition, is challenged to demonstrate that she really cares for that patient and is not just looking for the cure of a disease.

Is it ethically permissible to withhold an antibiotic from a child who is severely afflicted, say, with a genetic disease such as spina bifida? The child's situation is not parallel to that of the elderly person who is at the end of their life, the child still has much life ahead of him/her. But does that difference make a difference in the moral argument? There may be a parallel with the infamous Johns Hopkins' case in which a newborn child with Down's Syndrome was discovered to be also afflicted with duodenal atresia. A relatively straight forward operation would correct the latter condition. However, the parents decided against the corrective surgery and the child was allowed to starve to death at the hospital over a period of 15 days. Subsequently, numerous commentators on the case concluded that the nontreatment was ethically inadmissible. The child with spina bifida in need of an antibiotic has a basic right to that treatment since the use of an antibiotic would be an ethically ordinary measure inasmuch as it would truly benefit the child whose life could continue on an ascending path (See chapter 15 for a fuller discussion of spina bifida).

A variation on the above is the child with multiple handicaps and especially one who is severely mentally retarded. According to present medical capabilities, such individuals will never gain full mental awareness and autonomy and so the question arises as to their medical treatment when ill. May it be substantially different from that of the normal child who has the same physical illness?

Because a child is afflicted with multiple handicaps and/or is mentally retarded in no way lessens his basic right to appropriate medical treatment. Nonetheless, there may be a difference in what is ethically ordinary treatment for such an individual. The critical question must be asked: does this treatment hold out reasonable expectations that it will truly benefit the child? Merely to prolong for a time the *dying process* is of itself of no benefit. But if the child otherwise is not dying but living and growing, it can truly benefit from the recovery of an otherwise fatal condition. Such treatment could be deemed as ethically ordinary and, therefore, obligatory.

In a significant article, [5] Fr. Richard McCormick explores the question of sustaining the life of a grossly deformed, but nondying, newborn infant. He argues from the following statement of Pope Pius XII regarding the obligation to employ ordinary means of sustaining life:[6]

> But normally one is held to use only ordinary means — according to circumstances of persons, places, times and culture — that is to say, means that do not involve any grave burden for oneself or another. A more strict obligation would be too burdensome for most men and would render the attainment of the higher, more important good too difficult. Life, health, all temporal activities are in fact subordinated to spiritual ends. On the other hand, one is not forbidden to take more than the strictly necessary steps to preserve life and health, as long as he does not fail in some more serious duty.

After exploring what might be meant by the Pope's words "higher, more important goods," Fr. McCormick concludes that these goods might be "human relationships, and the qualities of justice, respect, concern, compassion, and support that surrounds them."[7] Accordingly, if a child does not even have the *potential* for such human relationship, McCormick argues that the child has reached his maximum potential and any medical means used to continue that life would not be morally obligatory.

This approach to a complex and very agonizing problem has been received with mixed reactions. Even with the important caveats cited by Fr. McCormick, the proposed solution has been critized as introducing a quality of life standard into the determination of who should live. Properly understood and applied, it may provide another insight into the making of very difficult and painful decisions.

In situations where treatment of a dying person only serves to prolong the dying process, does the nurse have the freedom to tell the patient or family that he or she has other options? Not infrequently, the physician is not able appropriately to deal with death. Because some physicians are not ready to accept the fact of death, even when it is inevitable and when further therapy is of no benefit, they will continue to use what have become ethically extraordinary means to sustain life and put the patient and family through additional agony and expenses. The nurse who is seriously convinced that these means are ethically extraordinary should alert the physician, in one way or another, to an awareness of these options. If the physician does not respond to the nurse's objection or suggestion, the nurse then should seek whatever appropriate channels are available for the obtaining of the rights of the patient. At times, a suitable management decision could be to refer them to a hospice.

Not only physicians have trouble dealing with death, but so do many nurses. (Could the same be said of some pastoral care persons?)

Nursing care is oriented to the patient as a person, not merely to the cure of his diseased condition. That a person dies as a result of his disease or injury should not be seen as a consequence of a nursing care failure. Hence, the nurse — more readily, perhaps, than the physician — can view the patient's death as not challenging her nursing skills.

On the other hand, because nurses are in more frequent and personal contact with their patients, some degree of emotional involvement with the patient may be inevitable. In addition, if nurses have not worked out their attitudes and feelings regarding their own death, more difficulty will it be to deal well with the death of their patients.

Nursing Care

A common problem associated with nursing care, as practiced in intensive care units (ICU), is that because there is so much work to be done and so few people to do it, nurses do not have sufficient time to spend with individual patients. When the patient is not able to communicate with the nurse, that lack of time becomes all the more difficult to bear. In a particular case, for example, the patient could not speak because of oral surgery, and the only item wanted —but could not obtain for hours — was a piece of paper on which eventually he asked, "Am I gonna be all right?" What the patient needed was reassurance after a painful and frightening experience. But often the nurse is not able to spend much time with a patient or to be aware that such is necessary at a particular instant of time. Furthermore, because of the intensity of care in the ICU, there is often a lack of privacy, and the individual who is more alert is able to know in greater detail, but incompletely, what is occuring around him and what is happening to the other patients, including their deaths. Such partial knowledge can be very disturbing to the patient.

Another complaint of ICU patients is the constant stimulation — bright lights, sound, activity of all kinds. Still another problem in intensive care units is the inability or the lack of time during which the patient can receive visits from family or friends. Frequently, these persons were the source of great support and now, when patients need it the most, they are not able to get it. In that context, it may be opportune now for a hospital to review its policies with regard to visitation by a representative family member. It may be possible for pastoral care persons to come in and provide support to these intensive care patients, where, on the one hand, the family members are absent or are unable to enter and, on the other hand, the nurses are too busy ordinarily with immediate medical and nursing concerns to give much supportive time to each individual patient.

A major concern of patients is the control of pain. The impression of many nurses is that patients are not so much afraid of death itself, but afraid of the dying process and, in particular, of the pain associated with it. Within appropriate limits, the patient should receive what pain medication is necessary to control the pain.

In an address in 1957 to the Italian Society of Anesthesiology, Pope Pius XII discussed at some length the religious and moral dimensions of using analgesics to relieve severe pain. He stated:[8]

> To sum up, you ask Us: "Is the removal of pain and consciousness by means of narcotics (when medical reasons demand it) permitted by religion and morality to both doctor and patient even at the approach of death and if one foresees that the use of narcotics will shorten life?" The answer must be: "Yes — provided that no other means exist, and if, in the given circumstances, that action does not prevent the carrying out of other moral and religious duties."

As We have already explained, the ideal of Christian heroism does not require — at least in general — the refusal of narcosis justified on other grounds, even at the approach of death. Everything depends on the particular circumstances. The most perfect and most heroic decision can be present as fully in acceptance as in refusal.

Increasingly, the hospice concept is being accepted in this country. Some hospitals now have a few beds reserved for hospice care. The basic principle is that the imminent death of the patient is accepted and the focus of attention of medical and nursing staff is on *care* rather than cure. By providing a pleasant "home-life" atmosphere, family and friends are encouraged to visit. Pain medication is administered as needed but a common experience is that, in a hospice environment, *less* analegisic is required to control the pain, especially if the patient has control over the administration of the pain medication and does not have to wait for a fixed hour. Similarly, a patient is less anxious if orally administered analgesic is given at a sufficient dosage to keep the patient pain free until the next scheduled medication. The more personalized atmosphere of the hospice appears to respond more adequately to the real needs of the dying patient. A nurse working in such an atmosphere finds the task of ministering to such patients more tolerable than is generally experienced in the usual hospital setting.

An often overlooked or underestimated nursing resource is the sense of touch. Not only is it soothing to be gently touched but also reassuring. It communicates the message that someone cares in a way which words often are not able to do. Another aspect of touch that is being increasingly employed is its healing potential. While some charismatic healers make great claims for the healing power of the "laying on of hands," such sweeping pronouncements need to be received with caution. Ultimately, God can choose to heal through someone's touch — as with Jesus — but more often God works through secondary causes. Whatever healing which may take place through touch does so through the natural recuperative powers of the body. The precise nature of the interaction between touch and those recuperative powers is poorly understood at present.

Christian nurses, in addition, can enhance their nursing effectiveness if they unite their professional skills and faith by praying with and for their patients. In touching the patients in their charge during the daily nursing routine, they can perceive their skilled touching as an extension of Jesus' healing mission on earth.

In summary, it would seem that a nurse has many wonderful opportunities to be a channel of God's healing grace. Furthermore, the physician, generally speaking, is more focused on the patient's disease or injury — what is wrong and how to treat it — whereas the nurse is more concerned about the patient as a whole, more concerned about his personhood and his health and rights. The nurse as part of a team needs to cooperate rather than compete with other health professionals.

An important rule to consider and remember is that nurses have a ministry one to the other. They may have to stand alone and without support in very difficult situations, so nurses should not forget one another. The nurse has changed some of her tasks — the carrying of bed pans and taking of temperatures, for example — which now are often delegated to others. On the other hand, the nurse is now doing procedures —such as starting an IV — which physicians appear to have abdicated in many instances. The challenge is to keep skilled nursing care as human as possible, notwithstanding all the technology which may have to be employed for the proper nursing and medical care of such patients. If nurses and other health-care providers develop an ability to *care*, then when cure is no longer possible, they can certainly care and help ease the patient's journey home.

Notes

1. American Nurses' Association, *Code for Nurses* with interpretive statements. American Nurses' Association, 1976.

2. For example, see the following:

American Journal of Nursing. "Special American Journal of Nursing Feature: Ethics." *American Journal of Nursing*, May 1977, pp. 845-876.

American Nurses' Association. *Code for Nurses with Interpretive Statements*. Kansas City, MO: American Nurses' Association, 1979.

Aroskar, Mila A. "Anatomy of An Ethical Dilemma: The Theory and Practice." *American Journal of Nursing* 80(4):658-663, April, 1980.

Chinn, Peggy L., R.N., Ph.D., ed. *Ethics and Values*: Volume 1, No. 3 of *Advances in Nursing Science*, April, 1979.

Nursing Clinics of North America. I. *Bioethical Issues in Nursing*, edited by Mary Lou de Leon Siantz, R.N.; II. *Care of the Patients with Neuromuscular Disease*, edited by Katharine Donohoe. Volume 14, No. 1, March 1979. Philadelphia: W. B. Saunders Company, 1979.

Stanley, Sister Teresa, "Ethics as a Component of the Curriculum." *Nursing and Health Care*, September 1980, pp. 63-72.

3. Doona, M. E. "The Ethical Dimension in 'Ordinary Nursing Care'," *Linacre Quarterly* Volume 44, November 1977, pp. 320-327.

4. Mullins, A. C. and Barstow, R. E. "Care for the Caretakers," *American Journal of Nursing*, August, 1979, Vol. 79, pp. 1425-7.

5. McCormick, Richard A. "To Save or Let Die," *Journal of the American Medical Association*, 229(2), July 8, 1974, pp. 172-176.

6. Pope Piux XII, "The Prolongation of Life," English Translation, *The Pope Speaks* Vol. 4, Spring 1958, p. 395-6.

7. *Op. Cit.* p. 174.

8. Pope Piux XII, "Anesthesia: Three Moral Questions" English Translation, *The Pope Speaks*, Vol. 4(1), Summer 1957, pp. 48-49.

Chapter 20

Responsibilities of
Pastoral Care Persons

The Reverend Donald G. McCarthy, Ph. D.

The discussions among pastoral care persons concerned with prolonging life decisions revealed the fact that they approach these decisions from a different perspective from that of administrators, physicians, and nurses. Three aspects of their work will be listed here and then discussed in this chapter. First, pastoral care persons can exercise a leadership role regarding medico-moral education in their institutions. Secondly, they usually bring an ethical perspective in the whole broad spectrum of prolonging life decisions along with their spiritual assistance to patients and their families. And, finally, those who provide pastoral care from the Catholic tradition include the Sacraments and sacramental liturgy in their ministry.

Medico-Moral Education

Pastoral care persons are expected to be aware of ethical pluralism. In one of the seminars the question was asked whether the increased acceptance of abortion in the United States will lead to increased acceptance of mercy-killing. The theologian who responded to this question, Father Benedict Ashley, did not merely link abortion and mercy-killing, but raised a more basic point. He suggested that proponents of the religious tradition opposing abortion and mercy-killing need to recognize that secular humanism in the United States must be seen as a kind of secular religion with its own beliefs and ethical teaching. Secular humanism tends to take a permissive view of abortion and mercy-killing and would expect its view to be reflected in public laws and policies.

While Judaeo-Christian ethics and secular humanist ethics are not two totally distinct and contradictory systems, they are independent systems. Many people do not appreciate their differences. Hence, religiously sponsored health care institutions cannot ignore the difficult educational task of distinguishing the practical implications of these two systems.

Therefore, pastoral care persons who explicitly represent the Judaeo-Christian ethical tradition have a major educational responsibility within the health care institutions which reflect that tradition. For example, pastoral care persons in Catholic hospitals are expected to witness to and teach the Catholic medical-moral tradition within their own institutions. Obviously, they are not policy-makers or even specially trained in moral theology but they are representatives of a value system which needs to be better understood by staff and patients alike.

The trend to establish medical-moral committees in Catholic hospitals over the past decade grows out of the need for continuing ethical leadership. Pastoral care persons almost invariably serve on these interdisciplinary committees because of their understanding of moral and religious values. Faced with the confusion between various ethical systems and the complexity of ever-expanding medical-moral issues, these committees cannot merely issue policy statements, even though they have studied the issues exhaustively and acted responsibly. They also have the responsibility of explaining these policy statements, and, more broadly, educating the entire staff of a health care facility to understand and accept them.

In fact, Fathers Ashley and O'Rourke, in their scholarly *Health*

Care Ethics, A Theological Analysis,[1] review the need for "Christian Identity Committees" to assume a broad role of assuring the religious value orientation of Christian health care facilities. They see that ethical and religious values go far beyond the issues of prolonging life decisions discussed in this volume. Some idea of that scope can be found in the eight principles presented in the *Evaluative Criteria for Catholic Health Care Facilities.*[2]

Pastoral care persons neither can nor should attempt to carry out such vast responsibilities in ethical and religious education single-handedly within a health care facility. But they are often the catalysts for collective effort and they do have specific opportunities to influence orientation programs for new employees, to insert discussion of ethical and religious questions in hospital publications, and to contribute their insights in interdisciplinary meetings and continuing medical and nursing education programs. They also bring both an ethical perspective and spiritual assistance to patients and their families faced specifically with prolonging life decisions.

Prolonging Life Decisions

Father Ashley, author of Chapter 8 above, introduced his comments in one of the seminars with pastoral care persons by distinguishing ethical and spiritual questions. In the book mentioned above, which he co-authored with Kevin O'Rourke, O.P., this distinction is presented succinctly:

> Spiritual counseling deals with the ultimate, existential questions, the problems of commitment to certain fundamental values or life goals. Ethical counseling in the strict sense, on the other hand, deals with the decisions that have to be made about actions that have to be taken to achieve these goals. In brief, the former deals with *ends,* the latter, with the *means.*[3]

The pastoral care counselor normally focuses particularly on spiritual questions — helping the patients relate their present situation of sickness and suffering to their understanding of human life and destiny. Christians approach the mystery of suffering in the awareness that Jesus not only bore the burden of human infirmities but called upon His followers to do likewise. "If a man wishes to come after me, he must deny his very self, take up his cross, and follow in my steps" (Mk. 8:34). Jesus taught that there is no entrance into messianic glory without suffering.

In addition to this spiritual counseling, the pastoral care person must often be prepared for ethical counseling. Fr. Ashley pointed out in his remarks that patients may be so ovewhelmed by an overload of anxiety and related feelings that they are not free enough to think about duties, obligations, and their own ultimate goal in life. If so, this overload must be diminished, perhaps with expert psychological help if necessary, before ethical and spiritual counseling can take place properly.

Pastoral care persons who have grasped the stewardship of life model of making prolonging life decisions presented in this volume can provide patients and families with a perspective which evaluates whether a life prolonging procedure should be counted as ordinary or extraordinary, obligatory or optional. This presumes they understand as fully as possible both the medical aspects of the procedure and the kind of burden, including the financial burden, it represents to specific patients and families.

At one of the seminars for pastoral care persons, Father Timothy Toohey, Executive Director of the National Association of Catholic Chaplains, pictured the pastoral care person as a catechist or teacher in dialogue with physicians, nurses, and therapists, as well as patients and families. In a sense the pastoral care person facilitates the ethical decision-making of the patient or family by assuring adequate understanding and consideration of all factors. By their professional expertise physicians tend to look almost exclusively at the medical aspects of these procedures. Yet it is clear from the preceding chapters that in some instances a procedure may be medically routine or ordinary but ethically extraordinary and optional.

Furthermore, physicians themselves do not always agree in their own medical judgments about the risks or burdens of given procedures or the appropriate medical approach to reach a specific goal — as in the determination of death by brain criteria. Father Ashley commented on such situations in terms of what Catholic theology has called "probabilism." In this systematic approach to resolving differences of opinion people may follow the less burdensome opinion provided it is solidly probable and does not offer risk of serious damage to others or to themselves.[4]

Sister Loretta Geringer, C.D.P., a member of the pastoral care staff of the St. Louis University Hospitals, described in one of our seminars her vision of the mediator role pastoral care staff often can play when patients and families do not seem to be adequately informed to make life-prolonging decisions:

> In speaking with patients and families, I find their expectations can be very unrealistic regarding the expected outcome of a particular medical or surgical procedure, or relative to their understanding of a patient's condition or prognosis.

> I cannot and should not assume from this, that they have not been adequately informed by the physician, since we all tend to hear at times what we want to hear.

> My first procedure would be to ask the nurse or doctor what the physician has actually told the patient and/or family. If they relate that the patient and/or family was given a more complete picture than first indicated to me by the patient or family, I believe our role could be to reinforce with them that which was perhaps too painful for them to assimilate the first time.

> If, on the other hand, the nurse gives any indication that maybe the doctor didn't spell out enough to the patient or family, I will then relate to the nurse what the patient's or family's present understanding is. If she tells me *she* will relate this to the doctor, I will at a later time try to ascertain from the patient or family if their understanding is any better.

> If the nurse does *not* assure me she will speak to the doctor, I myself will relate to the doctor the misrepresentation on the part of the patient or family. I might add that I limit myself to misunderstandings about very serious matters. If a patient or family indicates a lack of informed consent of a lesser consequence — perhaps misconceptions about a medical or surgical procedure — I encourage them to ask for clarification from the doctor or nurse.

Sister Loretta's description outlines a role for pastoral care persons within an acute care hospital when patient or family are giving consent to a life-prolonging procedure, such as radiation therapy or a radical surgical procedure like amputation. In one of our seminars, the chaplain of an extended care facility cited cases of two elderly priests who went to acute care hospitals and received heart pacemakers, which might easily have been considered ethically extraordinary, without proper safeguarding of consent procedures.

One was the case of Father Ed, 84 years of age, experiencing continually deteriorating health and quite fully prepared for death for the previous two years. He suffered a heart attack. The chaplain of the nursing home called the priest who was handling Father Ed's temporal affairs to alert him that Father Ed would not wish extraordinary procedures, and to suggest that in the circumstances a pacemaker would be ethically extraordinary. Nonetheless, the device was implanted and Father Ed was brought back to the nursing home without ever truly consenting to what was done.

In the same context of prolonging life decisions in nursing homes, a pastoral care person raised the difficult case of persons who are comatose or semi-comatose and nourished artificially with nasogastric tubes. Father Connery responded with the basic principle that such feeding tubes, as well as IV's and oxygen supplies, are ethically ordinary procedures when used on a temporary basis to assist a patient through a health crisis. On the other hand, he pointed out, they can easily become ethically extraordinary, and therefore not morally obligatory, if they become a way of life on a permanent basis.

This basic principle suggests that these procedures may sometimes be withdrawn without violating respect for life and without the withdrawal involving moral negligence. Yet, this very sensitive question cannot be taken lightly. The legal status of such actions does not seem as clear as the ethical status. The actual decision to forego an ethically optional procedure should be made by a patient or at least by the proper proxy who reflects the patient's own wishes. Sometimes no actual proxy can be found to represent a patient's interests. The law traditionally respects patients' own decisions to refuse a treatment or procedure, except in exceptional cases, but the law tends to protect patients' rights by great caution when proxies are acting in behalf of patients. Hence a proxy's decision may be ethically acceptable and still legally questionable. Refusal of treatment was discussed above in this volume by Dennis Horan in chapter 11.

A more directly pastoral question concerns the spiritual care of comatose or semi-comatose persons. Unless such persons can actually be declared dead by reason of reliable criteria, they are not dead and may not be ignored or treated as "vegetables." Pastoral care persons can influence the attitude of nursing staff to such persons by their own respect and concern. As mentioned above in chapter 13, such patients can often still hear and sense the presence of people attending to them without being able to respond or communicate.

In one of the seminars, a pastoral care person told of Albert V., a

20-year-old college student who was comatose for three weeks in November, 1979. When Alfred regained consciousness he told of knowing when he had visitors even though he could not respond to them. "In fact," he said, "you were here on Thanksgiving Day, and no one bothered to wish me a Happy Thanksgiving!"

Hence the recommendation is often made that comatose persons be treated just as if they were conscious, and never be spoken about in their rooms as if they were not present. Prayers can be offered aloud in much the same way as prayers for the dying are offered in their presence. The pastoral suggestion was made that, in cases of those who are comatose over an indefinite period, a prayer service be held periodically with family and friends present, if possible.

Pastoral care persons should make contact with the families of comatose persons, who are usually grieving and experiencing guilt because they cannot be reconciled with that person or cannot seem to communicate their love and concern. An important dimension of pastoral ministry centers on stress and helping people deal with it. In the case of comatose persons, both staff and family undergo extreme stress so that pastoral care persons have a clear responsibility to them.

The pastoral care seminars also discussed the particular urgency of providing pastoral support at the time when death occurs. While the factual pronouncement and announcement that a patient has died remains the responsibility of a physician, most physicians welcome the presence and support of pastoral care persons when the family receives the sad news. If there has been previous contact with family members, this pastoral presence becomes even more precious to the family. In the seminars, examples were given of follow-up ministry to grieving families through phone calls and visits and even periodic memorial Masses for those who have died in the previous month or two.

Pastoral care always creates a sharing of burdens and anxieties. In the Christian vision of common belonging to the body of Christ this sharing includes a mutual experience of Christ. Christians believe that Sacraments are experiences of the presence of Christ. Hence pastoral care within the Catholic tradition always incorporates the experience of sacramental rituals and prayer.

Sacramental Ministry

Discussions about sacramental ministry to persons facing life-prolonging decisions revealed the dual theological perspective of the recipient's disposition and the promised grace of the Sacrament. Those who emphasize the promised grace tend to an almost routine multiplication of sacramental experiences. Those who emphasize the recipient's disposition tend to delay the Sacraments in favor of better preparation.

Thus, in one of our seminars the following interesting question was raised. Suppose someone neglected to receive the Eucharist before their admission to the hospital, perhaps even neglected to attend Mass regularly. Can a pastoral care person presume that such a patient is now suddenly prepared for daily reception of the Eucharist?

Obviously, such a person, now burdened with grave illness, might well be disposed for daily Communion. The sick person may have devoutly received the Sacrament of Penance and have experienced a genuine conversion which daily Communion will strengthen. But this disposition must not be presumed, although the pastoral care person should offer assistance and encouragement to achieve it. The practice of many hospital chaplains of offering a convenient opportunity for the Sacrament of Penance to every newly admitted Catholic patient seems highly appropriate for the sacramental ministry in the hospital or nursing home.

In his comments to pastoral care persons, Father Ashley emphasized the importance of administering the Sacraments with dignity and with the fullest possible participation and liturgical celebration. Thus, he questioned the very abbreviated administration of Holy Communion where the distributor rapidly visits room after room with only the simple phrase, "Body of Christ," pronounced in each room. He encouraged efforts to schedule group Communions on given floors for those patients who can assemble. When this happens, a more appropriate Communion service can be held, including penitential rite, Scripture reading, and common prayer.

Such group gatherings can pose practical problems. Another alternative was proposed: common preparation for Holy Communion over hospital video or audio communication systems followed by simultaneous room visits by several distributors, depending on the size of the hospital and availability of lay persons to assist.

The proposal of group Holy Communion rests on a basic liturgical principle: the communal nature of the Sacraments in the Church. Christ gave the Sacraments to the Church as community and they should be received in community as far as possible. The communal Penance services which have become popular in the last decade exemplify this principle, even though group absolution of sins is reserved for special circumstances. Nursing home chaplains, especially, and even hospital chaplains may find ways of scheduling communal penance services for the convenience of residents or patients.

Father Ashley also emphasized group experience of the Sacrament of Anointing of the sick. Even though only one person is anointed, the Church should be represented, when possible, by family, friends, and nursing staff. Even the patient's physician, who is the professional healer, should be invited and perhaps a prayer be added for the physician during the service.

The practical question of which patients should be anointed came up in one of the seminars. The present practice of the Catholic Church does not reserve anointing for an extreme or lasting anointing, so a person need not be dangerously ill. Some patients still think this sacrament indicates that death is near and they are still frightened when it is offered to them. In one hospital, all Catholic patients over the age of 65 are offered the Sacrament of the Sick, as well as younger patients admitted for serious surgery, and all patients with terminal illness, even though not yet critically ill.

The Sacrament of the Sick can be administered to unconscious persons who have sufficient dispositions for its valid reception. But it cannot validly be administered to one who has died. In cases of sudden death, a priest may still administer the Sacrament conditionally, but the past custom of extending this period of conditional administration for two to three hours after sudden death is considered extreme by many pastoral theologians today.

Two other very practical questions about administering the Sacraments to the sick concern recipients who are Christian but not Catholic, or who are Catholic, but living in marriages considered invalid by the Church. With regard to Christians who are not Catholic, there are questions of both differences of belief and lack of expressed unity with the Catholic community. However, this does not absolutely rule out every possible instance of administering the Sacraments to Christians separated from the Church. If the minister of the Sacrament is satisfied that the person's faith is substantially that of the Church in regard to the Sacrament, and if there is a good reason not to deny the Sacrament, as when the persons ask for it in good faith or their own minister is not reasonably available, the Sacrament may be licitly administered.

The question of administering the Sacraments to a Catholic living in an invalid marriage raises numerous possibilities. For example, if the couple are elderly and living as brother and sister, a pastoral judgment may be made to give the Sacraments with a provision to avoid giving scandal, if such a reminder seems necessary. If the marriage can be readily validated since only the canonical form of marriage is lacking, the Sacraments may be administered with the understanding that the couple will not exercise their marital privileges until the validation takes place.

If the obstacle to validating the marriage is a previous marriage bond by one of the partners, the hospital chaplain may be able to give only limited assistance, unless the couple are disposed to live as brother and sister. There are at least three canonical outcomes of examining such situations. One is that a declaration of nullity can be granted, but a minimum of 6 to 18 months will be necessary for the Tribunal procedure. Another is that true grounds exist for an ecclesiastical declaration of nullity, but testimony is unavailable. Another is that a declaration has already been denied by a Tribunal or no realistic grounds exist. It would seem that in all three of these instances the chaplain should refrain from administering the Sacraments unless there is genuine and proximate danger of death and a sincere spirit of repentance by the patient.

In the first instance, the chaplain should give the patient as much guidance and encouragement as possible in presenting to a Tribunal the case for a declaration of nullity of the previous marriage. In the second instance, the chaplain might raise the possibility of an "internal forum" approach to returning to the Sacraments, but normally this presumes an effort first to verify the alleged grounds and consult with a Tribunal priest or someone specializing in marriage cases. In the third instance, the chaplain does not have the authority to administer the sacraments if the couple are going to continue to live as man and wife in the invalid marriage.

In all these cases where the Sacraments cannot be administered, there is not less, but more, need for pastoral care for patients. It should be made abundantly clear to the patient that, although the Church must maintain its discipline for the guidance of the Christian community and a witness to others, it fully recognizes that only God can judge the heart of the individual. Consequently, the Church continues to love and pray for those who are not ready to accept this discipline and stands ready to give them every support they are ready to accept. They should, therefore, be encouraged to turn to God in prayer and repentance so they will be properly disposed in their hearts, whether or not they are ever able to receive the Sacraments. The very disposition to hunger and thirst for the Sacraments should be seen as a sign of faith and a reason for great support and encouragement from pastoral care persons.

In summary, the Sacraments of Reconciliation, Anointing, and Holy Eucharist (or Viaticum if the patient is dying) represent peak experiences in Catholic pastoral ministry within health care facilities. They deserve all the care and liturgical preparation that can be afforded. They are public acts of the Church in which the sacramental minister represents the entire Church as well as Christ Himself. The living Church comes together in community as far as possible for all the Sacraments. Yet the life of faith undergirds the sacramental life and must be nourished through prayer and penance even when the Sacraments are not available.

Conclusion

This chapter did review, in its middle section, the special role of pastoral care persons assisting patients and families in making ethically responsible decisions about prolonging life procedures. No one is as uniquely equipped for both ethical and spiritual counseling as an experienced pastoral care person.

Yet this chapter began with the much broader role of leadership within health care institutions in matters of moral and religious values which falls upon the shoulders of pastoral care persons. And the chapter concluded with a much more specific discussion, the sacramental ministry which Christian, and especially Catholic, pastoral care persons are privileged to exercise. This is the last, but obviously not the least important, chapter of this volume.

Notes

1. St. Louis, MO: Catholic Hospital Association, 1978, pp. 151-154.
2. St. Louis, MO: Catholic Health Association, 1980, 62 pp.
3. *op. cit.*, p. 415.
4. *op. cit.*, pp. 68-69.

Declaration on Euthanasia

Vatican Congregation for the Doctrine of the Faith
June 26, 1980

Introduction

The rights and values pertaining to the human person occupy an important place among the questions discussed today. In this regard, the Second Vatican Ecumenical Council solemnly reaffirmed the lofty dignity of the human person, and in a special way his or her right to life. The council therefore condemned crimes against life "such as any type of murder, genocide, abortion, euthanasia, or wilful suicide" (pastoral constitution, *"Gaudium et Spes"* no. 27).

More recently, the Sacred Congregation for the Doctrine of the Faith has reminded all the faithful of Catholic teaching on procured abortion.[1] The congregation now considers it opportune to set forth the church's teaching on euthanasia.

It is indeed true that, in this sphere of teaching, the recent popes have explained the principles, and these retain their full force;[2] but the progress of medical science in recent years has brought to the fore new aspects of the question of euthanasia, and these aspects call for further elucidation on the ethical level.

In modern society, in which even the fundamental values of human life are often called into question, cultural change exercises an influence upon the way of looking at suffering and death; moreover, medicine has increased its capacity to cure and to prolong life in particular circumstances, which sometimes give rise to moral problems.

Thus people living in this situation experience no little anxiety about the meaning of advanced old age and death. They also begin to wonder whether they have the right to obtain for themselves or their fellowmen an "easy death," which would shorten suffering and which seems to them more in harmony with human dignity.

A number of episcopal conferences have raised questions on this subject with the Sacred Congregation for the Doctrine of the Faith. The congregation, having sought the opinion of experts on the various aspects of euthanasia, now wishes to respond to the bishops' questions with the present declaration, in order to help them to give correct teaching to the faithful entrusted to their care, and to offer them elements for reflection that they can present to the civil authorities with regard to this very serious matter.

The considerations set forth in the present document concern in the first place all those who place their faith and hope in Christ, who, through his life, death and resurrection, has given a new meaning to existence and especially to the death of the Christian, as St. Paul says: "If we live, we live to the Lord, and if we die, we die to the Lord" (*Romans* 14:8; cf. *Philippians* 1:20).

As for those who profess other religions, many will agree with us that faith in God the creator, provider and lord of life — if they share this belief — confers a lofty dignity upon every human person and guarantees respect for him or her.

It is hoped that this declaration will meet with the approval of many people of good will, who philosophical or ideological differences notwithstanding, have nevertheless a lively awareness of the heights of the human person. These rights have often in fact been proclaimed in recent years through declarations issued by international congresses;[3] and since it is a question here of fundamental rights inherent in every human person, it is obviously wrong to have recourse to arguments from political pluralism or religious freedom in order to deny the universal value of those rights.

I. The Value of Human Life

Human life is the basis of all goods, and is the necessary source and condition of every human activity and of all society. Most people regard life as something sacred and hold that no one may dispose of it at will, but believers see in life something greater, namely a gift of God's love, which they are called upon to preserve and make fruitful. And it is this latter consideration that gives rise to the following consequences:

1. No one can make an attempt on the life of an innocent person without opposing God's love for that person, without violating a fundamental right, and therefore without committing a crime of the utmost gravity.[4]

2. Everyone has the duty to lead his or her life in accordance with God's plan. That life is entrusted to the individual as a good that must bear fruit already here on earth, but that finds its full perfection only in eternal life.

3. Intentionally causing one's own death, or suicide, is therefore equally as wrong as murder; such an action on the part of a person is to be considered as a rejection of God's sovereignty and loving plan. Furthermore, suicide is also often a refusal of love for self, the denial of the natural instinct to live, a flight from the duties of justice and charity owed to one's neighbor, to various communities or to the whole of society — although, as is generally recognized, at times there are psychological factors present that can diminish responsibility or even completely remove it.

However, one must clearly distinguish suicide from that sacrifice of one's life whereby for a higher cause, such as God's glory, the salvation of souls or the service of one's brethren, a person offers his or her own life or puts it in danger (cf. *John* 15:14).

II. Euthanasia

In order that the question of euthanasia can be properly dealt with, it is first necessary to define the words used.

Etymologically speaking, in ancient times euthanasia meant an easy death without severe suffering. Today one no longer thinks of this original meaning of the word, but rather of some intervention of medicine whereby the sufferings of sickness or of the final agony are reduced, sometimes also with the danger of suppressing life prematurely. Ultimately, the word euthanasia is used in a more particular sense to mean "mercy killing," for the purpose of putting an end to extreme suffering, or saving abnormal babies, the mentally ill or the incurably sick from the prolongation, perhaps for many years, of a miserable life, which could impose too heavy a burden on their families or on society.

It is therefore necessary to state clearly in what sense the word is used in the present document.

By euthanasia is understood an action or an omission which of itself or by intention causes death, in order that all suffering may in this way be eliminated. Euthanasia's terms of reference, therefore, are to be found in the intention of the will and in the methods used.

It is necessary to state firmly once more that nothing and no one can in any way permit the killing of an innocent human being, whether a fetus or an embryo, an infant or an adult, an old person, or one suffering from an incurable disease, or a person who is dying. Furthermore, no one is permitted to ask for this act of killing, either for himself or herself or for another person entrusted to his or her care, nor can he or she consent to it, either explicitly or implicitly. Nor can any authority legitimately recommend or permit such an action. For it is a question of the violation of the divine law, an offence against the dignity of the human person, a crime against life, and an attack on humanity.

It may happen that, by reason of prolonged and barely tolerable pain, for deeply personal or other reasons, people may be led to believe that they can legitimately ask for death or obtain it for others. Although in these cases the guilt of the individual may be reduced or completely absent, nevertheless the error of judgment into which the conscience falls, perhaps in good faith, does not change the nature of this act of killing, which will always be in itself something to be rejected.

The pleas of gravely ill people who sometimes ask for death are not to be understood as implying a true desire for euthanasia; in fact it is almost always a case of an anguished plea for help and love. What a sick person needs, besides medical care, is love, the human and supernatural warmth with which the sick person can and ought to be surrounded by all those close to him or her, parents and children, doctors and nurses.

III. The Meaning of Suffering for Christians and the Use of Painkillers:

Death does not always come in dramatic circumstances after barely tolerable sufferings. Nor do we have to think only of extreme cases. Numerous testimonies which confirm one another lead one to the conclusion that nature itself has made provision to render more bearable at the moment of death separations that would be terribly painful to a person in full health. Hence it is that a prolonged illness, advanced old age, or a state of loneliness or neglect can bring about psychological conditions that facilitate the acceptance of death.

Nevertheless the fact remains that death, often preceded or accompanied by severe and prolonged suffering, is something which naturally causes people anguish.

Physical suffering is certainly an unavoidable element of the human condition; on the biological level, it constitutes a warning of which no one denies the usefulness; but, since it affects the human psychological makeup, it often exceeds its own biological usefulness and so can become so severe as to cause the desire to remove it at any cost.

According to Christian teaching, however, suffering, especially suffering during the last moments of life, has a special place in God's saving plan; it is in fact a sharing in Christ's Passion and a union with the redeeming sacrifice which he offered in obedience to the Father's will. Therefore one must not be surprised if some Christians prefer to moderate their use of painkillers, in order to accept voluntarily at least a part of their sufferings and thus associate themselves in a conscious way with the sufferings of Christ crucified (cf. *Matthew* 27:34).

Nevertheless it would be imprudent to impose a heroic way of acting as a general rule. On the contrary, human and Christian prudence suggest for the majority of sick people the use of medicines capable of alleviating or suppressing pain, even though these may cause as a secondary effect semi-consciousness and reduced lucidity. As for those who are not in a state to express themselves, one can reasonably presume that they wish to take these painkillers, and have them administered according to the doctor's advice.

But the intensive use of painkillers is not without difficulties, because the phenomenon of habituation generally makes it necessary to increase their dosage in order to maintain their efficacy. At this point it is fitting to recall a declaration by Pius XII, which retains its full force; in answer to a group of doctors who had put the question: "Is the suppression of pain and consciousness by the use of narcotics — permitted by religion and morality to the doctor and the patient (even at the approach of death and if one foresees that the use of narcotics will shorten life)?"

The Pope said: "If no other means exist, and if, in the given circumstances, this does not prevent the carrying out of other religious and moral duties: Yes."[5] In this case, of course, death is in no way intended or sought, even if the risk of it is reasonably taken; the intention is simply to relieve pain effectively, using for this purpose painkillers available to medicine.

However, painkillers that cause unconsciousness need special consideration. For a person not only has to be able to satisfy his or her moral duties and family obligations; he or she also has to prepare himself or herself with full consciousness for meeting Christ. Thus Pius XII warns: "It is not right to deprive the dying person of consciousness without a serious reason."[6]

IV. Due Proportion in the Use of Remedies

Today it is very important to protect, at the moment of death, both the dignity of the human person and the Christian concept of life, against a technological attitude that threatens to become an abuse. Thus, some people speak of a "right to die," which is an expression that does not mean the right to procure death either by one's own hand or by means of someone else, as one pleases, but rather the right to die peacefully with human and Christian dignity. From this point of view, the use of therapeutic means can sometimes pose problems.

In numerous cases, the complexity of the situation can be such as to cause doubts about the way ethical principles should be applied. In the final analysis, it pertains to the conscience either of the sick person, or of those qualified to speak in the sick person's name, or of the doctors, to decide, in the light of moral obligations and of the various aspects of the case.

Everyone has the duty to care for his or her own health or to seek such care from others. Those whose task it is to care for the sick must do so conscientiously and administer the remedies that seem necessary or useful.

However, is it necessary in all circumstances to have recourse to all possible remedies?

In the past, moralists replied that one is never obliged to use "extraordinary" means. This reply, which as a principle still holds good, is perhaps less clear today, by reason of the imprecision of the term and the rapid progress made in the treatment of sickness. Thus some people prefer to speak of "proportionate" and "disproportionate" means.

In any case, it will be possible to make a correct judgment as to the means by studying the type of treatment to be used, its degree of complexity or risk, its cost and the possibilities of using it, and comparing these elements with the result that can be expected, taking into account the state of the sick person and his or her physical and moral resources.

In order to facilitate the application of these general principles, the following clarifications can be added:

— If there are no other sufficient remedies, it is permitted, with the patient's consent, to have recourse to the means provided by the most advanced medical techniques, even if these means are still at the experimental stage and are not without a certain risk. By accepting them, the patient can even show generosity in the service of humanity.

— It is also permitted, with the patient's consent, to interrupt these means, where the results fall short of expectations. But for such a decision to be made, account will have to be taken of the reasonable wishes of the patient's family, as also of the advice of the doctors who are specially competent in the matter. The latter may in particular judge that the investment in instruments and personnel is disproportionate to the results foreseen; they may also judge that the techniques applied impose on the patient strain or suffering out of proportion with the benefits which he or she may gain from such techniques.

— It is also permissible to make do with the normal means that medicine can offer. Therefore one cannot impose on anyone the obligation to have recourse to a technique which is already in use but which carries a risk or is burdensome. Such a refusal is not the equivalent of suicide; on the contrary, it should be considered as an acceptance of the human condition, or a wish to avoid the application of a medical procedure disproportionate to the results that can be expected, or a desire not to impose excessive expense on the family or the community.

— When inevitable death is imminent in spite of the means used, it is permitted in conscience to take the decision to refuse forms of treatment that would only secure a precarious and burdensome prolongation of life, so long as the normal care due to the sick person in similar cases is not interrupted. In such circumstances the doctor has no reason to reproach himself with failing to help the person in danger.

Conclusion

The norms contained in the present declaration are inspired by a profound desire to serve people in accordance with the plan of the creator. Life is a gift of God, and, on the other hand, death is unavoidable; it is necessary therefore that we, without in any way hastening the hour of death, should be able to accept it with full responsibility and dignity. It is true that death marks the end of our earthly existence, but at the same time it opens the door to immortal life. Therefore all must prepare themselves for this event in the light of human values, and Christians even more so in the light of faith.

As for those who work in the medical profession, they ought to neglect no means of making all their skill available to the sick and the dying; but they should also remember how much more necessary it is to provide them with the comfort of boundless kindness and hearthfelt charity. Such service to people is also service to Christ the Lord, who said: "As you did it to one of the least of these my brethren, you did it to me." (Matthew 25:40)

At the audience granted to the undersigned prefect, His Holiness Pope John Paul II approved this declaration, adopted at the ordinary meeting of the Sacred Congregation for the Doctrine of the Faith, and ordered its publication.

Rome, the Sacred Congregation for the Doctrine of the Faith, 5 May 1980.

Franjo card. Seper
Prefect
Jerome Hamer, O.P.
Tit. Archbishop of Lorium, secretary.

Notes

1. *Declaration on Procured Abortion*, 18 November 1974: AAS 66 (1974), pp. 730-747.

2. Pius XII, address to those attending the Congress of the International Union of Catholic Women's Leagues, 11 September 1947: AAS 39 (1947), p. 2483, *Address to Midwives*, 29 October 1951: AAS 43 (1951), pp. 835-854, *Speech to the Members of the International Office for Documentation*, 19 October 1953: AAS 45 (1953), pp. 744-754, address to those taking part in the ninth Congress of the Italian Anæsthesiological Society, 24 February 1957: AAS 49 (1957) p. 146. Cf. also address to the members of the United Nations Special Committee on Apartheid, 22 May 1974: AAS 66 (1974), p. 346. John Paul II: address to the bishops of the United States of America, 5 October 1979: AAS 71 (1979), p. 1225.

3. One thinks especially of recommendation 779 (1976) on the rights of the sick and dying, of the Parliamentary Assembly of the Council of Europe at its 25th ordinary session; cf. Sipeca, no. 1 March 1977, pp. 14-15.

4. We leave aside completely the problems of the death penalty and of war, which involve specific considerations that do not concern the present subject.

5. Pius XII, address of 24 February 1957: AAS 49 (1957) p. 147.

6. Pius XII, *ibid* p. 145, Cf. address of 9 September 1958: AAS 50 (1958), p. 694.

Hospital Policies on
Prolonging Life Decisions

In this appendix we have included suggestions on no-code orders from a lawyer's perspective and three sample policies presently in use in hospitals in the United States.

A. Suggestions for Hospital Policies on No-code Orders

There's little question legally that under appropriate circumstances an order not to institute cardiopulmonary resuscitation is a legally permissible treatment option. On the other hand, in today's modern hospital the utilization of specialty teams of nursing staffs and physicians to respond to "code blue" calls is more and more routine. The calling of a code blue is the standard of care by which the medical profession or the hospital is judged in the absence of clearly articulated decisions not to institute CPR.

Accordingly, the following suggestions are made:

- *No-code orders must be recorded in writing on the patient's chart.* Written documentation establishes professional review of the patient's condition, and that resuscitative measures were determined to be medically inappropriate. Without a written order, the failure to respond with the crash cart in a

297

situation of cardiac or respiratory arrest could be considered negligence. While some physicians are reluctant to write no code orders, preferring instead to give the order orally or in some clandestine fashion, this is clearly inappropriate legally. Failing to write such orders in the chart not only does not protect the physician but in fact will compromise what might otherwise be a legally appropriate course of action. JCAH requires orders to be entered in writing on the patient's chart, and this factor would undoubtedly be raised by one claiming negligent care in a lawsuit. Furthermore, the chances of error are greatly increased by not having clearly documented orders. Without a written order, the nursing staff finds itself pitted against the doctor to explain why no CPR efforts were undertaken.

- *Second opinions or committee evaluations should be obtained.* The treating physician must consult with at least one other physician who is familiar with the patient and who concurs in the decision not to resuscitate. Consultation should be fully documented on the patient's chart. Some hospitals have formed physician committees to assist in the evaluation of such matters, but ultimately it is the burden of the attending physician to render the appropriate decision in light of the patient's medical condition.

- *Consultation with the family and obtaining their approval is essential.* The patient's family must be completely informed as to the action being taken. They must be informed *throughout* the decision-making process, for in the last analysis it is for the family members to decide, in close consultation with the physician, after assessing all the medical factors in the case. (Of course if the patient's wishes are known, those wishes should be followed.) Where the physician concludes that CPR should be withheld, it is better for the physician to inform the family the reasons why that decision is recommended rather than approaching them by asking whether they want CPR to be attempted. In any event, however, if the family does not concur in the physician's recommendation, then the no-code order should not be implemented.

- *No-code orders must be constantly updated.* They should be reconsidered at least every 24 hours to determine if they are in fact still appropriate. Provision must be made to notify the physician in the event of any change in the patient's condition.

- *Support of the patient and the family must be maintained.* During the entire process and until the inevitable death of the patient, the care rendered to comfort the patient and provide for the ordinary means of care must not diminish. Likewise, family members must be supported and comforted to the fullest extent possible by all members of the hospital staff including pastoral care personnel, nursing personnel, physicians and others.

If these points are followed and the family is fully informed and given objective medical reasoning why such a course of action is being carried out, the likelihood of any exposure for alleged medical malpractice is extremely remote. In fact, most families of dying loved ones in these situations will recognize that the facility and its medical and nursing staff are providing the best of care in a professional way and with genuine compassion.

J. Stuart Showalter, J.D.
Director, Division of Legal Services
Catholic Health Association
St. Louis, MO

B. Sample Administrative Policy I

Withdrawal of Patient From Life-Support Equipment

Ed. Note: This policy, in use in the state of Massachusetts, limits itself to the incompetent, terminally ill patient who is comatose and in a medically hopeless condition.

Policy: A patient shall not be suddenly and totally withdrawn from a mechanical life support system except under the following procedures:

Procedures:

1. When a physician has previously pronounced the patient dead based on ordinary and accepted standards of medical practice for determining death, the mechanical respirator may be withdrawn.

2. When, after receiving a written consult from a staff neurologist, the physician is of the opinion that all of the following criteria have been met, the physician may request that the Medical Morals Committee be convened in accordance with paragraph 3 below. The criteria are as follows:

   (a) The patient is incompetent and terminally ill; and

   (b) The patient is in an irreversible, permanent or chronic vegetative coma; and

   (c) The patient is in a medically hopeless condition and has no reasonable prospects of regaining cognitive brain function such that the maintenance of the patient on the life support system is not medical treatment which has any reasonable likelihood of benefitting the patient; and

   (d) After consultation with the patient's next of kin who concur in, or request that the life support system be withdrawn, it is evident that the patient, on the basis of his or her own expressions on the subject or on his or her actual interest and preferences, would, in the present circumstances choose to have the life support system withdrawn if he or she were competent to make such decision, taking into account his or her present and future incompetency.

3. When a physician is of the opinion that all of the criteria set forth in paragraph 2 above have been met, the physician may, if he/she is of the opinion that the life support system should be withdrawn, request that the Medical Morals Committee be convened to review the ethical considerations of the case. If the Medical Morals Committee finds no ethical objections to the withdrawal of the life support system for such a patient, the life support system may be withdrawn.

4. The sudden and total withdrawal of a patient from a mechanical life support system must be performed by a physician.

C. Sample Administrative Policy II

Policy Guidelines for Withholding or Withdrawing
Medical Treatment for Terminally Ill Patients

Ed. Note: This policy was published by Robert L. Heath, J.D., in Health Law Trends *(Vol. 11, No. 5, May 1980), a newsletter published monthly in Wichita, KS, by Stephen M. Blaes and Robert L. Heath. It proposes a Declaration which may be made available to patients by a hospital and used by the hospital in cases of withholding or withdrawing medical treatment for the terminally ill.*

I. Policy Regarding Treatment.
A. It is the policy of the Medical Staff to render to each patient in the Hospital the appropriate type and level of care consistent with good medical practice and the resources of this Medical Staff and Hospital.
B. All decisions to render or withhold treatment and all decisions regarding the selection of treatment shall be based upon sound medical principles reflecting the appropriate level of care.
C. Patients and families will be involved in decisions concerning care and treatment. The rights of the patient shall be respected.

II. Patients Executing Declarations Concerning Life Sustaining Procedures.
A. It is recognized that adult persons have the right to execute a Declaration instructing the physician to withhold or withdraw life-sustaining procedures in the event of a terminal condition. This Declaration will be recognized under the following conditions:
  1. The Declaration must be in writing, dated and signed by the declarant or by another person at the declarant's direction and in his or her presence.
  2. The Declaration must be signed in the presence of two or more witnesses 18 years of age or older neither of whom shall be the person signing on behalf of the declarant or be related by blood or marriage, have any financial interest in declarant's estate or have any responsibility for the medical care of declarant.
B. Upon receipt of such a Declaration, the attending physician shall make the Declaration, or a copy thereof, part of the patient's medical record.
C. The Form of Declaration should conform substantially to Exhibit A attached to this guideline.

III. Procedure For Patients With Valid Declarations On File.
A. The attending physician who is notified of a Declaration shall, without delay, provide for written confirmation of the patient's terminal condition, which should conform to Exhibit B attached to this guideline.
B. A second physician shall be notified who shall personally examine the patient and certify in writing whether he agrees with the diagnosis of a terminal condition. If both physicians concur, life-sustaining procedures shall be withheld or withdrawn pursuant to the patient's Declaration.

IV. **Revocation By The Patient.**
   A. A Declaration may be revoked at any time by the declarant by any of the following methods:
      1. By obliterating, burning, tearing or otherwise destroying the executed Declaration.
      2. By a written revocation signed and dated by the declarant, or person acting at his or her direction.
      3. By verbal expression of intent to revoke the Declaration in the presence of a witness 18 years of age or older who signs and dates a writing confirming such expression.
   B. The revocation shall become effective upon receipt by the attending physician. The physician shall record in the patient's chart the time, date and place of when notification of the revocation was received in a form complying substantially with Exhibit C attached to this guideline.
   C. Physicians shall still provide those ordinary measures of patient care to all patients including those executing a Declaration as described above. Should a physician refuse to comply with a Declaration, he or she shall transfer the patient to another physician.

V. **Responsibility of Patient.**
   A. It shall be the responsibility of the patient to notify the physician of the existence of the Declaration.
   B. A patient is presumed to be of sound mind to execute a Declaration absent actual notice to the contrary.
   C. The desires of a patient shall at all times be paramount and shall supercede the effect of the Declaration.

VI. **Competent Patients Not Executing Declarations.**
   In the case of patients who are competent and desire to have life-sustaining procedures withheld or withdrawn in the event their condition becomes terminal, such patients shall be informed concerning the execution of a Declaration. However, such Declaration shall not be a requirement in every case where the physician and patient have discussed and agreed to the withholding or withdrawal of extraordinary measures of care, provided the patient's rights are fully protected and appropriately respected as required by law and suitable documentation thereof is recorded in the medical chart.

EXHIBIT A

DECLARATION

Declaration made this _____ day of _____,
19 _____ . I, _____ being of sound
mind, willfully and voluntarily make known my desire that my dying shall
not be artificially prolonged under the circumstances set forth below. I
hereby declare:

If at any time I should have an incurable injury, disease, or illness
certified to be a terminal condition by two physicians who have personally
examined me, one of whom shall be my attending physician, and the physicians
have determined that my death will occur whether or not life-sustaining
procedures are utilized, and that such procedures would serve only to artificially prolong the dying process, I direct that such procedures be withheld
or withdrawn, and that I be permitted to die naturally with only the administration of medication or the performance of any medical procedure deemed
necessary to provide me with comfort care.

In the absence of my ability to give directions regarding the use of such
life-sustaining procedures, it is my intention that this Declaration shall be
honored by my family and physician(s) as the final expression of my legal
right to refuse medical or surgical treatment and accept the consequences
from such refusal.

I understand the full import of this Declaration and I am emotionally
and mentally competent to make this Declaration.

Signed _____

City, County and State of Residence _____

_____

The declarant has been personally known to me and I believe him or
her to be of sound mind. I did not sign the declarant's signature above for or
at the direction of the declarant. I am not related to the declarant by blood or
marriage, entitled to any portion of the estate of the declarant according to
the laws of intestate succession or under any will of declarant or codicil thereto,
or directly financially responsible for declarant's medical care.

Witness _____

Witness _____

EXHIBIT B

CERTIFICATION OF TERMINAL CONDITION

We hereby certify:

1. That the undersigned are duly licensed to practice medicine and surgery in this State.

2. That the above patient is diagnosed as having a terminal condition, namely: _____

   _____.

3. That the above patient has supplied the attending physician with a directive concerning the withholding or withdrawal of life-sustaining procedures which shall be carried out without delay upon our signing this Certification.

DATED this _____ day of _____, 19 _____ .

_____ A.M.   P.M.

_____	_____
Attending Physician	Consulting Physician

_____
Witness

_____
Witness

D. Sample Administrative Policy III

Policy and Procedure Regarding
No Code Orders and Orders Not to Provide
Therapeutic or Emergency Medical Treatment
of Terminally Ill Patients

Ed. Note: This lengthy and complex policy was adopted by the Board of a large municipal teaching hospital. It carefully protects patients' rights and insists on medical judgements to determine the Medical Criteria in Part II, which limit the writing of a "No-Code Order" or the withdrawing of treatment.

Part I. Policy Regarding Treatment

In order to maintain and improve the quality of care available to patients at this hospital, the medical staff of this hospital adopts the following statement of policy with regard to treatment generally and with regard to treatment and procedures in specific instances.

A. Definitions

1. The term "No Code Order" refers solely to the withholding of the automatic initiation of cardio-pulmonary resuscitation (CPR) by written and signed order in the medical record in accordance with the procedure outlined herein.

2. "Death is imminent" shall mean "near at hand"; "impending"; "hanging threateningly over one's head"; "menacingly near" and as determined by the attending physician in accordance with accepted standards of medical practice and the procedures outlined herein.

3. "Life sustaining procedure" shall mean any medical procedure or intervention which utilizes mechanical or other artificial means to sustain, restore or supplant a vital function, which, when applied to a terminally ill patient, would serve only to artificially prolong the moment of death and where, in the judgment of the attending physician, death is imminent whether or not such procedures are utilized. "Life-sustaining procedure" shall not include the administration or the performance of any medical procedure deemed necessary to alleviate pain.

4. "Terminal condition" means an incurable condition caused by injury, disease or illness, which, regardless of the application of life-sustaining procedures, would, within reasonable medical judgment, produce death and where the application of life-sustaining procedures serves *only* to postpone the moment of death of a patient.

5. "Attending physician" shall mean the attending physician or senior resident authorized by the bylaws to be ultimately responsible for the treatment of the patient.

B. General Policy

It is the policy of the medical staff:

1. To render to each patient in the hospital the appropriate type and level of care consistent with good medical practice and the resources of this medical staff and hospital.

2. To base all decisions to render or to withhold treatment and all decisions regarding the selection of treatment on sound medical principles reflecting the appropriate level of care.
3. To involve patients and families in decisions concerning the patient's care and treatment and respect the rights of all patients.
4. To seek appropriate assistance from consultants and colleagues.
5. To refrain from rendering or ordering care which is not medically warranted.

C. **Treatment of Patients with Terminal Conditions**
   In the case of patients with incurable terminal conditions for whom death is imminent, it is the policy of the medical staff that:
   1. A "No Code Order" and other orders not to provide therapeutic or emergency procedures, intervention or medical treatment, shall not be considered unless there is an underlying incurable terminal condition and death is imminent. Nothing in this policy and procedure shall be construed to condone, authorize or approve mercy killing or to permit any affirmative or deliberate act or omission to end life other than to permit the natural process of dying as provided in this policy and procedure.
   2. CPR shall be initiated automatically if there is no written and signed "No Code Order" on the medical record in accordance with the procedure outlined herein. A specific written and signed "No Code Order" in compliance with the procedure herein is necessary if CPR is not to be initiated.
   3. In the case of a question regarding a "No Code Order" or other question regarding an order not to provide therapeutic or emergency procedure or care, all other hospital personnel or non-physician health care providers involved should immediately notify Risk Management.
   4. Terminally ill patients shall be involved in decisions regarding their care and treatment to the extent reasonably possible as determined by the attending physician.
   5. Terminally ill patients shall continue to receive all medically necessary care, treatment and attention consistent with the patient's condition and the ordinary standards of medical practice.
   6. Terminally ill patients may be comforted through the use of pain-relieving drugs and analgesics with their consent, notwithstanding that the administration of such drugs or analgesics, while providing comfort to the patient, may hasten the moment of death.
   7. Consents or refusals given by such patients while they are lucid and competent shall be respected and acted upon if and when such patients lapse into coma or incompetency because of their condition.
   8. "No Code Orders" or other orders not to provide treatment may not be entered, initiated or ordered orally. Such orders must be *written* on the medical record *before* the actual initiation of the order and shall not be written for such patients unless:
      a. The proper therapeutic or emergency care is refused by the patient or one recognized by law as authorized to refuse this treatment on behalf of such patient (Note: the Hospital Refusal of Treatment form must be

executed by the patient or by a legally authorized person on behalf of such patient); but such refusal may be revoked by the patient or such person orally or in *writing* at any time; *or*

b. Such "No Code Order" or other order not to provide further therapeutic or emergency treatment is made pursuant to this policy and procedure; *or*

c. The order is entered with respect to a patient who is pronounced dead in accordance with law.

9. The family or next of kin of a patient who has not himself refused further therapeutic or emergency treatment may not require such an order on the patient's behalf unless the attending physician exercising ordinary medical standards, concurs that the patient's condition meets the medical criteria contained in Part II of this policy and procedure. Furthermore, if a competent patient disagrees or, in those cases where the patient is incompetent, if the family, next-of-kin, the patient's guardian, or conservator disagrees, a "No Code Order" or other orders not to provide therapeutic or emergency care will not be written or initiated.

Part II: Medical Criteria

A. Before a "No Code Order" or other order not to provide further therapeutic or emergency treatment may be entered in the medical record, the attending physician, or consultant(s), as provided in this policy, must have reached a conclusion, based on ordinary medical standards, as understood and practiced in this hospital and community with a reasonable degree of medical certainty, that each of the following criteria has been met.

1. The patient's condition is terminal and death is imminent; and

2. There is no course of therapeutic or emergency care which offers any reasonable expectation of remission or cure of the patient's terminal condition; and there is no course of treatment which offers any reasonable alternative to certain death; and

3. There is no basis found in the ordinary standards of medical practice to render further or additional therapeutic or emergency treatment or to undertake new or additional procedures; and

4. The rendition of additional therapeutic or emergency services in the case of the specific patient is medically unwarranted and said services would be only life-sustaining procedures as defined herein.

Part III: Procedure

Except in cases of orders entered at the request of, or based upon the refusal of a patient with a terminal condition or one possessing legal authority to request such an order on behalf of a patient with a terminal condition (Note: the Hospital Refusal of Treatment form *must* be executed by the patient or by a legally authorized person on behalf of such patient), no such order may be written until the following procedure has been complied with:

A. The attending physician shall have reached a medical opinion that the patient's condition meets each and every medical criteria contained in Part II of this policy and procedure and shall have documented his opinion as to each criteria in the medical record in accordance with Part II of this policy.

B. The opinion of the attending physician shall have been concurred in by at least one consulting physician:

A consulting physician's opinion that the patient's condition meets each and every one of the medical criteria contained in Part II of this policy will be sufficient if the consulting physician(s) has personally examined the patient and reviewed the patient's medical records, and has concluded that the patient's condition meets each of the medical criteria contained in Part II of this policy and procedure and has documented that conclusion in the medical record.

C. The patient's condition and prognosis and the decision of the attending physician and concurring opinion of the consulting physician(s) that further therapeutic or emergency treatment is medically unwarranted, shall be communicated to the patient's family or next-of-kin (if any are located), except in the unusual case in which the attending physician enters his written opinion that the decision should not be communicated to the family or next-of-kin out of concern for the physical or mental health of any such individual(s). All such communication or lack thereof shall be documented in the medical record by the attending physician.

D. Thereafter, the attending physician shall continue to examine the patient at least once every twenty-four (24) hours. All documentation, "No Code Order" or other orders not to provide therapeutic or emergency treatment *must* be written and each such order and documentation must be signed by the attending physician. Such orders must be renewed in writing and signed by the attending physician every twenty-four (24) hours. The use of "Renew," "Repeat," and "Continue Orders" is not acceptable. If not renewed every twenty-four (24) hours, such orders shall become null and void. Verbal orders are not sufficient and not acceptable. The signature and order of the attending physician must be legible. Significant changes in the patient's condition observed by the nursing staff shall be brought to the attention of the attending physician. Any "No Code" order or other order not to provide therapeutic or emergency treatment may be cancelled at any time by the attending physician. Such cancellation must be in writing and signed by the attending physician.

Selected Bibliography

Books

Ashley, Benedict M., O.P., and O'Rourke, Kevin D., O.P. *Health Care Ethics: A Theological Analysis*. St. Louis: The Catholic Hospital Association, 1978. A thorough and current textbook which reflects magisterial teaching and contemporary scholarship.

Grisez, Germain, and Boyle, Joseph M. *Life and Death with Liberty and Justice: A Contribution to the Euthanasia Debate*. University of Notre Dame Press, 1979. A recent study which raises serious objections to all deliberate taking of human life.

Death, Dying, and Euthanasia, edited by Dennis J. Horan and David Mall. Washington, DC: University Publications of America, 1977. A thorough anthology of articles from various points of view.

Lamerton, Richard, *Care of the Dying*. London: Priory Press LTD, 1973; Westport, CT: Technomic Publishing Company, 1976. A classical description of the hospice approach to terminal illness.

May, William E. *Human Existence, Medicine and Ethics*. Chicago: Franciscan Herald Press, 1977. A short textbook written from the perspective of a contemporary personalism which reflects the natural moral law tradition of the Church.

New Technologies of Birth and Death, Medical, Legal, and Moral Dimensions. St. Louis, MO: Pope John XXIII Medical-Moral Research and Education Center, 1980. The second half of this book, "Death Issues," contains articles relevant to prolonging life decisions by Vincent J. Collins, M.D.; Dennis J. Horan, J.D.; Rev. Donald G. McCarthy, Ph.D.; and Thomas J. O'Donnell, S.J.

Ramsey, Paul. *The Patient as Person*. New Haven: Yale University Press, 1970. Almost a classic despite the difficulty of Ramsey's style. Reflections on the prolonging life issue very similar to Catholic tradition although the author is not a Catholic Christian.

Ramsey, Paul. *Ethics at the Edges of Life*. New Haven: Yale University Press, 1978. Part Two (pp 143-336) offers Ramsey's response to issues of the 70's such as the Quinlan and Saikewicz cases.

Weber, Leonard. *Who Shall Live?* New York: Paulist Press, 1976. A useful small book dealing with the dilemma of care for severely handicapped children in the light of the ethical tradition of ordinary and extraordinary means.

(Continued)

Articles

Bayley, Sr. Corrine, C.S.J., "Terminating Treatment: Asking the Right Questions," *Hospital Progress,* Sept. 1980, pp. 50-53 and 72.

Boyle, Joseph M. Jr., "The Concept of Health and the Right to Health Care"' *Social Thought,* 3 (1977), pp. 5-17.

Boyle, Joseph M. Jr., "On Killing and Letting Die," *The New Scholasticism,* 51 (1977), pp. 433-452.

Byrne, Paul A., MD; O'Reilly, Sean, MD, FRCP; Quay, Paul M., SJ, PhD, "Brain Death — An Opposing Viewpoint," *Journal of the American Medical Association,* Nov. 2, 1979, Vol. 242, No. 18, pp. 1985-1990.

Connery, John R., S.J., "Court's Guidelines on Incompetent Patients Compromise Their Rights," *Hospital Progress,* Sept. 1980, pp. 46-49.

McCarthy, Rev. Donald G., "The Use and Abuse of Cardiopulmonary Resuscitation," *Hospital Progress,* Ap. 1975, pp. 64-68 and 80.

McCartney, James J., O.S.A., "The Development of the Doctrine of Ordinary and Extraordinary Means of Preserving Life in Catholic Moral Theology before the Karen Quinlan Case," *Linacre Quarterly,* 47 (1980), pp. 215-224.

McCormick, Richard A., S.J., and Veatch, Robert, "Preservation of Life," *Theological Studies,* June 1980, pp. 390-396.

McCormick, Richard A., S.J., "The Preservation of Life," *Linacre Quarterly,* 43 (1976), pp. 94-100.

Pius XII, "The Prolongation of Life," *The Pope Speaks,* Vol. 4, No. 4, (Spring, 1958), pp. 393-398.

Ramsey, Paul, "Prolonged Dying: Not Medically Indicated," *Hastings Center Report,* 6 (1976), 14-17.

Pope John Center Publications

The Pope John XXIII Medical-Moral Research and Education Center has dedicated itself to approaching current and emerging medical-moral issues from the perspective of Catholic teaching and the Judeo-Christian heritage. Previous publications of the Pope John Center include:

HUMAN SEXUALITY AND PERSONHOOD, Proceedings of the Bishops Workshop in Dallas, February, 1981, 254 pp., $9.95.

GENETIC COUNSELING, THE CHURCH AND THE LAW, edited by Albert S. Moraczewski, OP, and Gary Atkinson, 1980, 259 pp., $9.95.

NEW TECHNOLOGIES OF BIRTH AND DEATH: Medical, Legal, and Moral Dimensions. A volume containing lectures presented by 9 scholars at the Workshop for Bishops in Dallas, January, 1980, 196 pp., $8.95.

A MORAL EVALUATION OF CONTRACEPTION AND STERILIZATION, A Dialogical Study, by Gary Atkinson and Albert S. Moraczewski, OP, 1980, 115 pp., $4.95.

ARTFUL CHILDMAKING, Artificial Insemination in Catholic Teaching, by John C. Wakefield, 1978, 205 pp., $8.95.

AN ETHICAL EVALUATION OF FETAL EXPERIMENTATION, edited by Donald McCarthy and Albert S. Moraczewski, OP, 1976, 137 pp., $8.95.

These books may be ordered from: The Pope John Center, 4455 Woodson Road, St. Louis, Missouri 63134. Telephone (314) 428-2424. Prepayment is encouraged. Please add $1.00 for shipping and handling for the first book ordered and .25¢ for each additional book.

Subscriptions to the Pope John Center monthly newsletter, *Ethics and Medics*, may be sent to the same address, annual subscriptions are $10.00.